Coronary Circulation in Nonsmokers and Smokers

Aurelio Leone

Nova Biomedical Books
New York

For permission to use material from this book please contact us:
Telephone 631-231-7269; Fax 631-231-8175
Web Site: http://www.novapublishers.com

NOTICE TO THE READER

The Publisher has taken reasonable care in the preparation of this book, but makes no expressed or implied warranty of any kind and assumes no responsibility for any errors or omissions. No liability is assumed for incidental or consequential damages in connection with or arising out of information contained in this book. The Publisher shall not be liable for any special, consequential, or exemplary damages resulting, in whole or in part, from the readers' use of, or reliance upon, this material.

Independent verification should be sought for any data, advice or recommendations contained in this book. In addition, no responsibility is assumed by the publisher for any injury and/or damage to persons or property arising from any methods, products, instructions, ideas or otherwise contained in this publication.

1005774197

This publication is designed to provide accurate and authoritative information with regard to the subject matter covered herein. It is sold with the clear understanding that the Publisher is not engaged in rendering legal or any other professional services. If legal or any other expert assistance is required, the services of a competent person should be sought. FROM A DECLARATION OF PARTICIPANTS JOINTLY ADOPTED BY A COMMITTEE OF THE AMERICAN BAR ASSOCIATION AND A COMMITTEE OF PUBLISHERS.

Library of Congress Cataloging-in-Publication Data

Leone, Aurelio.
Coronary circulation in nonsmokers and smokers / Aurelio Leone (author).
     p. ; cm.
Includes bibliographical references and index.
ISBN 978-1-60456-608-6 (hardcover)
1. Coronary heart disease--Etiology. 2. Coronary heart disease--Pathophysiology. 3. Smoking. 4. Coronary circulation. I. Title.
[DNLM: 1. Coronary Circulation. 2. Coronary Disease--etiology. 3. Myocardial Ischemia. 4. Smoking--adverse effects. WG 300 L583c 2008]
RC685.C6L46 2008
616.1'23071--dc22   2008013222

Published by Nova Science Publishers, Inc. ≃ *New York*

Contents

Preface

The knowledge of coronary artery tree characteristics is basic to interpret both baseline heart function and function under different stimuli that can affect the heart and, by so doing, modify its physiological response. The whole cardiovascular homeostasis depends deeply on coronary circulation. Moreover, each arterial segment in the coronary tree has specific properties and functions although a close interaction exists among adjacent arterial segments which, therefore, act strictly together and in series to supply blood flow to the heart.

It is worthwhile to underline that coronary artery disease is, still nowadays, the major health problem in the civilized countries, even if an increase in its appearance has been seen in countries yet far from either an industrially clear development or social and economic progress. These countries are, however, addressed regarding this lifestyle.

Efforts have been conducted in an attempt to reduce either mortality or morbidity from coronary heart disease worldwide.

Mortality would seem to be reduced by using a "cocktail" of medical, surgical and diagnostic measures that could be able to decrease mainly the incidence of cardiovascular attacks in those individuals who are suffering from ischemic heart disease. On the contrary, morbidity from ischemic heart disease could be better controlled by a large series of measures which reduce the negative effects of those factors, not yet fully known, that are, generically, defined coronary risk factors. Among these, there are some, such as increased LDL-cholesterol concentrations, hypertension, cigarette smoking and diabetes mellitus, usually defined as major coronary risk factors which are frequently associated with the appearance of ischemic pathology for the heart. They may act isolatedly or all together by different combinations causing a wide spectrum of coronary artery alterations mainly of thrombotic or thrombogenic type. There is prevailing, sometimes, the first type, sometimes, the second type of damaging mechanism with regard to a stronger activity of one factor having a determined effect rather than another with a different pathogenetic mechanism. However, the final step of the damage due to major coronary risk factors is an acceleration in atherosclerotic plaque formation with consequent narrowing of arterial lumen which are responsible for coronary blood flow impairment with reduced adaptability to adjust blood flow supply to functional and metabolic demands of the heart. It is particularly true that the final coronary alteration makes it hard to distinguish structurally what is due to one risk factor rather than to another, unless one can be sure that only the single factor analyzed gave the observed effect. Such a condition may be more easily obtained by experimental studies conducted on animals.

The type of alterations caused to coronary arteries by major coronary risk factors, although similar, does not follow, however, at least initially, the same ways. The analysis of these ways could permit us to identify the specific characteristics due to the responsible factor and, therefore, interpret those differences that exist in the context of coronary artery lesions. Moreover, assessing the appearance and progression of coronary artery lesions due to single or multiple risk factors is basic to establish the degree of impairment of coronary circulation. There are lesions, namely those caused by a thrombogenic mechanism, that develop earlier than those due to thrombotic mechanisms which may develop, usually, later.

To clarify further this concept, it is worthwhile mentioning, among other things, the association between cigarette smoking with oral contraceptive drugs in women. These two factors associated in a premenopausal woman can have thrombogenic effects, whereas post-menopausal women usually display atherothrombotic coronary artery alterations as a possible result of cigarette smoking and contraceptive drug interaction. The main reason for that is due to the fact that a pre-menopausal woman usually activates a mechanism of lesion that is a consequence of arterial wall, platelet and coagulation-fibrinolysis function impairment with earlier coronary artery changes. On the contrary, smoking alone acts particularly by a chronic mechanism of damage that involves all aforesaid factors although by a prevalence of arterial wall and platelet changes that form, more slowly, atherosclerotic plaque with no influence of contraceptive drugs, when administered in post-menopause. Such a condition well shows the different types of alterations that a risk factor, namely smoking, may cause as well as the possibility of recognizing the characteristics of induced lesion on the coronary arteries.

From this example (one could identify a large series of others), there is evidence that the type of alterations caused by a specific risk factor on the coronary circulation may be followed throughout its development and progression, and each risk factor may act differently according to the peculiar events that it may influence. Therefore, a careful observation of coronary circulation changes may help to interpret the   causative mechanism and possibly a single factor of lesion, if any. It is known that the latter parameter is often misinterpreted since the global burden of damage due to coronary risk factors is, usually, assessed. Therefore, in the search for the mechanisms that can cause coronary artery disease, attention should be focused on the variations between the characteristics of those subjects who suffer attacks of coronary artery disease and those who do not with regard to the number and type of coronary risk factors. Those individuals with increased risk have, usually, more evident coronary alterations without, necessarily, imputing a direct causal relationship between risk factors and coronary circulation changes.

The purpose of this volume is to provide the readers with a comprehensive description of the state of coronary circulation in healthy and diseased nonsmokers and smokers analyzing the characteristics of artery lesions, when observed, in both groups, their possible relationship with those coronary alterations resulting from different combinations of smoking with other major coronary risk factors, and the type and incidence of cardiac pathology observed. A brief attempt to interpret why some coronary lesions in nonsmokers and smokers are followed by cardiovascular events in some cases and not in other similar cases will be also described.

The volume consists of thirteen chapters grouped into three main sections: the first one is related to anatomical and functional patterns of coronary circulation, the second section to the mechanisms by which smoking – either active smoking or passive smoking – usually alters coronary circulation, and the third section is built to assess the incidence and type of cardiac pathology that affects individuals who are current smokers, ex- smokers or nonsmokers.

The first three chapters describe the anatomy, physiology and metabolism of coronary circulation under normal conditions. Chapter 4, specifically, analyzes the physiology and response of coronary endothelium to different stimuli. Chapters 5 to 9 discuss the biochemical smoking compounds capable of harmful effects on coronary arteries, type of damage observed as a consequence of smoking exposure, and coronary changes, particularly of the atherosclerotic type, in nonsmokers and smokers. Finally, chapters 10, 11, and 12 contain a comparison between coronary alterations due respectively to active smoking and passive smoking exposure, ischemic cardiac pathology closely related to smoking, and post-surgical cardiac pathology influenced by cigarette consumption. A conclusion with the basic remarks that must be carefully kept in mind to assess the specific type of alterations due to smoking, their interaction, and consequences on coronary circulation will come at the end of the book.

This volume was written primarily for the cardiologists, researchers, and, generally, physicians, although students in medicine, nurses, and social operators may find interesting up-to-date data.

The book should be seen as a source of current information about the damaging effects of cigarette smoking on coronary artery circulation since the knowledge of existing characteristic alterations is basic to better understand the problems related to the subject of the volume.

Aurelio Leone

Dedication

To :
my wife Elena Archilli-Leone,
the sweet "flower" of my life.

Chapter I

Anatomy of the Coronary Arteries

Abstract

Anatomic features of the coronary circulation show some interesting data which have been obtained by both in vivo and postmortem studies.

Firstly, the greater majority of myocardial muscle is under the control of the left coronary arteries: the left main coronary artery and its branches, the left anterior descending artery, and circumflex artery, which provide several arterial vessels particularly to the left anterior ventricular wall, interventricular septum and apex of the heart. Also a large portion of the posterior left ventricular wall is supplied by left coronary circulation. The right coronary artery supplies blood flow, mainly, to the posterior wall of the heart and right atrium.

Secondly, a complex system of coronary anastomoses has been demonstrated, so that coronary arteries must not be interpreted as end-arteries but as arteries widely communicating among themselves.

Thirdly, from the network that forms capillary bed a series of cardiac veins of different size and caliber takes back the blood to the coronary sinus located in the right atrium.

Differences in coronary circulation may exist between men and animals as a lot of studies seem to show. However, generally, also animal hearts have left coronary circulation usually prevailing.

Keywords: Coronary circulation, left main artery, left anterior descending artery, circumflex artery, right coronary artery, perforator vessel(s), diagonal artery, anastomoses, intracoronary anastomoses, homocoronary anastomoses, intercoronary anastomoses, capillary network, postmortem angiography, cast(s), coronary venous system, great cardiac vein, posterior cardiac vein, anterior cardiac vein, left anterior vein, small coronary vein, Thebesii venae, coronary sinus, coronary wall ultrastructure, histology, coronary blood volume, geometrical distribution.

Coronary arteries supply blood flow to the heart either under physiologic conditions or pathologic state. Benchmark of the coronary circulation is not to provide the heart with a constant amount of blood volume, but, otherwise, to adjust blood volume to metabolic demand of cardiac muscle since this parameter is changing with regard to the degree of cardiac work being performed.

Since both a hypoxic mechanism and direct damage due to smoking compounds cause those structural alterations of coronary circulation that usually have been well identified, the obvious consequence is that there is an involvement of the arterial anatomy that will depend on the degree and type of smoking exposure.

Among coronary vessels which are damaged by smoking, particularly extramural (epicardial) coronary arteries, intramyocardial vessels, and vascular endothelium are the target organs. Indeed, these structures are those which particularly feel hypoxia as well as changes in blood flow and blood components [1–3] capable of inducing cellular alterations and atherosclerotic lesion progression [4–7].

In this chapter, gross and microscopic characteristics of extramural coronary arteries and intramyocardial vessels as well as normal endothelium are reviewed in an attempt to better understand those changes that they experience as a consquence of tobacco smoke exposure.

Epicardial Coronary Arteries and Intramyocardial Circulation

A description of the main characteristics of epicardial and intramyocardial circulation of the coronary arteries sets together to explain possibly different mechanisms which can cause cardiovascular damage due to smoking exposure. Usually, alterations are related to hypoxia that triggers anatomical and/or functional changes on vessel structures with a reduction in lumen diameter because of the presence of isolated or multiple stenoses of different size and degree.

Similar to what characterizes artery vessels deputed to provide blood and metabolites to body organs, coronary circulation, at least for its epicardial portion, is formed by conduit vessels. On the contrary, intramyocardial coronary arteries play, particularly, a leading role as resistance vessels due to the complex interaction with myocardial fibers where they are elapsing.

Conduit vessels are segments of arteries of a cylinder shape that reduce progressively their caliber along the entire length from their origin to the end. This geometrical characteristic allows them to carry out basic functions.

A cylinder (figure 1.1.), geometrically, is an uniform and hollow three-dimensional solid with straight sides and a circular section. It arises from a complete rotation of a side of a plane figure, a rectangle, giving a tridimensional solid.

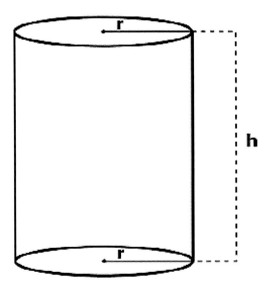

Figure 1.1. Longitudinal section of a hollow cylinder. One can see the height and radius that are those parameters that permit us to calculate the volume according to the formula: $V = \pi r^2 h$, where $\pi = 3.14$, r = radius, and h = height. Volume must be considered a certain parameter since the shape and dimension of the solid are the same for the whole figure.

As one can see, putting fluid into a cylinder allows us to calculate its volume when we know the basal circumference of the solid as well as its major parameter that can be, indifferently, named height or length according to the direction of the geometric figure. Moreover, in case of stiff sides the volume is easier to be assessed since influences due to the shape changes are quite lacking. On the contrary, blood flow into an arterial vessel is influenced by different factors, some of these due to structural characteristics of the wall, primarily the progressive reduction in circumference (internal diameter) observed from the origin of the vessel to its end (figure 1.2.), some others to heart function, and, finally, some more to blood rheology. Results of that may consist of arterial dilation or constriction, change in blood permeability, modifying a normal response to applied stimuli. These different circumstances make it hard to determine the blood volume in the coronary arteries since their caliber, physiologically, undergo different changes. However, this concept will be further discussed more widely in the next chapter on the physiology of coronary circulation because of the fact that possible coronary alterations can induce increased arterial stiffness.

Resistance vessels must include all arteries of the body just as they leave their origin, although particularly intramyocardial segments and their anastomoses play a basic role for what concerns coronary circulation. Indeed, heart function by its systolic and diastolic phases influences intramyocardial coronary vessels more than all other biochemical metabolites and, so doing, contributes to regulate coronary blood flow and intramyocardial metabolic changes. Major changes in resistance of coronary circulation are mediated primarily by those intramyocardial coronary vessels having a diameter from 10 mμ to 140 mμ [8–9].

Reciprocating clearance of pulling and compressing strengths due to the cardiac cycle makes it difficult to give a carefully tridimensional architecture to resistance intramyocardial vessels, and, consequently, calculate isolated segment volume, whereas, as it will be described more detailedly, the distribution volume to specific myocardial areas may be determined.

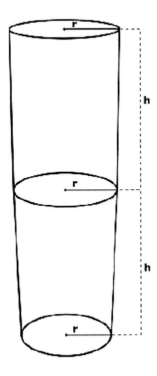

Figure 1.2. Longitudinal section of two consecutive hollow cylinders which reduce progressively their radius (r) from the origin to their end. Arterial coronary vessels are cylindric conduits formed by consecutive segments that reduce progressively their caliber from the origin to their end. There is evidence that the volume of the larger segments of the cylinder will be greater than that of the smaller segments since radius (r), a basic measure to calculate the volume, reduces its length progressively along its course.

Finally, capacitance and metabolic vessels are those artery-arteriolar structures deputed to reach myocardial metabolic units to carry active metabolites to heart cells.

Anatomically, a specific type of gross and histologic structure characterizes conduit, resistance, and capacitance-metabolic coronary arteries.

Table 1.1. summarizes the different coronary artery types.

Table 1.1. Anatomo-functional vessel types in the coronary tree

Type of vessel	Coronary tree
Conduit artery vessels	Epicardial arteries and first intramyocardial coronary arteries
Resistance artery vessels	Intramyocardial coronary arteries, anastomoses (intercoronary and intracoronary anastomoses)
Capacitance artery vessels	Arteriolar anastomoses, Capillary bed
Metabolic artery-arteriolar vessels	Capillary bed

The knowledge of how normal heart and the proximal portions of the great vessels originating beyond of aortic and pulmonic valves receive their physiologic blood supply needs a description of coronary arteries.

Epicardial Coronary Arteries

Two major coronary arteries and their branches provide blood flow to the heart.

The coronary arteries arise within the sinuses of Valsalva behind the aortic valve leaflets. The two main coronary arteries are the left main coronary artery and right coronary artery. Inconstantly, a third coronary artery, named conus artery, originates from a separate ostium in the right sinus in about 50 percent of individuals [10–11]. Additional small ostia have been described to be into the right sinus.

The left main coronary artery that arises from the left posterior sinus of Valsalva and then courses between the pulmonary artery and the left auricolar appendix, after a short distance that usually can vary from 0.5 cm. to 2 cm., branches, usually, into two vessels, called respectively the anterior descending artery and the circumflex artery. Left main coronary artery may branch in 60 percent of cases [12–13] in three or, very rarely, four small arteries. Among these, it is worthwhile to mention the diagonal artery. The right coronary artery branches more distally from its arising compared to what characterizes the left main coronary artery. Functionally, the coronary arteries were believed to be, in the past, end arteries, although, anatomically, numerous intercoronary and intracoronary (or homocoronary) anastomoses up to 40 μm in diameter, differently filled, in most normal hearts exist, and that will be described.

The left and right coronary arteries supply different myocardial areas, and the knowledge of blood flow distribution needs to explain both the localization and course of myocardial alterations as well as the relationship between vascular lesions and degree of cardiac lesions.

The anterior descending artery arises vertically 1 to 1.5 cm from the left main coronary artery. It courses down into the anterior interventricular groove, reaches the anterior portion of cardiac apex rounding the acute margin of the heart and, then, ascends up the posterior interventricular groove for about 1 cm. The left coronary artery supplies (table 1.2.) particularly the anterior wall of the left ventricle, the bordering third of the anterior surface of the right ventricle, the anterior two-thirds of the interventricular septum and most of the heart apex. Along its course, the left anterior descending artery gives off, in an usual order of origin, the first diagonal coronary artery, that can arise, as it will be described, from the left main coronary artery, the first septal perforator branch, and three to four septal perforator arteries as well as some other diagonal branches.

The right coronary artery, after its arising from the right anterior Valsava sinus of the aorta, courses the right atrioventricular sulcus, rounds the acute margin reaching the crux in a large majority of subjects and, then, provides a variable number of branches distributed to the anterior right ventricular wall. A branch (marginal branch), usually, courses the acute margin of the heart, while another branch, called posterior interventricular descending artery, courses down into the posterior interventricular groove reaching the posterior portion of the apex to about 1 cm. above. Along its course the right coronary artery provides a small branch to supply atrioventricular node as well as branches originating shortly after its take-off, to reach atrial myocardium and sinoatrial nodus. So doing, the right coronary artery supplies the remaining wall of the right ventricle anteriorly and posteriorly, the posterior third of both left ventricular wall and interventricular septum and most of atrial myocardium. Moreover, a little branch (infundibular coronary artery) arises from this vessel to ramify into the anterior portion of the arterious conus of the right ventricle.

The circumflex artery, usually a smaller branch if compared to the left anterior descending artery arising from the left main coronary artery, runs in the left ventricular sulcus after its origin and supplies a small portion of the lateral myocardium of the left ventricle together with a small portion of left ventricle anteriorly and posteriorly and left atrium by giving small branches to these areas. Usually, the circumflex artery ends at the obtuse margin of the heart although, in somes occurrences, it can reach the crux – namely the junction of the posterior interventricular sulcus and posterior atrioventricular groove. When this anatomical distribution occurs, allof the left ventricle and ventricular septum are supplied by blood from the left coronary arteries relieving the flow into the right coronary artery.

Finally, the diagonal artery that, usually, arises near the bifurcation of the left main coronary artery, courses inferiorly along an angle of the anterior wall of the left ventricle initially between the circumflex and the left anterior descending artery and then between the left descending artery and obtuse marginal artery. The diagonal artery supplies little branches to the interventricular septum, anterior wall of the left ventricle, and anterior papillary muscle.

Subepicardial portion of the coronary arteries is embedded by various amounts of subepicardial fat until entering coronary artery deeply into myocardial mass.

An excellent and complete description of the anatomy of coronary arteries may be examined in a fairly recent report [14].

Indeed, from these considerations there is evidence that variations in branching patterns may be seen in the human heart making dominant, sometimes, the right coronary circulation, sometimes the left coronary circulation, or a balanced coronary circulation according to the type and distribution of the coronary tree. Also different locations of lesions may be influenced by the characteristics of coronary artery variations. Since smoking affects preferably some coronary artery segments rather than others, as it will be described widely in the next chapters, one can understand the absolute need to know the coronary anatomy to interpret the significance of possible alterations.

Schematic figures 1.3. to 1.5, obtained by drawing the heart after pericardium removal, display anatomical course of the coronary arteries.

The course and branching of coronary arteries may be shown either by in vivo coronary angiography or by postmortem coronary angiography (figure 1.6.) [15-16] as well as necropsy techniques. These methods of study provide detailed data on the anatomical and pathological characteristics of the coronary tree allowing us to identify the relationship that exists between metabolic demand of the heart and blood flow supply.

Table 1.2. Different myocardial areas supplied by coronary arteries

Anterior descending coronary artery	Anterior wall of the left ventricle
	Bordering third of the anterior surface of right ventricle
	Two-third anterior of interventricular septum
	Almost total heart apex
Right coronary artery	Reminder anterior and posterior right ventricle wall
	Posterior third of left ventricular wall
	Posterior third of interventricular septum
Circumflex coronary artery	Small portion of lateral wall of left ventricle
	Small portion of left ventricle anterior wall
	Small portion of left ventricle posterior wall
Diagonal artery	Interventricular septum
	Anterior wall of the left ventricle
	Anterior papillary muscle

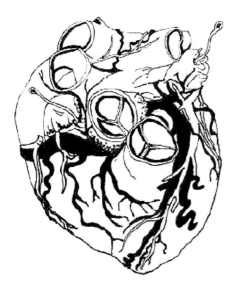

Figure 1.3.

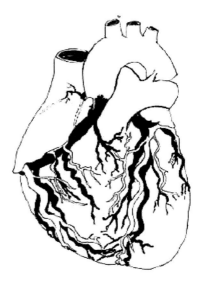

Figure 1.4.

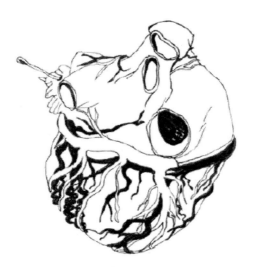

Figure 1.5.

Figures 1.3 to 1.5 showing schematic drawings of the heart carried out from different projections. Cephalic view (figure 1.3.), ventral view (figure 1.4.), and dorsal view of the heart after removing pericardium to see the coronary tree injected in black. One can see, respectively the left coronary distribution, particularly in figure 1.3. and 1.4, and right coronary distribution, particularly in figure 1.5. White color characterizes the accompaning coronary veins which reach, at their end, the coronary sinus into the right atrium (figure 1.5.).

Intramyocardial Circulation

Intramyocardial circulation (table 1.3.) is formed by: 1. Intramyocardial coronary arteries; 2. Coronary arterioles; 3. Intercoronary and intracoronary (homocoronary) anastomoses; 4. Capillary bed.

Coronary vessels enter into myocardial mass perpendicularly. They have different length and caliber going from up to 6 cm, the longest branches (usually arising from left anterior descending artery), to about one millimeter, the smallest arterioles proximally to capillary bed. Similarly, the artery caliber also diminishes progressively from arterial entering into myocardial mass to its branching in the capillary network.

Table 1.3. Intramyocardial coronary artery vessels

Large intramyocardial coronary arteries
Small intramyocardial coronary arteries
Intramyocardial coronary arterioles
Intercoronary anastomoses
Intracoronary (homocoronary) anastomoses
Coronary capillary bed

Intramural coronary circulation feels deeply either the anatomical integrity of extramural coronary arteries or myocardial mass since these vessels are respectively stressed and released during systole and diastole of the cardiac cycle. In case of a poor availability of oxygen, intramyocardial vessels suffer chronically and show in time hyperplastic and degenerative changes with evident impairment of their metabolic function. The basic function of intramural circulation includes providing anastomoses among adjacent branches. In normal hearts, usually the communications between various arteries are particularly developed among vessels of small diameter like arterioles and prearterioles. Anastomoses can undergo a gradual enlargement or also become functionally of significant caliber if their wall does not show alterations in presence, particularly, of narrowing epicardial artery pathology. Finally, intramural vessels branch into a capillary bed and may be also connected directly with cardiac chambers as arterioluminal vessels [17–19].

Anastomoses, which may be observed also in normal hearts, show that, at least from an anatomic point of view, coronary arteries are not end-arteries, as believed in the past, but a network structurally organized in any intramyocardial area. Moreover, anastomoses, independently from the development of coronary collaterals, are developed at any level of myocardial mass although their maximum development has been demonstrated to occur distally.

Differences exist about the characteristics of the intramyocardial coronary vessels according to the fact of left or right dominant coronary circulation. Such a feature can determine variations in the blood supply to certain parts of the myocardium which become more clearly evident in case of coronary vessel pathology.

Atrial Circulation

Finally, the atria are supplied by small branches arising from those coronary trunks of the corresponding side.

Pathological narrowings or occlusion of the coronary arteries can cause severe damage to ventricular muscle, but much less to atrial muscle. Therefore, also those myocardial lesions due to smoking prefer a ventricular localization rather than an atrial site.

Geometrical Distribution of Coronary Tree

Techniques of study carried out by using postmortem coronary injection with a radiopaque mass associated with a chemical diaphaneity of myocardial mass permitted to obtain heart casts which give three-dimensional pictures of the coronary tree (figure 1.6.).

Briefly, the postmortem method consists, for what concerns coronary injection, of removing the heart [20] by severing the pulmonary artery and aorta about 5 cm from the free margin of the semilunar valves. After observing the external aspect of the heart to identify possible areas of myocardial damage, without opening the coronary vessels, a plug is placed through the aorta into the aortic orifice and then the coronary arteries are injected at a pressure of 130 mmHg using a barium-iodine-gelatin radiopaque mass by a cannula tied into the aorta. When a good degree of contrast is noted in x-rays, the heart undergoes cast building by a chemical procedure. Also direct injection by radiopaque mass of each single coronary artery through a cannula into its orifice of origin may be used.

After the injection, that can be carried out also by using different radiopaque masses, maceration and corrosion of the heart follow to produce vascular casts. Customarily, the injection mass must be of material that resists corrosive techniques. Myocardial mass is destroyed by strong alkaline or acid solutions. In the past years, numerous substances have been used [21–26] to visualize the coronary tree for producing casts. Among them, there were methacrylate and plexiglass [21], vinylite – probably the most used medium- [22], resins [23], nylon [24], neophrene and different types of latex [25–26]. Rubber latex [16] has been well associated with barium sulphate injection to obtain a good contrast of coronary vessels.

Casts permitted to identify particularly some spatial (three-dimensional) characteristics of the coronary artery system that could better explain the relationship existing between coronary tree and strongly related blood flow supply.

Firstly, there is evidence that numerous anastomoses different with regard to type, caliber, and distribution may be documented into intramyocardial mass. These anastomoses occur between branches of the same coronary artery (called intracoronary or homocoronary anastomoses) as well as branches of different intramyocardial coronary arteries (called intercoronary anastomoses). Anastomoses appear to be either functioning structures or empty structures in relation to the metabolic demand of the heart. Therefore, they may be observed transiently or, on the contrary, permanently, but they exist with no doubt. Usually, a diffuse anastomotic network may be seen in any intramyocardial area. This network plays a significant role in the transport of the oxygen and those active metabolites that diffuse into the myocardial cells to influence their function.

Secondly, the course of the main subepicardial coronary arteries may be carefully established. The left coronary tree, that arise from the posterior aortic ostium, goes anteriorly towards the anterior wall of the left ventricle, while right coronary artery from the anterior aortic ostium reaches the posterior wall of the left ventricle. This running is in relation to the portion of heart that the coronary tree supplies.

Finally, not yet well classified stimuli and heavy coronary pathology, that will be described in the next chapters, determine, in a significant number of patients, the development of the coronary collateral circulation [27].

Usually, in individuals the development of coronary collaterals is related to significant coronary artery narrowings [28]. The number and type of these collaterals, as shown by plastic casts of the heart, vary widely being, sometimes, so high that it is very difficult to determne their real amount; on the contrary, sometimes, collaterals are poorly developed in the case of small or no coronary artery narrowings or in the presence of cardiac atrophy.

Spatially, within the myocardium collaterals have an oblique or parallel course with respect to muscular layers and endocardial surface where, usually, parallel distribution is furtherly stressed.

These spatial shapes permit the improvement of coronary collateral function during systolic and diastolic phases of the cardiac cycle with positive influence on heart demand.

Casts, similar to what in vivo or postmortem angiography by radiopaque mass without heart corrosion shows, provide detailed data about the development of coronary collaterals although, geometrically, information about three-dimensional distribution of these arterial branches are more evident by casts than isolated postmortem angiographic studies.

Nowadays, postmortem coronary injection by radiopaque mass and casts to identify the anatomical status of the coronary arteries are used even less since the development of refined instrumental techniques of study in vivo of the heart like three-dimensional echocardiography, computed tomography and nuclear magnetic resonance permit one to obtain selective images of the different cardiac structures which are completely similar to those that one can observe by necropsy examination. Thus, the above diagnostic instrumental techniques are used even more frequently because of the progress in therapeutic treatment of coronary artery disease for those patients who are at risk.

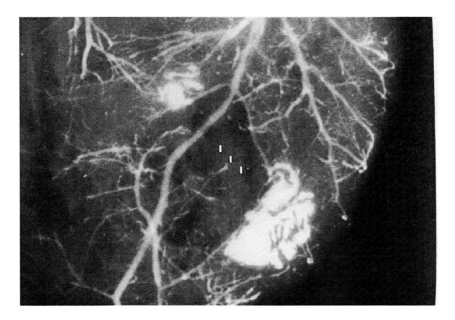

Figure 1.6. An angiographic view obtained by using barium sulphate combined with bacto-gelatin of a part of myocardial mass in a heart cast. There is a clear evidence of coronary collaterals, intercoronary and intracoronary anastomoses as well as an avascular area in the central zone of the left ventricular wall due to an old myocardial infarction (white arrows).

Histology of Coronary Artery Wall

Similar to what characterizes all arteries in different tissues of the body, the coronary artery wall in conduit vessels, namely epicardial coronary vessels and large intramural coronary vessels, consists of three coats differently developed with respect to artery course: tunica intima, tunica media, and tunica adventitia.

The intima, the inner luminal layer, consists of a lining of cells called endothelial cells, and a subendothelial layer where there are connective tissue and smooth muscle cells. All these structures form the endothelium which is a selective barrier of diffusion between the blood and other wall coats. Spatially, endothelial cells follow the major dimension of the coronary artery and, therefore, are oriented longitudinally along the vessel and attached among them by junctions of two types: occluding junctions and gap junctions.

The vascular endothelium has been long interpreted as a simply physical separation between blood and tissue [29] , a lining of the arterial intima to protect passively this structure from the mechanical injuries coming through the blood.

Over the last twenty years, experimental and clinical results have shown that the endothelium is not only a lining structure of vessels and the heart (endocardium) , but particularly a widely distributed organ among and within tissues [30–31] deeply involved in regulating vascular physiology and its pathophysiologic changes. These functions, that will be widely discussed in the next chapter, are strictly related to its position at the interface between blood and tissue. Moreover, the progression of the knowledge on endothelial function has demonstrated that, similar to the heart [32], the vascular endothelium also can be considered a target organ of smoking damage [33–38] since smoking is capable of inducing earlier endothelial dysfunction and, then, later, after several years, structural alterations.

There is growing evidence that endothelium, among the different structures of the body, is capable of better harmonizing its anatomical shape with function.

The intima is separated from the medial coat by the internal elastic membrane, called internal elastic lamina, which may be differently structured in relation to its integrity or harm due to injuring phenomena. The large majority of its composition is elastic tissue with a sinusoid orientation. Internal elastic lamina is not a continuous structure, but it is fenestrated and so smooth muscle cells of media can migrate to the intima coat.

Endothelium is the coronary artery structure that tends to keep its shape along the entire coronary network.

Medial coat consists of multiple layers of smooth muscle cells, collagen and elastic fibers. There is evidence that the amount of each of the above components varies widely with regard to coronary course, having less elastic material and a greater number of smooth muscle cells in the epicardial coronary arteries compared with elastic arteries of different locations [14] of the body.

Spatially, the media may consist of up to 40 layers of smooth muscle cells oriented in a circle or helix. Smooth muscle cells are embedded in a connective glycoprotein mix which, chemically, reacts with periodic acid-Schiff giving a stain PAS-positive [39]. This stain method permits one to identify glycogen and, generally, glycoproteins in those tissues where these substances are present by oxidizing glucose residues and forming aldehydes which react with the Schiff reagent.

An external elastic lamina, considerably thinner than the internal elastic lamina and composed particularly of elastin, separates the medial from adventitial coat. Closely in contact to the outer border of this lamina unmyelinated nervous axons may be identified.

Medial coat is that structure which more deeply feels pathologic injuries from what concerns arterial stiffness due to the effects of the major coronary risk factors, smoking included.

Adventitial coat consists of a significant amount of fibrous tissue, particularly collagen and elastic fibers oriented longitudinally. In its context vasa vasorum, lymphatic vessels and nerves exist. The thickness of the coat may vary widely going from 300 to 500 μm.

Figures 1.7. to 1.10. show the main features of the arteries for what concerns arterial coats.

Some interesting characteristics, that may be seen in the coronary tree, must be kept in mind: progressive structural changes along coronary artery course and changes that occur, physiologically, with age.

From the origin to intramyocardial coronary network, there is a progressive reduction up to lacking of the thickness of adventitial and medial coats whereas the endothelium improves more and more its metabolic and functional properties.

Age [40] determines a progressive sclerosis of the coronary vessels with changes of structural orientation of elastic and smooth muscle cells as a consequence of hemodynamic changes that characterize advancing age. On the contrary, intimal and adventitial coats in fetal coronary arteries are not well developed, but media consists of a well-defined presence of smooth muscle cells and elastic fibers. Therefore, aging determines increased arterial stiffness, although endothelial cells, which develop their function progressively after birth, tend to be preserved for a longer time.

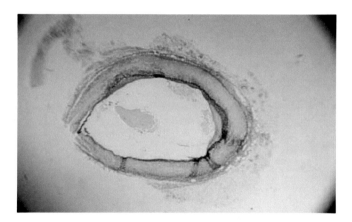

Figure 1.7.

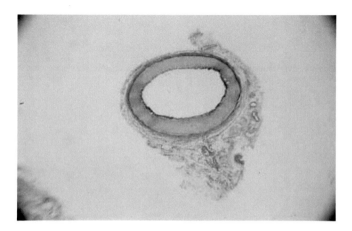

Figure 1.8.

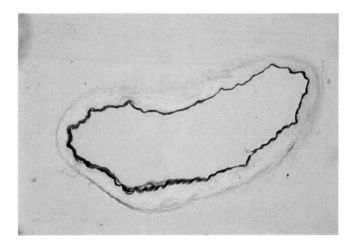

Figure 1.9.

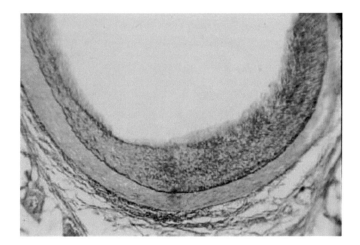

Figure 1.10.

Figures from 1.7. to 1.10. showing patterns of arteries of different caliber and size where the three vessel coats (intima, media, and adventitia) are evident. One can see that difference in thickness of the three coats exists at different levels of the arterial tree while internal elastic lamina is clearly more developed than external elastic lamina in all segments of all the arteries.

The Coronary Veins

Venous drainage of the coronary circulation is the result of the combined action of a rich venous network and cardiac veins.

The venous systems which return the blood from capillary bed are listed in table 1.4.

Table 1.4. The venous system of the heart

Great cardiac vein		Anterior cardiac vein
Posterior cardiac vein		Right or small coronary vein
Left cardiac vein		Coronary sinus
	Venae Thebesii	

The great cardiac vein, also called coronary vein, is a vessel of great size. From the apex of the heart, the vessel ascends along the anterior interventricular groove to the base of the ventricles, reaches the atrio-ventricular groove, and, then, opens into the coronary sinus.

The posterior cardiac vein – also called middle cardiac vein – from the apex of the heart, where small tributary branches flow together, ascends along the posterior interventricular groove to the base of the heart terminating in the coronary sinus.

Three to four small venous branches, which collect the blood from the posterior surface of the left ventricle, form the left cardiac vein that opens into the lower border of the coronary sinus. Similarly, three to four small branches collect the blood from the anterior surface of the right ventricle forming the anterior cardiac vein. They open separately into the inferior portion of the right auricle.

The small coronary vein, which receives blood from the posterior portion of the right ventricle and auricle, runs along the right portion of the atrio-ventricular groove to reach the coronary sinus.

The coronary sinus, located in the posterior part of the left atrio-ventricular groove, anatomically belongs to the anterior cardiac vein but receives blood from all other veins. The coronary sinus opens into the right auricle between the inferior vena cava and auriculo-ventricular aperture by an orifice limited by the Thebesian valve.

Finally, venae Thebesii are the smallest venous branches with no relation to the venous system which returns blood directly from the myocardial mass, opening by thin orifices, called foramina Thebesii, into the inner surface of the right auricle.

Table 1.5 summarizes blood venous distribution.

From the examination of table 1.5, there emerges clearly that the reservoir of the coronary circulation return is the coronary sinus which is the cardiac structure that is more strictly linked to the right atrium similarly to what occurs for the systemic venous circulation that flows venous blood into the right atrium.

Table 1.5. Coronary vein course and opening into the heart

Coronary vein	Course	Opening
Great cardiac vein	Anterior interventricular groove	Coronary sinus
Posterior cardiac vein	Posterior interventricular groove	Coronary sinus
Left cardiac vein	Posterior left ventricular surface	Coronary sinus
Anterior cardiac vein	Anterior right ventricular surface	Right auricle
Small coronary vein	Right atrio-ventricular groove	Coronary sinus
Coronary sinus	Between vena cava and Thebesian valve	Right auricle
Venae Thebesii	Myocardium	Right auricle

Ultrastructural Features of the Coronary Arteries

In electron microscopy, the structure of epicardial coronary arteries is similar to that of all other arteries of the body which are of the same anatomical type and have a conduit function. However, vascular endothelium of the coronary tree needs special attention since damaging mechanisms which are a result of the effects of the major risk factors have, usually, a strong impact on endothelial cells causing early endothelial dysfunction [34, 38].

For the most part, results concerning ultrastructural characteristics of the coronary arteries were coming from experimental studies conducted on animals which analyzed, particularly, pathological patterns [41–42] under the effects of major coronary risk factors, primarily cigarette smoking.

By electron miscroscopy findings [43], one can establish that the basic constituents of the coronary wall are the endothelial cells, smooth muscle cells and an extracellular matrix particularly composed of connective material that includes elastic fibers, collagen and proteoglycans. Usually, the intima is a concentric monolayer of poligonal cells which are in contact with arterial lumen. Minimal underlying subendothelial connective tissue is also present. Media shows particularly smooth muscle cells oriented circularly or spirally. Elastin is usually arranged near the internal and external elastic laminae. Nervous components and metabolic granules of vasoactive substances are also present. A significant amount of elements belonging to connective tissue characterizes the adventitia where vasa vasorum and nerve fibers are dispersed. An electron microscopy pattern of the wall of a coronary artery of a rat, the picture of which was taken by also using a green polarized light filter, may be seen in figure 1.11. All the main components which form the arterial coats may be seen to have a regular series of elements oriented along the main course of the vessel.

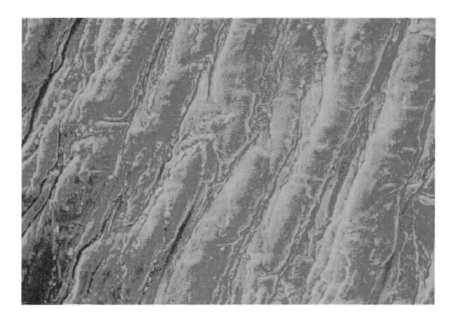

Figure 1.11. Ultrastructural pattern of the wall of a coronary artery. Picture was taken by using a green light polarized filter. One can see a regular series of cellular components formed by smooth muscle fibers, elastic fibers, and some connective structures.

Blood Volume of the Coronary Circulation

In normal hearts, the total volume of the left ventricular coronary vessels related to coronary arteries, capillary bed, and venules less than 100 μm in diameter has been calculated, experimentally, to be from 6 to 15 ml per 100 grams of the left ventricle myocardial mass [44–45]. These measures were carried out by using instrumental diagnostic techniques associated with chemical substance injection since the geometrical formula to calculate the volume in a cylinder constant in dimensions, as shown in the paragraph concerning conduit vessels, could not be used because of the different caliber and shape of the coronary vessels estimated.

The knowledge of the amount of blood volume in coronary circulation permits one to establish some interesting observations.

The stiffness of the left ventricular wall is influenced by intracoronary blood flow volume [46–47]. Moreover, the volume into coronary vessels plays a transient reservoir function. Indeed, each cardiac cycle pumps an amount of about 15 percent of the total volume in the system into coronary vessels. In so doing, the blood which is stored in the vessels could deaden, theoretically, with the possible sudden reduction in coronary flow for a few cardiac cycles providing a transiently limited protection to heart muscle demand.

Finally, the estimate of blood volume of coronary circulation as well as its changes under different stressing events permit one to establish if coronary vessels are able to warrant metabolic demand of the heart or fail with regard to this function. Such information can provide interesting data about anatomical features of the coronary vessels.

Differences in anatomy of coronary arteries as well as myocardial distribution may be seen among animal species [48–52]. That should be kept in mind since partial or total occlusions of a specific vessel may cause a myocardial infarction in some animals but not in others. Moreover, development of coronary collaterals may be lacking in some species.

Experimentally, the most used animals to assess cardiac and coronary pathology (like rats, rabbits, dogs) were markedly predisposed to develop a massive myocardial infarction following an acute occlusion of the left anterior descending artery because of morphologic differences in the coronary circulation with a significant prevailing in the left arterial distribution.

References

[1] Leone A. Cardiovascular damage from smoking: a fact or belief? *Int. J. Cardiol.* 1993; 38: 113 – 7.

[2] Hammond EC, Garfinkel L. Coronary heart disease, stroke and aortic aneurysm. *Arch. Environ. Health.* 1969; 19: 167 – 82.

[3] Auerbach O, Carter HW, Garfinkel M, Hammond EC. Cigarette smoking and coronary heart disease, a macroscopic and microscopic study. *Chest.* 1976; 70: 697 – 705.

[4] Leone A, Lopez M. Oral contraception, ovarian disorders and tobacco in myocardial infarction of woman. *Pathologica.* 1986; 78: 237 – 42.

[5]   Strong JP, Richards ML. Cigarette smoking and atherosclerosis in autopsied men. *Atherosclerosis.* 1976; 23: 451 – 76.

[6]   Auerbach O, Hammond EC, Garfinkel L. Smoking in ralation to atherosclerosis of the coronary arteries. *New Engl. J. Med.* 1965; 273: 775 – 9.

[7]   Glantz SA, Parmley WW. Passive smoking and heart disease. *JAMA.* 1995; 273: 1047 – 53.

[8]   Nellis SH, Liedtke AJ, Whitessel L. Small coronary vessel pressure and diameter in an intact beating rabbit heart using fixed-position and free-motion techniques. *Circ. Res.* 1981; 49: 342 – 53.

[9]   Tillmans H, Steinhausen M, Leimberger H, Thederan H, Kubler W. Pressure measurements in the terminal vascular bed of the epimyocardium of rats and cats. *Circ. Res.* 1981; 49: 1202 – 11.

[10]   Waller BF. Anatomy, histology, and pathology of the major epicardial coronary arteries relevant to echocardiographic imaging techniques. *J. Am. Soc. Echocardiogr.* 1989; 2: 232 – 52.

[11]   Waller BF. Five coronary ostia: Duplicate left anterior descending and right conus coronary arteries. *Am. J. Cardiol.* 1983; 52: 126 – 37.

[12]   Crainicianu A. Anatomische studien uber die koronararterien und experimentelle untersuchungen uber ihre durchgangigkeit. *Virch. Arch. Pat. Anat.* 1922; 238: 1 – 13.

[13]   Smith GT. The anatomy of the coronary circulation. *Am. J. Cardiol.* 1962; 9: 327 – 42.

[14]   Baroldi G. Diseases of the coronary arteries. In: Silver MD, ed, *Cardiovascular Pathology.* 1. Churchill Livingstone, New York, USA, 1983: 317 – 91.

[15]   Schlesinger MJ. An injection plus dissection study of coronary artery occlusions and anastomoses. *Am. Heart J.* 1938; 15: 528 – 68.

[16]   Salans AH, Tweed P. A preliminary study of the coronary circulation post-mortem. *Am. Heart J.* 1947; 33: 477 – 89.

[17]   Wearn JT. The extent of the capillary bed of the heart. *J. Exp. Med.* 1928; 47: 273 – 91.

[18]   Wearn JT. The role of the thebesian vessels in the circulation of the heart. *J. Exp. Med.* 1928; 47: 293 – 316.

[19]   Wearn JT, Mettier SR, Klump TG, Zschiesche LJ. The nature of the vascular communications between the coronary arteries and the chambers of the heart. *Am. Heart J.* 1933; 9: 143 – 64.

[20]   Leone A. L'angiografia coronarica postmortem nello studio anatomo-patologico del cuore. *G. Ital. Cardiol.* 1972; 2: 688 – 92.

[21]   Van der Ghinst M. L'injection du système coronarien par des matières plastiques. *Acta Cardiol.* 1949; 4: 274 – 9.

[22]   Stern H, Ranzenhofer ER, Liebow AA. Preparation of vinylite casts of the coronary vessels and cardiac chambers. *Lab. Invest.* 1954; 3: 337 – 47.

[23]   Zugibe FT, Bourke DW, Brown KD. A plastic injection method for grading atherosclerosis of the coronary arteries. *Am. J. Clin. Pathol.* 1961; 35: 563 – 71.

[24]   Wagner A, Poindexter CA. Demonstration of the coronary arteries with nylon. *Am. Heart J.* 1949; 37: 258 – 66.

[25]   Smith JR, Henry MJ. Demonstration of the coronary arterial system with neophrene latex. *J. Lab. Clin. Med.* 1945; 30: 462 – 6.

[26] Baroldi G, Mantero O, Scomazzoni G. The collaterals of the coronary arteries in normal and pathological hearts. *Circ. Res.* 1956; 4: 223 – 9.

[27] Schaper W, Bernotat-Danielowski S, Nienaber C, Schaper J. Collateral circulation. In: Fozzard HA, Haber E, Jennings RB, Katz AM, Morgan HE, eds. *The Heart and Cardiovascular System.* 2nd ed, Raven, New York, USA, 1991: 1427 – 64.

[28] Gregg DE, Patterson RE. Functional importance of the coronary collaterals. *N. Engl. J. Med.* 1980; 303: 1404 – 6.

[29] Fishman AP. Endothelium: a distributed organ of diverse capabilities. *Ann. N.Y. Acad. Sci.* 1982; 401: 1 – 8.

[30] Cines DB, Pollak ES, Buck CA, Loscalzo J, Zimmerman GA, McEver RP, Pober JS, Wick TM, Konkle BA, Schwartz BS, Barnathan ES, McCrae KR, Hug BA, Schmidt AM, Stern DM. Endothelial cells in physiology and in the pathophysiology of vascular disorders. *Blood.* 1998; 91: 3527 – 61.

[31] Stevens T, Rosemberg R, Aird W, Quertenous T, Johnson FL, Garcia JG, Hebbel RP, Tuder RM, Garfinkel S. NHLBI workshop report : endothelial cell phenotypes in heart, lung, and blood diseases. *Am. J. Physiol. Cell Physiol.* 2001; 281: C1422 – 33.

[32] Leone A. The heart: a target organ for cigarette smoking. *J. Smoking-Related Dis.* 1992; 3: 197 – 201.

[33] Celermajer DS, Adams MR, Clarkson P, Robinson J, McRedie R, Donald A, Deanfield JE. Passive smoking and impaired endothelium-dependent arterial dilatation in healthy young adults. *N. Engl. J. Med.* 1996; 334: 150 – 4.

[34] Sumida H, Watanabe H, Kugiyama K, Ohgushi M, Matsumura T, Yasue H. Does passive smoking impair endothelium-dependent coronary artery dilation in women? *J. Am. Coll. Cardiol.* 1998; 31: 811 – 5.

[35] Davis J, Shelton L, Watanabe I, Arnold J. Passive smoking affects endothelium and platelets. *Arch. Intern. Med.* 1989; 149: 386 – 9.

[36] Raitakari OT, Adams MR, McRedie RJ, Griffiths KA, Celermajer DS. Passive-smoke related arterial endothelial dysfunction is potentially reversible in healthy young adults. *Ann. Intern. Med.* 1999; 130: 578 – 81.

[37] Celermajer DS, Sorensen KE, Georgakopoulos D. Cigarette smoking is associated with dose-related and potentially reversible impairment of endothelium-dependent dilation in healthy young adults. *Circulation.* 1993; 88: 2149 – 55.

[38] Deedwania PC. Endothelium: a new target for cardiovascular therapeutics. *J. Am. Coll. Cardiol.* 2000; 35: 67 – 70.

[39] Bangle R Jr, Alford WC. The chemical basis of the periodic acid Schiff reaction of collagen fibers with reference to periodate consumption by collagen and by insulin. *J. Histochem. Cytochem.* 1954; 2: 62 – 76.

[40] Neufeld HN, Schneeweiss A. *Coronary artery disease in infants and children.* Lea and Febiger, Philadelphis, USA, 1983: 1 – 22.

[41] Lough J. Cardiomyopathy produced by cigarette smoke. Ultrastructural observations in guinea pigs. *Arch. Pathol. Lab. Med.* 1978; 102: 377 – 80.

[42] Kjeldsen K, Thomsen HK, Astrup P. Effects of carbon monoxide on myocardium. Ultrastructural changes in rabbits after moderate, chronic exposure. *Circ. Res.* 1974; 34: 339 – 48.

[43] Schoen FJ, Cotran RS. Blood Vessels. In: Cotran RS, Kumar V, Collins T, eds. *Pathologic Basis of Disease*. 6th Ed, WB Saunders Company, Philadelphia, USA, 1999: 493 – 541.

[44] Crystal GJ, Downey HF, Bashour FA. Small vessel and total coronary blood volume during intracoronary adenosine. *Am. J. Physiol.* 1981; 241: H 194 – 201.

[45] Gaasch WH, Bernard SA. The effect of acute changes in coronary blood flow on left ventricular end-diastolic wall thickness. An echocardiographic study. *Circulation.* 1977; 56: 593 – 8.

[46] Salisbury PF, Cross CE, Rieben PA. Influence of coronary artery pressure upon myocardial elasticity. *Circ. Res.* 1960; 8: 794 – 800.

[47] Olsen CO, Attarian DE, Jones RN, Hill RC, Sink JD, Lee KL, Wechsler AS. The coronary pressure-flow determinants of left ventricular compliance in dogs. *Circ. Res.* 1981; 49: 856 –65.

[48] Borer JS, Harrison LA, Kent KM, Levy R, Goldstein RE, Epstein SE. Beneficial effect of lidocaine on ventricular electrical stability and spontaneous ventricular fibrillation during experimental myocardial infarction. *Am. J. Cardiol.* 1976; 37: 860 – 3.

[49] Astrup T. The hemostatic balance. *Thromb. Diath. Haemorrh.* 1958; 2: 347 – 57.

[50] Grant RT. Development of the cardiac coronary vessels in the rabbit. *Heart.* 1926; 13: 261 – 71.

[51] Provenza DV, Scherlis S. Coronary circulation in dog's heart. Demonstration of muscle sphincters in capillaries. *Circ. Res.* 1959; 7: 318 – 24.

[52] Bajusz E. Experimental pathology and histochemistry of heart muscle. *Meth. Achievm. Exp. Path.* 1967; 2: 172 – 223.

Chapter II

Physiology of the Coronary Circulation

Abstract

Coronary circulation is deputed to provide the supply of oxygen for heart function. Therefore, coronary blood flow increases when the work of the heart increases its demand for oxygen. Coronary blood flow can increase its rest measures up to five times.

Different factors regulate coronary blood flow changes: autoregulation (myogenic regulation), metabolic and humoral regulation, physical regulation, and autonomic regulation. Some of these determinants like myogenic factor and physical factors regulate coronary blood flow by changes in perfusion pressure, whereas metabolic regulation occurs maintaining perfusion pressure at constant values and coronary blood flow increases as a consequence of active metabolite release. Autonomic regulation involves both heart parameters - heart rate, blood pressure and myocardial contractility -and receptor structures of the coronary arterial wall.

All these parameters are, usually, described separately because of didactic reasons. Really, they are closely inter-related to permit those adjustments in coronary blood flow to meet the heart's continuous demand for oxygen, needed for a correct function.

Keywords: Physiology, coronary circulation, regulation, myocardial oxygen consumption, physical regulation, humoral regulation, metabolic regulation, autonomic regulation, myogenic regulation, autonomic nervous system, coronary blood flow, endothelial dysfunction, aerobic metabolism, heart, anaerobic metabolism , coronary reserve, coronary wall receptor(s), sympathetic system, parasympathetic system, vagus, vascular tone, bradycardia, myocardial contractility, perfusion pressure, systemic blood pressure, carotid baroreceptor(s), physical force.

Physiologically, artery vessels play a dynamic function – to transport blood oxygen and active metabolites to the organs of the whole body. To do that, vessels are influenced by several factors, mainly cardiac inotropism, myocardial mass, peripheral vascular resistance, and blood rheology. Physical strength, mechanical factors and biochemical substances interact among themselves to permit artery function to be performed correctly.

Table 2.1. summarizes basic elements that influence artery function.

Table 2.1. Main factors which are able to influence artery vessel function

1. Determinants of heart function	Inotropic state
	Heart rate
	Left ventricular wall tension
2. Determinants of peripheral vascular resistance	Vasoconstriction factors
	Vasodilation factors
	Blood oxygen concentration
	Neurohormonal factors
	Pharmacological agents
3. Blood rheology	Blood volume
	Blood viscosity

The majority of these determinants which control the arterial function are able to change their level of response with regard to body organ demands for oxygen. Arteries which supply blood to muscular structures like skeletal muscle and the heart differ deeply in their function to transport oxygen in view of the fact that skeletal muscle and the heart have different functional properties, although vessels are related to structurally similar tissues. Thus, the heart is a muscle that works continuously and, therefore, cannot accumulate oxygen debt to restore later, and, moreover, the heart is an aerobic organ. On the contrary, skeletal muscle may have an oxygen imbalance after exercise that will be restored later during rest following its active function. In so doing, skeletal muscle alternates exercise phases with rest phases to restore its metabolism. Moreover, anaerobic glycolysis, as it has been seen even under experimental conditions of maximum exercise, plays a limited role to provide active metabolites, like adenosine triphosphate, to the heart [1].

Myocardial oxygen consumption (MVo2) is the parameter most strongly related to myocardial oxygen demand [2–4] and, consequently, to the capacity of coronary circulation in changing its blood flow to face this need [5].

MVo2 may be well calculated by using the Fick principle [6] by applying the formula:

MVo2 = Total CBF (coronary blood flow) x Arteriovenous oxygen difference

Simply, MVo2 may be estimated by an empirical method using the product between heart rate and systolic blood pressure, two of the basic determinants of oxygen demand required by the working heart [4, 7–9]. Both heart rate and systolic blood pressure are two parameters which can be easily deduced by a clinical exam of an individual.

Before analyzing in detail the function of coronary circulation, it should be worthwhile to discuss briefly what either aerobic or anaerobic metabolism can provide to the myocardial muscle, what these two pathways demand back, which relationship with MVo2 exists, and the main chemical reactions that permit a correct interpretation of the phenomena.

Aerobic Metabolism of the Heart

As mentioned, the heart is a body organ with an aerobic metabolism under physiological demands. However, in some occurrences anaerobic glycolysis may be transiently utilized.

Aerobic pathways require a series of biochemical reactions that utilize different substrates. Reactions are aimed to provide biochemical energy, which needs cellular respiration and, consequently, cellular function.

Cellular respiration is the result of a balance between processes that take place into a cell to produce, particularly, adenosine triphosphate (ATP), energetic intracellular substrate, and processes that release waste products.

Energy is released by oxidation processes, while the reactions involved in intracellular respiration are the catabolic phase of metabolism.

Molecules commonly used by cells for respiration include chemical components belonging to the whole chain of metabolism like glucose, amino acids and fatty acids, and a common oxidizing agent that is molecular oxygen (O_2). Indeed, aerobic respiration requires oxygen in order to generate energy (ATP). Glucose metabolism is the basic substrate to obtain an optimized heart function under physiologic conditions.

Biochemical reactions of the aerobic metabolism require preferably pyruvate breakdown from glycolysis. Then, pyruvate enters the mitochondria to be fully oxidized by the Krebs cycle, also called citric acid cycle [10]. The product of this process is energy in the form of ATP (Adenosine Triphosphate), by substrate-level phosphorylation, NADH and $FADH_2$. The reducing potential of NADH and $FADH_2$ is converted to more ATP through an electron transport chain with oxygen as the "terminal electron acceptor". Most of the ATP produced by cellular respiration is by oxidative phosphorylation. Therefore, respiration and, consequently, a correct function is the process by which cells obtain energy when oxygen is present in the cell. These processes permit a normal heart function.

ATP molecules that can be obtained by glucose during cellular respiration arise from glycolysis, from the Krebs cycle, and, in a large majority, from the electron transport system.

The energy conversion reaction may be expressed as follows:

$$C_6H_{12}O_6 + 6O \rightarrow 6CO_2 + 6H_2O + energy (ATP).$$

Thus, two processes, one a chemical process, the Krebs cycle, and another a physical process, the electron transport chain, linked by a chemiosmotic phosphorylation, produce ATP.

A large series of enzymatic reactions characterizes aerobic metabolism and Krebs cycle [11–13]. Firstly, pyruvate is converted into acetylCoA. Then, citrate is formed by a combination of acetylCoA with oxaloacetate of the previous Krebs cycle. A process of isomerism forms isocitrate that is oxidized into 5-carbon α-ketoglutarate with release of carbon dioxide. Alpha-ketoglutarate meets a process of oxidation to form succinyl CoA that releases coenzyme A and phosphorylates ADP (adenosine diphosphate) into ATP. Figure 2.1. summarizes the main steps of Krebs cycle.

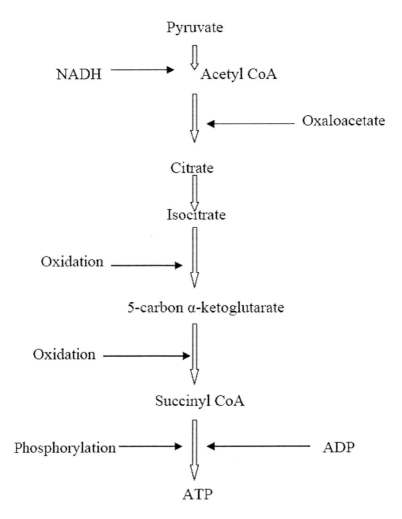

Figure 2.1. Pathways of Krebs cycle to produce ATP necessary for cardiac muscle metabolism.

Under moderate exertion, carbohydrate metabolism is of an aerobic type. Moreover, if there is availability of plenty of oxygen and required function is of a low or moderate degree, the pyruvate from glucose metabolism is converted to carbon dioxide and water into the mitochondria. Moreover, alternative pathways of carbohydrate metabolism may be followed during physical training or body organ demands [14]. However, there is a strong difference among various body organs in utilizing alternative pathways to develop their function.

Anaerobic Metabolism

When oxygen is almost absent or lacking, pyruvate, the basic substrate in carbohydrate metabolic chain, does not undergo cellular respiration to produce energy but a process that follows different pathways with the end production of lactic acid. Moreover, all cells can obtain a more limited amount of energy from glucose without oxygen availability, although with difference in duration and type of function. In mammalians, this process is the glycolysis which is characterized by a series of chemical reactions that occur in anaerobiosis [15]. Glycolysis is a metabolic pathway that occurs in the cytoplasm of cells in all living organisms and does not require oxygen. The process converts one molecule of glucose into two molecules of pyruvate, and produces energy in the form of two net molecules of ATP. Usually, four molecules of ATP per glucose are produced. However, this phase is characterized by a partial loss of produced energy since two molecules of ATP are consumed for the preparatory phase. Glycolysis takes place in the cytoplasm of the cell where the pyruvate is converted to waste products that may be removed from the cell by the venous network. Waste products vary depending on the organism. In skeletal muscles, the waste product is lactic acid.

Glycolysis provides rapidly an amount of ATP in relatively anaerobic organs such as a skeletal muscle that requires intense energy for vigorous contractility during exercise. The heart muscle may benefit anaerobic glycolysis although for a very limited time. Final waste product of glycolysis, as mentioned, is lactic acid that derives from a large series of reactions which are summarized in figure 2.2.

A large series of enzymes, particularly of the fermentation chain instead of oxidative chain, are involved in the different pathways that characterize glycolysis. This phase, metabolically, should be considered to start from the glucose 6-phosphate rather than from glucose itself.

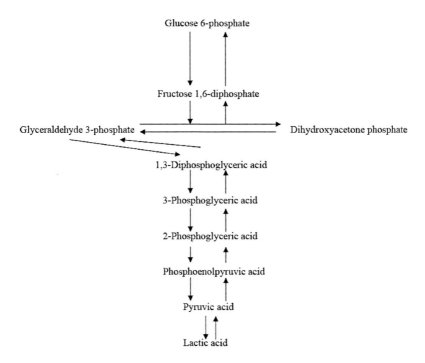

Figure 2.2. Main chemical reactions that characterize anaerobic glycolysis. One can see that phosphate compounds participate widely to the various metabolic pathways.

The cardiac muscle requires oxygen for its physiological function, but, in some circumstances and for a very limited time, anaerobic glycolysis occurs to preserve cell viability when availability of oxygen falls. Therefore, it is worthwhile to know the basic concepts, just explained, of metabolic pathways that can take part in interpreting correctly the type of physiological response of the heart related to the amount of oxygen that coronary circulation, time by time, is capable of providing.

Compensatory Mechanisms of the Coronary Circulation

As a consequence of the metabolic characteristics of the heart, which are almost completely of the aerobic type, coronary circulation may undergo up to five compensatory mechanisms (table 2.2.) to supply blood flow to meet the demands of the myocardium when there are conditions of inappropriate oxygen availability.

Table 2.2. Compensatory mechanisms of coronary circulation

Increase in number and size of capillary network
Increase in small coronary anastomoses
Consumption of stored glycogen
Increased maximum diffusion (passively) of blood oxygen to interstitium
Reduced heart contractility

Mechanisms in table 2.2. may act transiently to preserve myocardial cell viability lasting a variable time according to the degree and intensity of oxygen demand of the myocardium. Therefore, a normal balance between coronary blood flow supply and myocardial demand must be shortly restored.

Normally, coronary circulation is able to increase its flow five-to-six times its rest value as a large series of experimental and clinical data seem to demonstrate [16–27].

At rest, coronary blood flow measures from approximately 70 to 90 mL/100 g per minute with an oxygen consumption of the cardiac muscle at rest of approximately 10 mL/100 g per minute [27]. However, these parameters may change widely also under physiological conditions and, customarily, the heart at rest often requires a greatest extraction of the oxygen contained in its blood supply. Thus, the content in oxygen measured in the coronary sinus, where the coronary venous return may be assessed, is poor and corresponds to approximately 30 percent saturation. The consequence is that any increase in oxygen demand by the heart may be obtained by an increase in coronary blood flow. Indeed, normal coronary circulation may support such a demand within some limits.

A series of factors, which are listed in table 2.3, influences coronary blood flow in an attempt to maintain oxygen demand for the heart at the required level and, consequently, permitting normal heart response.

Table 2.3. Factors that influence and regulate coronary blood flow

Physical factors	Arterial pressure gradient (aortic-left ventricular diastolic pressure)
	Time spent in diastole
	Decreased coronary perfusion
	Vasoconstriction
	Ventricular systole
	Ventricular myocardial mass
	Diffusion distance of oxygen from capillaries
	Blood viscosity
Metabolic factors	Chemical vasodilators
	Chemical vasoconstrictors
	Hormones
Humoral factors	Catecholamines
	Angiotensin II
	Prostaglandins
	Chemoreceptors
Neural factors	Sympathetic nerves
	Parasympathetic nerves
Myogenic regulation	

Perfusion pressure is one of the major determinants for the regulation of the coronary blood flow [5, 28].

Physical Factors

Perfusion pressure, otherwise to be meant as a filling pressure, of each vascular bed is a parameter which is, usually, controlled by a series of physical forces particularly related to those factors like gradient and velocity of blood flow, arterial elasticity or, in the opposite direction, arterial stiffness, diameter of the vessel conduits where blood runs, and peripheral artery resistances.

Under a physical point of view [29], the pressure of a solid column is due to application of an external force or weight (gravity) exerted on the column itself. It is well known that a force F loading on a specific area has a pressure defined by the ratio:

$$P = \frac{F\iota}{A}$$

where P is the pressure;

Fι is the weight of the applied forces;
A is the involved area.

On the contrary, physiologically, a running fluid like blood flow changes the degree of pressure along its course in relation to its velocity, vascular caliber, blood viscosity, and peripheral resistances. The property of changing the pressure force makes possible arrangements of the flow to the characteristics of vascular conduits, the opposite of what occurs as a consequence of a physical force applied on a solid surface. Moreover, the coronary circulation feels particularly some effects that are a consequence of heart function.

Two main external dominants influence coronary circulation: cardiac cycle and coronary vessel twisting that is a close consequence of the systolic phase of the cardiac cycle.

Coronary artery filling occurs during the diastole of cardiac cycle for the left ventricle. Right ventricle is perfused also during cardiac systole due to the fact of its significantly less ventricular mass.

During ventricular systole, intramyocardial pressure of the left ventricle exceeds ventricular cavity and intra-aortic pressure. This condition that is a result of a mechanical phenomenon like contraction of the heart, and a hemodynamic phenomenon like increase in intramyocardial pressure, determines both a compression and twisting of intramyocardial coronary arteries [30–32]. Moreover, the aorta is strongly impeded to fill major epicardial coronary vessels which originate from aortic coronary ostia.

Diastolic phase is the part of the cardiac cycle in which coronary artery perfusion obtains major impulse. Both diastolic pressure and total diastolic time per minute play a strong role in controlling coronary artery perfusion. Therefore, all those conditions that modify these two parameters, and there are a lot that will be discussed in the next chapters, determine important changes to coronary blood flow supply. Coronary blood flow must activate one or more of those compensatory mechanisms listed in table 2.2. Left ventricular diastolic pressure influences, and also it could reduce coronary blood flow, particularly to the subendocardium, when associated heart failure often added to hypotension, occurs.

Although the majority of the coronary blood flow occurs during the diastole, it has been demonstrated that up to 20 to 30 percent of coronary blood flow occurs during the systolic phase of the cardiac cycle [5].

As already mentioned, myocardial contractile function is closely related to coronary flow. A minimal reduction of coronary blood flow as little as 10 to 20 percent will impair systolic function, also acutely [33–34].

Blood viscosity is an additional mechanism that may influence coronary blood flow and heart function [35–42], although it interferes particularly when coronary vessel alterations are associated. The main effect of an increased blood viscosity greatly worsens coronary circulation via thrombi formation in smokers especially by changes of coagulation-fibrinolysis cascade and platelet function.

Metabolic and Humoral Factors

A large series of well-documented reports identifies a lot of chemical compounds that are able to induce changes in coronary blood flow by mechanisms of vasoconstriction or dilatation according to oxygen demand of the heart [43-60]. Among these, particularly adenosine is one of the most active mediators for coronary blood flow autoregulation. Also, compounds that usually are found to be constituents of cigarette smoking [57, 60] may influence coronary blood flow in different ways in relation to their environmental concentrations.

Compounds that regulate coronary blood flow differ widely in chemical structure and may be produced in various body structures even if they influence actively coronary circulation.

Their chemical properties and mechanism of action will be described detailedly in the next chapter.

Neural Factors

Although coronary vascular resistance is regulated primarily by metabolic and humoral factors, sympathetic and parasympathetic nervous systems play an important role that is usually mediated by baroreceptors located in the carotid sinus [61-63].

Carotid sinus chemoreceptors, which are usually stimulated by altered metabolic conditions like hypoxemia, acidosis or increased carbon dioxide concentrations, may feel particularly vagal effects that determine vasodilation, while they are influenced much less by sympathetic stimulation. However, coronary resistance may be changed by the functional status of the nerves that distribute their endings to coronary artery wall causing different types of responses.

Cigarette smoking components may influence particularly sympathetic nerves on the coronary circulation, causing transiently functional coronary alterations in smokers as well as in nonsmokers exposed passively to environmental tobacco. These functional alterations, that do not occur in the non-exposed who never smoked, are the "door" to the development of heavy anatomical damage in the long run [64–68]. Therefore, those smokers, who do not display, initially, coronary alterations, could be already affected by transient damage not yet evident.

Sympathetic nerves to the heart and coronary vessels arise from the three cervical and the first four or five thoracic sympathetic ganglia. Sympathetic stimulation of the coronary circulation is largely mediated by the release of norepinephrine. The parasympathetic innervation of the coronary vessels is under the influence of the right and left vagus nerves. Two sets of cardiac nerves originate from each vagus nerve: the superior cardiac nerves that arise from the vagi in the neck, and the inferior cardiac nerves, which arise from either the vagus nerves or branches of the vagi (recurrent branches). Cardiac parasympathetic impulses are mediated by acetylcholine.

Table 2.4. summarizes the anatomical distribution of vagus and sympathetic nerves.

The large epicardial coronary arteries and veins are primarily under sympathetic control as well as intramyocardial coronary arteries, capillary network, and venules [69–75]. Moreover, increases in coronary blood flow [74] in response to sympathetic stimulation well correlate with the regional norepinephrine content in the cardiac sympathetic nerve endings.

The vagi provide endings to heart and coronary circulation by efferent cholinergic fibers. Although vagal nerves are weakly distributed to ventricular myocardial mass, they are of abundant supply to both conduction system of the heart and coronary circulation [73, 76–80].

Table 2.4. Anatomical distribution of the vagi and sympathetic nerves

Vagus nerve	Left vagus	Superior cardiac nerves (superior and inferior cervical)
		Inferior cardiac nerves (thoracic)
	Right vagus	Superior cardiac nerves (superior and inferior cervical)
		Inferior cardiac nerves (thoracic)
Sympathetic nerves		Superior cardiac nerve (superior cervical ganglia)
		Middle cardiac nerve (middle cervical ganglia)
		Inferior cardiac nerve (inferior cervical ganglia)
		Thoracic nerves (first 4 or 5 thoracic ganglia)
	Stellate ganglion (fusion inferior cervical and first thoracic)	

Coronary vessels contain different types of receptors that are distributed variously in the segments of the coronary tree and determine different responses related to the type of stimulation that they usually induce [81–92]. Alpha-1, alpha-2, beta-1, beta-2, and muscarinic-cholinergic receptors have been demonstrated in the coronary artery wall.

Alpha adrenergic stimulation, mediated by norepinephrine, determines a strong increase in coronary resistance and a vasoconstriction of both large epicardial coronary vessels and intramural vessels. All those factors that increase sympathetic nerve stimulation can induce such type of changes in coronary arteries [91, 93–95] that are a consequence of alpha1-receptor activation. However, experimental findings would seem to show that sympathetic nervous ending stimulation produces coronary responses of a lower level than that due to the same chemical mediators which act by a metabolic regulation. This type of response should be partially due to the role of alpha2-receptors that, when activated in the coronary circulation, modulate the release of norepinephrine from sympathetic nerves. Thus, the selective in vivo stimulation of the alpha2-adrenoreceptors [96–98] would produce a reduction in coronary blood flow and diameter also in humans with angiographically normal coronary arteries [98]. Alpha2-adrenergic receptors are particularly distributed to arterioles and they could compete with alpha1-adrenergic receptors located throughout coronary microcirculation in modulating coronary blood flow. Moreover, the level of coronary vasomotor tone would regulate the alpha1 and alpha2- adrenoreceptor response that should be, however, of constriction type although with a different degree related to intrinsic autoregulatory mechanisms of vascular tone. The excellent paper of Chilian [97] underlines five basic observations about adrenergic activation: 1. If coronary vasomotor tone is intact, alpha1-adrenergic activation produces a sustained constriction of epicardial and intramural coronary arteries, but not arterioles; 2. Alpha2-adrenergic activation during baseline conditions does not produce vasoconstriction of arterioles or arteries; 3. When autoregulatory adjustments are blunted during coronary hypoperfusion, alpha1-adrenergic activation constricts both coronary arteries and arterioles by approximately the same degree; 4. During hypoperfusion, alpha2-adrenergic activation produces heavy constriction of coronary arterioles but not coronary arteries; 5. The magnitude of arteriolar constriction during hypoperfusion is significantly greater with alpha2-adrenergic activation than alpha1-adrenoreceptor stimulation.

Thus, when coronary autoregulatory mechanisms are related to an intact vasomotor tone, coronary arteries always feel vasoconstrictor effects of adrenergic stimulation, whereas arterioles could not feel the effects of both alpha1 and alpha2-adrenoreceptor stimulation.

For what concerns beta-receptors, vasodilation occurs secondary to activation of these receptors, which are located particularly where there is a rich autonomic innervation of the coronary wall - periadventitial and adventitial connective tissue and transition zone between medial and intimal coats.

Pharmacological stimulation [99–102] produces activation of both beta1 and beta2 – receptors with consequent vasodilation of coronary vessels and reduction in coronary resistance. Vasodilator effects may be obtained by using Isoproterenol.

Table 2.5. summarizes the main effects of coronary-wall receptor stimulation.

Table 2.5. Main responses of coronary-wall receptor stimulation

Type of receptor	Coronary response
Alpha1	Constriction
Alpha 2	Constriction/Dilation (Vascular Tone)
Beta 1	Vasodilation
Beta 2	Vasodilation
Cholinergic	Vasodilation

Both sympathetic stimulation and vagal stimulation compete with other mechanisms that can modify their type of response when it is not stimulated only by a single specific receptor. Thus, the typical response of the coronary artery, when sympathetic stimulation occurs, follows different phases: initially, a moderate constriction occurs; then, vasoconstriction is followed shortly by important coronary dilation. This apparently paradoxical response is due to the fact that sympathetic stimulation activates not only coronary responses but a global burden of responses that involve electrical, mechanical and metabolic phenomena of the heart. Thus, increased heart rate, myocardial contractility and blood pressure, that are a direct consequence of sympathetic stimulation, raise MVo2 that, consequently, produce coronary dilation [85, 103–104]. Following that, but almost simultaneously, sympathetic nerve stimulation activates alpha-adrenergic receptors, which promote coronary constriction (figure 2.3.).

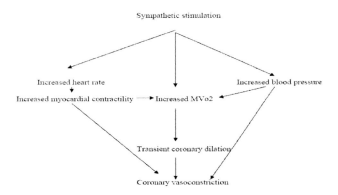

Figure 2.3. Physiological mechanisms of cardiovascular response to sympathetic stimulation.

Vagal stimulation [105–106], as it may be seen by intracoronary infusion of acetylcholine maintaining heart rate constant, determines a markedly coronary vasodilation. On the contrary, if the vagus is stimulated electrically, the changes in cardiac rate, consisting of a different degree of bradycardia, induce only a moderate vasodilation. Vasodilation due to direct vagal stimulation involves both epicardial and intramyocardial coronary vessels.

Vagal stimulation, in the intact coronary circulation, is followed immediately by coronary vasoconstriction since there is a decrease in myocardial metabolism. Simultaneously, those mechanisms that determine vasodilation are activated so that the final result is a coronary vasodilation of a different degree.

Figure 2.4. explains the main physiological mechanisms that regulate coronary circulation adjustment following vagal stimulation.

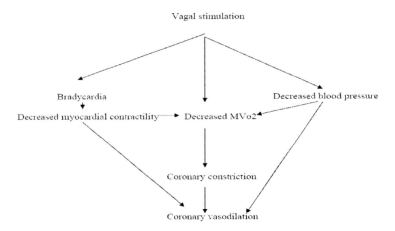

Figure 2.4 Physiological mechanisms of cardiovascular response to vagal stimulation.

Finally, muscarinic-cholinergic receptor stimulation usually produces almost the same effects of acetylcholine infusion or vagal stimulation.

Myogenic Regulation

Myogenic regulation plays a strongly controversial significance in coronary circulation since a large series of adjustment mechanisms is activated simultaneously when myocardial oxygen demand of the heart increases suddenly. However, a myogenic mechanism, or Bayliss phenomenon, would seem to regulate arterial smooth muscle cells even if a complex series of associated phenomena may be demonstrated [107–113].

The physical principle of the postulate of Bayliss was based on the hypothesis that the resistance in the coronary vessels was proportional to transmural microvascular pressure as a result of a direct effect of the intravascular pressure itself on arterial smooth muscle cells. Therefore, increases in intravascular pressure could cause vasoconstriction, whereas decreases of this parameter induced coronary vasodilation. Therefore, myogenic regulation is under the control of vascular tone that feels the effects of intrinsic mechanisms of the blood artery vessel. The arterial wall is sheared and struck repeatedly by the turbulence of the blood and also compressed and stretched by the pressure that exists into the vessels. These phenomena occur according to the demand for oxygen by the heart, and vary with amount or reduction of the oxygen demand.

Although myogenic tone is a major contributor to vascular resistance to blood flow, the mechanisms by which it occurs may be widely different. Some responses are characterized by an increase in vasomotor frequency, particularly when venous system or lymphatic conduits are involved [114–115]. On other circumstances, particularly when arterioles are involved, periodic contractions related to the duration in changes of intravascular pressure occur [116].

For the coronary arteries, whatever it might be morphological patterns caused by intravascular pressure changes, the difficulty in establishing the exact role of myogenic regulation, as just discussed, is impeded by the simultaneous activation of all those factors that control coronary blood flow in case of suddenly increased oxygen demand. However, mechanisms of vasoconstriction or vasodilation at different sites of the coronary tree could be induced by myogenic regulation.

Coronary Vascular Reserve

From the concepts just mentioned, there is evidence that a series of major and minor determinants may regulate coronary blood flow that, however, must supply oxygen demand to the heart for a correct function. Coronary vascular reserve is the capacity of coronary circulation to provide a further amount of oxygenated blood to the myocardium when it is required. Physiologically, coronary vascular reserve, which may be measured by intracoronary Doppler flow velocity method [117] or coronary thermodilution method [118], is characterized by a basal measure at rest and a maximal measure at working when a significant increase in oxygen demand occurs up a level beyond which there is no further physiological adjustment of coronary blood flow. Figure 2.5. explains physiological adjustments of coronary blood flow and its relationship with myocardial oxygen consumption (MVo2).

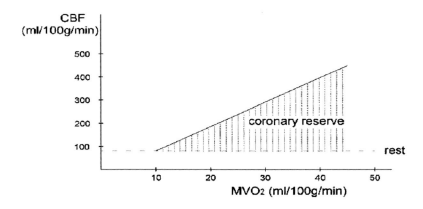

Figure 2.5. Physiologically, there is a linear relationship between CBF and MVO2 according to the fact that coronary reserve may increase CBF up to four to five times the rest value. CBF= coronary blood flow; MVO2= myocardial oxygen consumption.

In conclusion, several factors may control the supply of oxygen to the heart, modifying coronary blood flow. Some of these, like myogenic control and physical control, are closely related to changes of perfusion pressure; otherwise, neuroendocrine and metabolic control may require a constant perfusion pressure, and increased coronary blood flow, when there is an increase in work of the heart, is the consequence of release of active metabolites.

Finally, a brief observation is worthwhile to establish for the physiologic responses of coronary circulation in smokers, either active smokers or nonsmokers exposed to environmental tobacco. The subject will be widely discussed in the chapter on vascular endothelium. However, endothelial dysfunction following both long-term exposure or acute exposure to smoking, even passive smoking, has been well demonstrated to occur either in systemic arteries [67, 119–121] in healthy young individuals, or in coronary circulation [122–123]. Flow-mediated artery dilation, a parameter strongly related to endothelial function, was impaired to a different degree particularly because of reduced endothelial nitric oxide (NO) release. This type of abnormal physiological response involves primarily metabolic and humoral coronary vessel regulation. However, also those parameters related to physical regulation are simultaneously involved as it is shown by the increase in heart rate and systolic blood pressure during smoking exposure [124]. As one can see, this occurrence, too, is a clear manifestation of the close inter-relationship that links different determinants that control physiological regulation of the coronary circulation.

References

[1] Neely JR, Liedtke AJ, Whitmer JT, Rovetto MJ. Relationship between coronary flow and adenosine triphosphate production from glycolysis and oxidative metabolism. In: *Recent Advances in Studies on Cardiac Structure and Metabolism. The Cardiac Cytoplasm*, Roy PE, Harris P, eds., University Park Press, Baltimore, USA, 1975; 8: 301.

[2] Braunwald E, Control of myocardial oxygen consumption. *Am. J. Cardiol.* 1971; 27: 416 – 32.

[3] McKeever WP, Gregg DE, Canney PC. Oxygen uptake of the nonworking left ventricle. *Circ. Res.* 1958; 6: 612 – 23.

[4] Sarnoff SJ, Braunwald E, Welch G, Case RB, Stainsby WN, Macroz R. Hemodynamic determinants of oxygen consumption of the heart with special reference to the tension-time index. *Am. J. Physiol.* 1958; 192: 148 – 56.

[5] Gregg DE. Physiology of the coronary circulation. *Circulation.* 1963; 27: 1128 – 37.

[6] Berton C, Cholley B. Equipment review: New techniques for cardiac output measurement – oesophageal doppler, Fick principle using carbon dioxide, and pulse contour analysis. *Crit. Care.* 2002;6: 216 – 21.

[7] Sonnenblick EH, Skelton CL. Oxygen consumption of the heart: Physiological principles and clinical implication. *Mod. Concepts Cardiovasc. Dis.* 1971; 40: 9 – 16.

[8] Sonnenblick EH, Ross J Jr, Covell JW, Kaiser GA, Braunwald E. Velocity of contraction as a determinant of myocardial oxygen consumption. *Am. J. Physiol.* 1965; 209: 919 – 27.

[9] Neill WA, Levine HJ, Wagman RJ, Gorlin R. Left ventricular oxygen utilization in intact dogs: Effect of systemic hemodynamic factors. *Circ. Res.* 1963; 12: 163 – 9.

[10] Campbell NA, Reece JB. *Biology*, 7th edition, Benjamin Cummings Publisher, Pearson Education, Los Angeles, USA, 2005.

[11] Driedzic WR, Gesser H. Energy metabolism and contractility in ectothermic vertebrate hearts: hypoxia, acidosis and low temperature. *Physiol. Rev.* 1994; 74: 221 – 58.

[12] Kashiwaya Y, Sato K, Tsuchiya N, Thomas S, Fell DA, Veech RL, Passonneau JV. Control of glucose utilization in working perfused rat heart. *J. Biol. Chem.* 1994; 269: 25502 – 14.

[13] Mendez G, Gnaiger E. How does oxygen pressure control oxygen flux in isolated mitochondria? A methodological approach by high-resolution respirometry and digital data analysis. *Mod. Trends Biothermokinet.* 1994; 3: 191 – 4.

[14] Horecker BL. Alternative pathways of carbohydrate metabolism and their physiological significance. *J. Chem. Education.* 1965; 42: 244 – 5 3.

[15] Ashwell G. Carbohydrate metabolism. *Ann. Rev. Biochem.* 1964; 33: 101 – 38.

[16] Bassenge E, Heusch G. Endothelial and neuro-humoral control of coronary blood flow in health and disease. *Rev. Physiol. Biochem. Pharmacol.* 1990; 116: 77 – 165.

[17] Shipley RE, Gregg DE. The cardiac response to stimulation of the stellate ganglia and cardiac nerves. *Am. J. Physiol.* 1945; 143: 396 – 401.

[18] Parent R, Parè R, Lavallée M. Contribution of nitric oxide to dilation of resistance coronary vessels. *Am. J. Physiol.* 1992; 262 (Heart Circ Physiol 31): H10 – 16.

[19] Feigl EO. Coronary physiology. *Physiol. Rev.* 1983; 63: 1 – 205.

[20] Bassenge E, Busse R. Endothelial modulation of coronary tone. *Prog Cardiovasc Dis*, 1988; 30: 349 – 80.

[21] Lombardo TA, Rose L, Taeschler M, Tuluy S, Bing RJ. The effect of exercise on coronary blood flow, myocardial oxygen consumption and cardiac efficiency in man. *Circulation*, 1953; 7: 71 – 8.

[22] Dole WP. Autoregulation of the coronary circulation. *Prog. Cardiovasc. Dis.* 1987; 29: 293 – 323.

[23] Olsson RA, Bunger R. Metabolic control of coronary blood flow. *Prog. Cardiovasc. Dis.* 1987; 29: 369 – 87.

[24] Taylor RR, Cingolani HE, Graham TP, Clancy RL. Myocardial oxygen consumption, left ventricular fibre shortening and wall tension. *Cardiovasc. Res.* 1967; 1: 219 – 28.

[25] Rayford CR, Huvos A, Khouri EM, Gregg DE. Some determinants of coronary flow in intact dogs. *Physiologist.* 1961; 4: 92 .

[26] Young MA, Knight DR, Vatner SF. Autonomic control of large coronary arteries and resistance vessels. *Prog. Cardiovasc. Dis.* 1987; 30: 211 – 34.

[27] Berne RM, Rubio R. Coronary Circulation. In: Berne RM ed, *Handbook of Physiology*, sec 2: The cardiovascular System, vol 1: The Heart, Bethesda MD; American Physiological Society, USA, 1979; 873.

[28] Hanley FL, Messina LM, Grattan MT, Hoffman IE. The effect of coronary inflow
      pressure on coronary vascular resistance in the isolated dog heart. *Circ. Res.* 1984; 54:
      760 – 72.

[29] Cromer AH. *Physics for the life sciences.* Mc Graw-Hill, New York, 1974.

[30] Wiggers CJ. The interplay of coronary vascular resistance and myocardial compression
      in regulating coronary flow. *Circ. Res.* 1954; 2: 271 – 9.

[31] Panerai RB, Chamberlain JH, Sayers BM. Characterization of the extravascular
      component of coronary resistance by instantaneous pressure-flow relationship in the
      dog. *Circ. Res.* 1979; 45: 378 – 90.

[32] Bache RJ, Dymek DJ. Local and regional regulation of coronary vascular tone. *Prog.
      Cardiovasc. Dis.* 1981; 24: 191 – 212.

[33] Vatner SF.Correlation between acute reductions in myocardial blood flow and function
      in conscious dogs: *Circ. Res.* 1980; 47: 201 – 7.

[34] Gallagher KP, Kumada T, Koziol JA, McKown MD, Kemper WS, Ross J Jr.
      Significance of regional wall thickening abnormalities relative to transmural
      myocardial perfusion in anesthetized dogs. *Circulation.* 1980; 62: 1266 – 73.

[35] Kovacic JC. Further aspects of anemia, heart failure and erythropoietin. *J. Am. Coll.
      Cardiol.* 2005; 9: 1549 – 50.

[36] Shah PK. Plaque disruption and thrombosis: potential role of inflammation and
      infection. *Cardiol. Rev.* 2000; 8: 31 – 9.

[37] Feldman CL, Stone PH. Intravascular hemodynamic factors responsible for progression
      of coronary atherosclerosis and development of vulnerable plaque. *Curr. Opin.
      Cardiol.* 2000; 15: 430 – 40.

[38] Junker R, Heinrich J, Ulbrich H, Schulte H, Sconfeld R, Kohler E, Assmann G.
      Relationship between plasma viscosity and the severity of coronary heart disease.
      Arteriosclerosis, Thrombosis, and Vascular Biology. 1998; 18: 870 – 5.

[39] Lowe GD, Drummond MM, Lorimer AR, Hutton I, Forbes CD, Prentice CR, Barbenel
      JC. Relation between extent of coronary artery disease and blood viscosity. *BMJ.* 1980;
      280: 673 – 4.

[40] Dudaev VA, Evdokimov VV. Blood viscosity in ischemic heart disease with different
      types of hyperlipoproteinemia. *Kardiologiia.* 1977; 17: 79 – 82.

[41] Reinke W, Gaehtgens P, Johnson PC. Blood viscosity in small tubes: effect of shear
      rate, aggregation, and sedimentation. *Am. J. Physiol. Heart Circ. Physiol.* 1987; 253:
      H540 – 7.

[42] Leone A. Smoking, haemostatic factors, and cardiovascular risk. *Curr. Pharm. Design.*
      2007; 13: 1661 – 7.

[43] Schwartz GG, McHale PA, Greenfield JC. Coronary vasodilation after a single
      ventricular extra-activation in the conscious dog. *Circ. Res.* 1982; 50: 38 – 46.

[44] Rooke GA, Feigl EO. Work as a correlate of canine left ventricular oxygen
      consumption, and the problem of catecholamine oxygen wasting. *Circ. Res.* 1982; 50:
      273 – 86.

[45] Busse R., Trogisch G., Bassenge E. The role of endothelium in the control of vascular
      tone. *Basic Res. Cardiol.* 1985; 80: 475 – 90.

[46] Belardinelli L, Linden J, Berne RM. The cardiac effects of adenosine. *Prog. Cardiovasc. Dis.* 1989; 32: 73 – 97.

[47] Olsson RA, Snow JA, Gentry MK. Adenosine metabolism in canine myocardial reactive hyperemia. *Circ. Res.* 1978; 42: 358 – 62.

[48] Dunn RB, McDonough KM, Griggs DM Jr. High energy phosphate stores and lactate levels in different layers of the canine left ventricle during reactive hyperemia. *Circ. Res.* 1979; 44: 788- 95.

[49] Mubagwa K, Mullane K, Flameng W. Role of adenosine in the heart and circulation. *Cardiovasc. Res.* 1996; 32: 798 – 813.

[50] Vane JR, Anggard EE, Botting RM. Regulatory functions of the vascular endothelium. *N. Engl. J. Med.* 1990; 323: 27 – 36.

[51] Vanhoutte PM, Miller VM, Houston DS. Modulation of vascular smooth muscle contraction by the endothelium. *Annu. Rev. Physiol.* 1986; 48: 307 – 20.

[52] Ykoyama G, Goldman M, Henry PD. Supersensitivity of atherosclerotic arteries to ergonovine is partially mediated by a serotonergic mechanism. *Circulation.* 1979; 60 (Suppl 2):100A.

[53] Robertson RM, Robertson D, Roberts LJ, Maas RL, FitzGerald GA, Friesinger GC, Oates JA. .Thromboxane A2 in vasotonic angina pectoris. *N. Engl. J. Med.* 1981; 304: 998 – 1003.

[54] Berne RM. The role of adenosine in the regulation of coronary blood flow. *Circ. Res.* 1980; 47: 807 – 13.

[55] Driscol TE, Berne RM. Role of potassium in regulation of coronary blood flow. *Proc. Soc. Exptl. Biol. Med.* 1957; 96: 505 – 8.

[56] Dusting GJ, Moncada S, Vane JR. Prostaglandins, their intermediates and precursors: Cardiovascular actions and regulatory roles in normal and abnormal circulatory systems. *Progr. Cardiovasc. Dis.* 1979; 21: 405 – 29.

[57] Case RB, Felix A, Wachter M, Kyriakidis G, Castellana F. Relative effect of CO_2 on canine coronary vascular resistance. *Circ. Res.* 1978; 42: 410 – 8.

[58] Mudge GH Jr, Goldberg S, Gunther S, Mann T, Grossman W. Comparison of metabolic and vasoconstrictor stimuli on coronary vascular resistance in man. *Circulation.* 1979; 59: 544 – 50.

[59] Heistad DD, Armstrong ML, Marcus ML, Piegors DJ, Mark AL. Augmented responses to vasoconstrictor stimuli in hypercholesterolemic and atherosclerotic monkeys. *Circ. Res.* 1984; 54: 711 – 8.

[60] Leone A. Biochemical markers of cardiovascular damage from tobacco smoke. *Curr. Pharm. Design.* 2005; 11: 2199 – 208.

[61] Vatner SF, Franklin D, Van Citters RL, Braunwald E. Effects of carotid sinus nerve stimulation on the coronary circulation of the conscious dog. *Circ. Res.* 1970; 27: 11 – 21.

[62] Feigl EO. Carotid sinus reflex control of coronary blood flow. *Circ. Res.* 1968; 23: 223 – 37.

[63] Powell JR, Feigl EO. Carotid sinus reflex coronary vasoconstriction during controlled myocardial oxygen metabolism in the dog. *Circ. Res.* 1979; 44: 44 – 51.

[64] Leone A. Number of cigarettes, reinfarction/death in continuing smokers. *Il Cuore.* 1990; 7: 233 – 6.

[65] Leone A. The heart: a target organ for cigarette smoking. *J. Smoking-Related Dis.* 1992; 3: 197 – 201.

[66] Kritz H, Schmid P., Sinzinger H. Passive smoking and cardiovascular risk. *Arch. Intern. Med.* 1995; 155: 1942 – 8.

[67] Giannini D, Leone A, DiBisceglie D, Nuti M, Strata G, Buttitta F, Masserini L, Balbarini A. The effects of acute passive smoke exposure on endothelium-dependent artery dilation in healthy individuals. *Angiology.* 2007; 58: 211 – 7.

[68] Leone A. Passive smoking exposure and cardiovascular health. In: *Passive Smoking and Health Research*, Jeorgensen NA ed, Nova Science Publishers, Inc., New York, USA, 2007; 65 – 94.

[69] Dahlstrom A, Fuxe F, Mya-tu M, Zetterstrom BEM. Observation on adrenergic innervation of the dog heart. *Am. J. Physiol.* 1965; 209 : 689 – 92.

[70] Friedman WF, Pool PE, Jacobowitz D, Seagren SC, Braunwald E. Sympathetic innervation of the developing rabbit heart. *Circ. Res.* 1968; 23: 25 – 32.

[71] Malor R, Griffin CJ, Taylor S. Innervation of the blood vessels in guinea pig atria. *Cardiovasc. Res.* 1973; 7: 95 – 104.

[72] Forbes MF, Rennels ML, Nelson E. Innervation of myocardial microcirculation ; terminal autonomic axons associated with capillaries and postcapillary venules in mouse heart. *Am. J. Anat.* 1977; 149: 71 – 92.

[73] Saetrum Opgaard O, Gulbenkian S, Edvinsson L. Innervation and effects of vasoactive substances in the coronary circulation. *Eur. Heart J.* 1997; 18: 1556 – 68.

[74] Di Carli MF, Tobes MC, Mangner T, Levine AB, Muzik O, Chakroborty P, Levine B. Effects of cardiac sympathetic innervation on coronary blood flow. *N. Engl. J. Med.* 1977; 336: 1208 – 16.

[75] Hodgson JM, Cohen MD, Szentpetery S, Thames MD. Effects of regional alpha-and beta-blockade on resting and hyperemic coronary blood flow in conscious, unstressed humans. *Circulation.* 1989; 79: 797 – 809.

[76] Woollard HH. Innervation of the heart. *J. Anat.* 1926; 60: 345 – 73.

[77] Denison AB Jr, Green HD. Effects of autonomic nerves and their mediators on the coronary circulation and myocardial contraction. *Circ. Res.* 1958; 6: 633 – 43.

[78] Duncker DJ, Stubenitsky R, Verdouw PD. Autonomic control of vasomotion in the porcine coronary circulation during treadmill exercise. *Circ. Res.* 1998; 82: 1312 – 22.

[79] Cowan CL, McKenzie JE. Cholinergic regulation of resting coronary blood flow in domestic swine. *Am. J. Physiol.* 1990; 259: H109 – H115.

[80] Sanders M, White FC, Peterson TM, Bloor CM. Characteristics of coronary blood flow and transmural distribution in miniature pigs. *Am. J. Physiol.* 1978; 235: H601 – 9.

[81] Bassenge E, Kucharczyk M, Holtz J, Stolan D. Treadmill exercise in dogs under beta-adrenergic blockade: adaptation of coronary and systemic hemodynamics. *Pflugers. Arch.* 1972; 332: 40 – 55.

[82] Houk JC. Control strategies in physiological systems. *FASEB J.* 1988; 2: 97 – 107.

[83] Ekstrom-Jodal B, Haggendal E, Malmberg R, Svedmyr N. The effect of adrenergic beta-receptor blockade on coronary circulation in man during work. *Acta Med. Scand.* 1972; 191: 245 – 8.

[84] Miyashiro JK, Feigl EO. Feedforward control of coronary blood flow via coronary beta-receptor stimulation. *Circ. Res.* 1993; 73: 252 – 63.

[85] Hamilton FN, Feigl EO. Coronary vascular sympathetic beta-receptor innervation. *Am. J. Physiol.* 1976; 230: 1569 – 76.

[86] Cornish EJ, Miller RC. Comparison of the beta-adrenoreceptors in the myocardium and coronary vasculature of the kitten heart. *J. Pharm. Pharmacol.* 1975; 27: 23 – 30.

[87] Baron GD, Speden RN, Bohr DF. Beta-adrenergic receptors in coronary and skeletal muscle arteries. *Am. J. Physiol.* 1972; 223: 878 – 81.

[88] Schulz R, Oudiz RJ, Guth BD, Heusch G. Minimal alpha-1 and alpha-2 adrenoreceptor-mediated coronary vasoconstriction in the anaesthetized swine. Naunyn Schmiedebergs *Arch. Pharmacol.* 1990; 342: 422 – 8.

[89] Verdouw PD, Duncker DJ, Saxena PR. Poor vasoconstrictor response to adrenergic stimulation in the arteriovenous anastomoses present in the carotid vascular bed of young Yorkshire pigs. *Arch. Int. Pharmacodyn. Ther.* 1984; 272: 56 – 70.

[90] Williams DO, Most AS. Responsiveness of the coronary circulation to brief vs sustained alpha-adrenergic stimulation. *Circulation.* 1981; 63: 11 – 16.

[91] Gerovà M, Barta E, Gero J. Sympathetic control of major coronary artery diameter in the dog. *Circ. Res.* 1979; 44: 459 – 67.

[92] Heyndrickx GR, Vilaine JP, Moerman EJ, Leusen I. Role of pre-junctional alpha-2 adrenergic receptors in the regulation of myocardial performance during exercise in conscious dogs. *Circ. Res.* 1984; 54: 683 – 93.

[93] McRaven DR, Mark AL, Abboud FM, Mayer HE. Responses of coronary vessels to adrenergic stimuli. *J. Clin. Invest.* 1971; 50: 773 – 8.

[94] Bache RJ, Dai X, Herzog CA, Schwartz JS. Effects of non-selective and selective alpha1-adrenergic blockade on coronary blood flow during exercise. *Circ. Res.* 1987; 61 (Suppl II): 36 – 41.

[95] Holtz J, Mayer E, Bassenge E. Demonstration of alpha-adrenergic coronary control in different layers of canine myocardium by regional myocardial sympathectomy. *Pflugers. Arch.* 1977; 372: 187 – 94.

[96] Johansson UJ, Mark AL, Marcus ML. Alpha2-receptors modulate coronary responses to sympathetic nerve stimulation. *Circulation.* 1982; 66 (Suppl II): 153 A.

[97] Chilian WM. Functional distribution of alpha1 and alfa2- adrenergic receptors in the coronary microcirculation. *Circulation.* 1991; 84: 2108 – 22.

[98] Indolfi C, Piscione F, Villari B, Russolillo E, Rendina V, Gorlino P, Condorelli M, Chiariello M. Role of alpha2-adrenoreceptors in normal and atherosclerotic human coronary circulation. *Circulation.* 1992; 86: 1116 – 24.

[99] Klocke FJ, Kaiser GA, Ross J Jr, Braunwald E. An intrinsic adrenergic vasodilator mechanism in the coronary vascular bed of the dog. *Circ. Res.* 1965; 16: 376 – 82.

[100] Trivella MG, Brotean TP, Feigl EO. Beta-receptors sub-types in the canine coronary circulation. *Am. J. Physiol. Heart Circ. Physiol.* 1990; 259: H1575 – 85.

[101] Gross GJ, Feigl EO. Analysis of coronary vascular beta-receptors in situ. *Am. J. Physiol.* 1975; 228: 1909 – 13.

[102] Bilski A, Halliday SE, FitzGerald JD, Wale J. The pharmacology of a b2 selective adrenoreceptor antagonist ICI 118-551. *J. Cardiovasc. Pharmacol.* 1983; 5: 430 – 7.

[103] Feigl EO. Control of myocardial oxygen tension by sympathetic coronary vasoconstriction in the dog. *Circ. Res.* 1975; 37: 88 – 95.

[104] Mohrman DE, Feigl EO. Competition between sympathetic vasoconstriction and metabolic vasodilation in the canine coronary circulation. *Circ. Res.* 1978; 42: 79 - 86.

[105] Levy MN, Zieske H. Comparison of the cardiac effects of vagus nerve stimulation and of acetylcholine infusions. *Am. J. Physiol.* 1969; 216: 890 – 7.

[106] Gross GJ, Buck JD , Warltier DC. Transmural distribution of blood flow during activation of coronary muscarinic receptors. *Am. J. Physiol.* 1981; 240: H941 – 6.

[107] Bayliss WM. On the local reaction of the arterial wall to changes of internal pressure. *J. Physiol.* 1902; 28: 220 – 31.

[108] Folkow B. Intravascular pressure is a factor regulating the tone of the small vessels. *Acta Physiol. Scand.* 1964; 17: 289 – 310.

[109] Bevan JA. Vascular myogenic or stretch-dependent tone. *J. Cardiovasc. Pharmacol.* 1985; 7 (Suppl 3): S129 – 36.

[110] Nelson MT. Bayliss, myogenic tone and volume-regulated chloride channels in arterial smooth muscle. *J. Physiol.* 1998; 507: 629.

[111] Barcroft J Dixon WE. The gaseous metabolism of the mammalian heart. *J. Physiol.* 1907; 35: 182 – 204.

[112] Brayden JE, Nelson MT. Regulation of arterial tone by activation of calcium-dependent potassium channels. *Science.* 1992; 256: 532 – 5.

[113] Duan D, Winter C, Cowley S, Hume JR, Horowitz R. Molecular identification of a volume-regulated chloride channel. *Nature.* 1997; 390: 417 – 21.

[114] Wiederhielm CA. Effects of temperature and transmural pressure on contractile activity of vascular smooth cells. *Bibl. Anat.* 1967; 9: 321 – 7.

[115] Baez S, Laidlaw Z, Orkin LR. Localization and measurement of microvascular and microcirculatory responses to venous pressure elevation in the rat. *Blood Vessels.* 1974; 11: 260 – 76.

[116] Davignon J, Lorenz RR, Shepherd JT. Response of human umbilical artery to changes in transmural pressure. *Am. J. Physiol.* 1965; 209: 51 – 9.

[117] Kern M. Curriculum in interventional cardiology: Coronary pressure and flow measurements in the cardiac catheterization laboratory. *Cathet. Cardiovasc. Intervent.* 2002; 54: 378 – 400.

[118] Pijls NH, De Bruyne B, Smith L, Aarnoudse W, Barbato E, Bartunek J, Bech JW, Van de Vosse F. Coronary thermodilution to assess flow reserve: Validation in humans. *Circulation.* 2002; 105: 2482 – 6.

[119] Celermajer DS, Adams MR, Clarkson P, Robinson J, McCredie R, Donald A, Deanfield JE. Passive smoking and impaired endothelium-dependent arterial dilatation in healthy young adults. *N. Engl. J. Med.* 1996; 334: 150 – 5.

[120] Celermajer DS, Sorensen KE, Gooch VM, Spiegelhalter DJ, Miller OI, Sullivan ID, Lloyd JK, Deanfield JE. Non-invasive detection of endothelial dysfunction in children and adults at risk of atherosclerosis. *Lancet.* 1992; 340: 1111 – 5.

[121] Celermajer DS, Sorensen KE, Georgakopoulos D. Cigarette smoking is associated with dose-related and potentially reversible impairment of endothelium-dependent dilation in healthy young adults. *Circulation.* 1993; 88: 2149 – 55.

[122] Sumida H, Watanabe H, Kugiyama K, Ohgushi M, Matsumura T. Yasue H. Does passive smoking impair endothelium-dependent coronary artery dilation in women? *J. Am. Coll. Cardiol.* 1998; 31: 811 – 5.

[123] Otsuka R, Watanabe H, Hirata K, Tokai K, Muro T, Yoshiyama M, Takeuchi K, Yoshikawa J. Acute effects of passive smoking on the coronary circulation in healthy young adults. *JAMA.* 2001; 286: 436 – 41.

[124] Leone A, Bellotto C. Heart rate and ambulatory blood pressure monitoring in passive smoking. Role of autonomic system. *J. Clin. Hypertens.* 2007; 9 (Suppl A): P-538, A223.

Chapter III

Humoral and Metabolic Regulation of Coronary Circulation

Abstract

Many chemicals circulating in the blood and released by different tissues and organs of the body may metabolically influence coronary vascular tone. Two types of changes are the result of their action: a vasodilator response and a vasoconstrictor response. However, these two types of response may be easily identified when a vasodilator or vasoconstrictor substance may act directly on isolated segments of the coronary tree. More often, a paradoxical response may be obtained as a consequence of a balanced stimulation that is the result of a direct action of a chemical on coronary tone, or an indirect action due to heart and systemic vessel responses that the substance itself may induce, and, finally, compensatory mechanisms that can be activated.

Among vasodilators of the coronary tree, primarily adenosine, acetylcholine, histamine, PGE and PGI2 have the strongest effects, while catecholamines, angiotensin, vasopressin and thromboxane A2 are the most potent vasoconstrictors. However, a large series of other hormones, electrolytes, and amino-acids may regulate coronary vascular response although with weak and variable effects depending closely on their blood concentration.

Keywords: Coronary tone, vascular resistance, metabolic regulation, humoral regulation, coronary artery, myocardium, heart, endothelium, catecholamines, norepinephrine, epinephrine, dopamine, angiotensin, vasopressin, adenosine, acetylcholine, histamine, hormone (s), thyroid hormone, adrenal steroid(s), glucagon, vasoactive intestinal polypeptide, serotonin, ion(s), prostaglandins, PGE, PGI2, Thromboxane A2, arachidonic acid, smoking.

Humoral and metabolic control of the coronary circulation plays a significant role for the regulation of coronary blood flow.

Many chemicals have been tested to assess coronary responses to applied stimuli by using different substances as well as coronary blood flow adjustment. Of these chemicals, some induce significant coronary responses consisting, globally, of vasoconstriction, vasodilation or balanced changes in coronary blood flow as a consequence of compensatory mechanisms that may occur, some others may induce coronary circulation changes of weak intensity or, on the contrary, act when heart muscle meets, functionally, particular circumstances.

Strictly speaking, humoral regulation should be primarily attributed to those substances which are circulating continuously into the blood and can change, within certain limits, their concentrations with regard to physiological demands. On the contrary, metabolic regulation should be attributed to those organic compounds that are initial, intermediate or end-products of complex chemical reactions that lead to energetic material formation as well as catabolic products. Enzymatic chains take part to provide those substrates of reactions that modify small or simple chemical structures into more complex active metabolites. Thus, humoral substances primarily determine functional responses, whereas metabolic substances supply primarily energy to permit physiological effects.

However, although there are differences in the biochemical characteristics of the humoral and metabolic substrates, it is customary to consider their effects on coronary circulation together, since these compounds have a chemical structure and, moreover, they may influence directly coronary blood flow.

Table 3.1. lists the main chemicals able to induce coronary blood flow adjustments, although an enormous series of substances would seem to stimulate coronary blood flow even if, sometimes, without significant results. Moreover, it is very important to establish, when coronary blood flow is adjusted, the type and intensity of coronary response that may be influenced by different factors like anatomical status of the coronary tree, combined interference with other chemicals, health state of studied individuals, their lifestyle, and, particularly duration and need for a specific response.

These chemicals play their action at different levels of the coronary arteries and vasoactive response, depend on their blood concentrations as well as evoked compensatory mechanisms.

Table 3.1. Main humoral and metabolic substances that influence coronary blood flow

Catecholamines	Norepinephrine
	Epinephrine
	Dopamine
Angiotensin	
Vasopressin	
Adenosine	
Acetylcholine	
Histamine	
Hormones	Thyroid hormone
	Adrenal steroids
	Glucagon
	Vasoactive Intestinal Polypeptide (VIP)
Serotonin	
Cations	

Prostaglandins	PGA1
	PGE1
	PGE2
	PGH2
	PGI2
	Thromboxane A2

Catecholamines

The role of catecholamines as modulators of responses particularly of the sympathetic type to different organs and structures of the body has been well identified [1–3]. Moreover, heart and coronary circulation may be considered as target organs of these compounds [4–7]

Epinephrine, norepinephrine and dopamine are the only catecholamines of endogenous production. However, initially, only two chemical compounds have been isolated from adrenal medullary extracts, respectively epinephrine and norepinephrine. These substances are stored in separate cells of the medulla and are released by intercurrent events like accelerated metabolism or stimuli of different types. The release of catecholamines from the adrenal medulla is influenced by acetylcholine in the presence of calcium ions. Reaching this result is the final step of a complex series of changes that involve the autonomic system, endocrine glands and some biometabolites that separately or all together may be influenced by some compounds of tobacco smoke, primarily nicotine.

Catecholamines [1] are stored also in a large chromaffin tissue that develops in several structures of the body: sympathetic ganglions, located along the course of abdominal aorta, and all ganglionic sites that accompany sympathetic nerve endings. Moreover, there is an amount of intratissutal catecholamines which is produced in several organs.

The third natural catecholamine, dopamine, is also stored in a peripheral dopaminergic system not yet well identified.

Usually, catecholamines exert their effects where they are released or all around.

Epinephrine, norepinephrine and dopamine function as neurotransmitters in the central nervous system. Outside this structure, the activity of the catecholamines differs widely.

Epinephrine is a hormone of adrenal medulla with a prompt availability according to those events mostly linked to stress or acute stimuli which may cause stressing effects. On the contrary, norepinephrine acts primarily as a neurotransmitter of sympathetic postganglionic neurons; it is related to preganglionic neuron acetylcholine to regulate sympathetic activity. The third catecholamine, dopamine, has yet an unclear role and, probably, acts particularly as a neurotransmitter with a primary activity on cerebral structures that are strongly influenced by dopamine itself at a metabolic level throughout mechanisms of competition or facilitation with other nervous metabolites primarily serotonin.

Metabolically, catecholamines derive from the amino acid tyrosine by a complex process of hydroxylation, decarboxylation, and, again, hydroxylation. Figure 3.1. shows the main pathways that occur to synthesize catecholamines.

These main pathways develop in different structures like the liver, kidney, brain, but particularly the adrenal gland. A complex mechanism of feed-back that involves many structures as adrenoreceptors, peripheral tissues, metabolic and functional cell responses regulates catecholamine biosynthesis and release. Catecholamines lead their activity particularly to those structures like cardiovascular system which feel early stressing stimuli that increase the metabolism as well as create a major demand for oxygen. According to the different type of response, that catecholamines determine, an acute stimulation of cardiovascular system initiated by epinephrine could be prolonged by increased release and stimulation due to norepinephrine. Therefore, it is hard, sometimes, to establish what it is due to one hormone and what is due to the other, and such an occurrence explains how it could be complex to interpret coronary blood flow regulation due to these hormones.

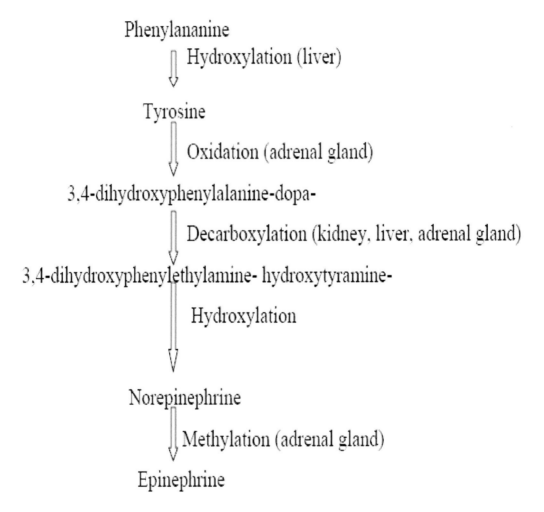

Figure 3.1. Main metabolic pathways for catecholamine biosynthesis.

Chemical formula of epinephrine and norepinephrine is as follows:

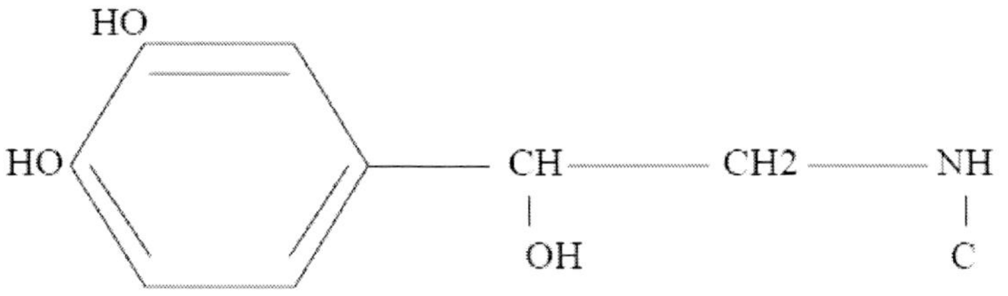

Epinephrine (C9 H13NO3)

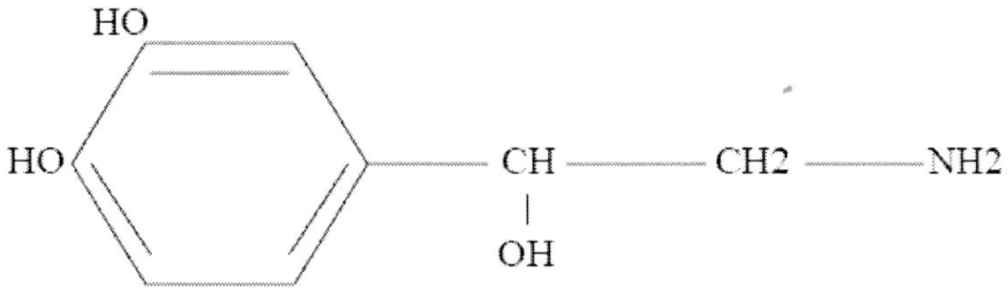

Norepinephrine (C8H11NO3)

Plasma concentrations of epinephrine and norepinephrine usually reflect respectively adrenal medullary secretion and sympathetic nerve activity. Several factors, which are, usually, related to exercise, mental stress, electrolyte balance, smoking and age [2–3], can stimulate the feed-back mechanism of catecholamine production, metabolism, uptake and excretion.

Dopamine, the third catecholamine with sympathomimetic vasopressor effects, is the immediate precursor of norepinephrine. Dopamine hydrochloride is a white to off-white crystalline powder, which may have a slight odor of hydrochloric acid. It is freely soluble in water and soluble in alcohol. Chemically it is designated as 4-(2-aminoethyl) pyrocatechol hydrochloride, and its structual formula is:

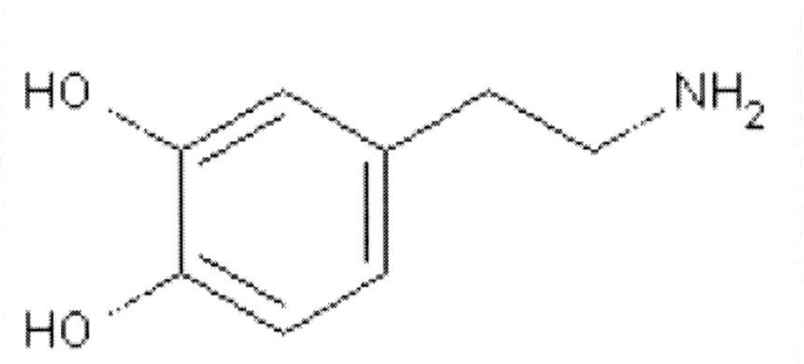

Dopamine (C8H11NO2)

Physiologically [7–10], catecholamines may be responsible for two effects: a direct effect, particularly towards cardiovascular system, and an indirect effect causing changes in hormone secretion and blood flow distribution (table 3.2.). Coronary blood flow regulation is, usually, under both types of control. With regard to these biochemical effects, catecholamines have a direct effect on vascular smooth cells, nonvascular smooth cells and cardiac muscle. The global results of these physiological effects consist of an activation of various cardiac reflexes as well as modulation of some metabolic responses that involve different pathways of metabolism, for instance glycogenolysis in the liver and muscle, that influence physiological responses at different levels of body organs and tissues.

Table 3.2. Physiological effects of catecholamines

Direct effect	- Cardiovascular system:	Vasoconstriction (CBF regulation)
		Increased heart rate
		Increased myocardial contractility
		Increased conduction velocity
		Enhanced cardiac output
		Venoconstriction
		Increased oxygen consumption
		Hypertension.
	- Central nervous system	
Indirect effect	- Endocrine system	
		Hormone release modulation
	- Blood flow redistribution	

The effects of catecholamines, primarily epinephrine, are very quick if compared with hormone activity of other endocrine glands. Therefore, changes in structure function may be seen acutely after exposure to a standard or harmful stimulus. Such a property tends to explain the negative effects of the catecholamines on target organs after acute exposure to smoking that must be considered a strong factor of adrenergic stimulation [11–13]. Moreover, increased levels of catecholamines can be dosed immediately before exercise since the mental stress that precedes exercise performance can induce a rise in these metabolites.

A large variety of hemodynamic and metabolic effects is the response of the cardiovascular system to those functional stimuli that cause catecholamine excess. Briefly, the result of the stimulus depends on the type of adrenoreceptor involved. Two types of adrenoreceptors primarily are influenced, α adrenoreceptors and β adrenoreceptors, the activity of which causes different responses in the cardiovascular system.

Catecholamines increase heart rate and myocardial contraction by a β stimulation. On the contrary, vasoconstriction is a result of α stimulation. However, vascular bed of the skeletal muscle undergoes vasodilation through the β adrenoreceptor effect. Norepinephrine induces an increase in both systolic and distolic blood pressure levels as a consequence of an amount in vascular tone, while epinephrine usually acutely raises only systolic blood pressure.

The direct effect of catecholamines causes changes in coronary blood flow and myocardium primarily by changes in vascular coronary tone, enhanced lipid mobility, calcium overload, free radical production, increased sarcolemmal permeability. Moreover, sustained increase in myocardial oxygen demand or decrease in myocardial oxygen availability induced by catecholamine release can cause myocardial damage. The first event occurs as a consequence of catecholamine stimulus, while the second recognizes primarily the effects of cigarette smoking [14] although catecholamines may also have a negative influence and potentiate the effects.

In short, catecholamines [15–23] stimulate α-receptors which determine coronary vasoconstriction as a consequence of a direct effect. Indirectly, however, catecholamine release increases coronary blood flow (CBF) by a phenomenon of coronary vasodilation due to markedly increased myocardial contractility and oxygen consumption. Dopamine seems to cause moderate coronary dilation although coronary response to dopamine stimulation seems to depend on dopamine levels in the blood. About β-receptor stimulation, there is clear evidence of a vasodilator effect at the beginning of the stimulation.

Finally, it is worthwhile, in my opinion, to give particular mention to some patterns that catecholamines could induce.

Toxically, foci of myocardial necrosis with contract bands have been observed as a response to catecholamines. These patterns are probably due to a direct effect of catecholamines on cardiac myocytes via calcium overload, although coronary vasoconstriction accompanied by increased heart rate may play an important role. Moreover, focal myocardial necrosis with contract bands has been described [24] in patients affected by intracranial lesions and elevated cerebrospinal fluid pressure. These manifestations are a response to acutely strong or prolonged catecholamine cardiotoxicity and are, therefore, not very likely to appear in coronary tone changes following, physiologically, coronary artery stimulation or exposure to smoking, unless in experimental cardiomyopathy of animals. However, this subject will be discussed in the section of the volume which concerns coronary pathology.

Angiotensin

Metabolically, angiotensin is one of the major stressing substances for coronary circulation since it influences coronary vasomotor tone either directly or indirectly by a series of changes in those cardiac parameters that, usually, contribute to stimulate coronary tone.

There are different types of angiotensin derived from a precursor called angiotensinogen modifying which originates all successors.

Angiotensinogen is an α-2-globulin produced and released into the circulation mainly by the liver, although other sites are thought to be involved. It is a member of the serpin family, which are a class of similar proteins able to inhibit protease, and the name of which is the result of the initial letters linked to their activity – serine protease inhibitors (serpin) –[25], although it is not known to inhibit other enzymes, unlike most serpins. Plasma angiotensinogen levels are increased by several hormones like plasma corticosteroid, estrogen, thyroid hormone concentrations as well as by its metabolite angiotensin II, which is the most potent pressor known [26-28].

Chemically, angiotensin II is an octapeptide formed by a sequence of eight amino-acids as follows:

Asp-Arg- Val-Tyr-Ile-His-Pro-Phe
Asp = asparagine (2-amino-4 succynil-amino acid)
Arg = arginine (2-amino –5-diaminomethylidene amino-pentoic acid)
Val = valine (α-amino-isovalerianic acid)
Tyr = tyrosine (ossiphenyl- propionic-amino acid)
Ile = isoleucine (2-amino-3-methylpentanoic acid)
His = histidine (2-amino-3-3H-imidazol-4-yl-propionic acid)
Pro = proline (s-pyrrolidine-2-carboxylic acid)
Phe = phenylalanine (phenylamino-propionic acid)

Some of these amino-acids like arginine, valine, isoleucine, histidine, phenylalanine are essential amino acids, namely those amino acids which cannot be synthesized by the organism and, therefore, must be supplied in the diet, whereas the remaining amino acids are not essential amino acids and, therefore, synthesized by several metabolic steps of organs and tissues of the body.

Angiotensin II originates from Angiotensin I, a decapeptide much less potent than angiotensin II, by the action of the enzyme ACE (angiotensin converting enzyme) present particularly in the pulmonary vascular endothelium, but also in other tissues, that determines splitting off the two C-teminal amino acids of angiotensin I, respectively histidine and leucine. In its turn, angiotensin I originates, metabolically, by its inactive precursor Angiotensinogen activated by active renine, a proteolytic enzyme, produced, stored, and released by the juxtaglomerular cells and cells of macula densa of the kidney. Figure 3.2. summarizes the main pathways to form angiotensin II. Therefore, production of angiotensin II involves many structures like the liver, kidney, vascular bed, particularly pulmonary vascular endothelium, sympathetic system, electrolyte balance. Moreover, a series of other chemicals, angiotensin III and angiotensin IV, which are much less potent than angiotensin II in the control of vascular coronary tone, originates from angiotensin II under the effects of enzymes like angiotensinases.

Many effects of angiotensin II are of a great importance to vascular blood control, particularly coronary circulation [29–40]. From the results derived by clinical and experimental studies on the subject, one can conclude that angiotensin II is one of the most potent substances in increasing coronary vascular resistance either by a direct action on the arterial wall, mediated by angiotensin II receptors, or by significant increase in myocardial oxygen consumption mediated by increased heart rate, systemic blood pressure and left ventricular wall stress. In its turn, increased cardiac metabolism tends to cause coronary vasodilation as a balanced and compensatory response to angiotensin II stimulation.

Stimulating effects due to angiotensin II involve both large and small coronary vessels [37]. Moreover, it has been hypothesized that there is more significant increase in vascular resistance of those vessels which run into the right ventricle than those arteries which supply left ventricular mass [41]. This type of response could be due to a different degree of stimulation that angiotensin II exerts on the right and left ventricle.

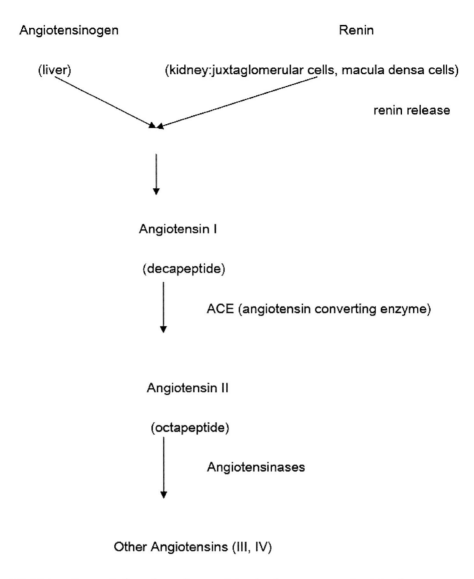

Figure 3.2. Main pathways to form the various angiotensins from precursor Angiotensinogen.

In conclusion, it is worthy to note that angiotensin II is the strongest vasoconstrictor that increases heavily vascular resistance primarily when it exerts its action on isolated structures or structures where antagonist responses have been blocked. On the contrary, different results may be observed when compensatory mechanisms are able to act. Moreover, there is strong evidence that a close and complex interaction links angiotensin II responses with the responses of other metabolites that modulate coronary vessel tone, either they are vasoconstrictor metabolites or metabolites which, usually, induce coronary dilation. Sympathetic stimulation also correlates its effects with angiotensin II effects originating an evident interaction of themselves.

Vasopressin

Vasopressin is a potent vasoconstrictor which is produced by the hypothalamus. It is stored and released by the posterior pituitary gland. Specifically, the hormone stimulates the absorption of the water from collecting ducts of the kidney [42–44].

Chemically, vasopressin is a peptide formed by a sequential series of amino-acids like:

Cys-Tyr- Phe-Gln- Asn- Cys-Pro-(Lys)-Gly---- NH2, with a chemical formula $C_{47}H_{66}N_{12}O_{12}S_2$ and chemical name of –4-(diaminomethylideneamino)butylpyrrolidine-2-carboxamide.

Spatial formula (figure 3.3.) may be seen as follows [45]:

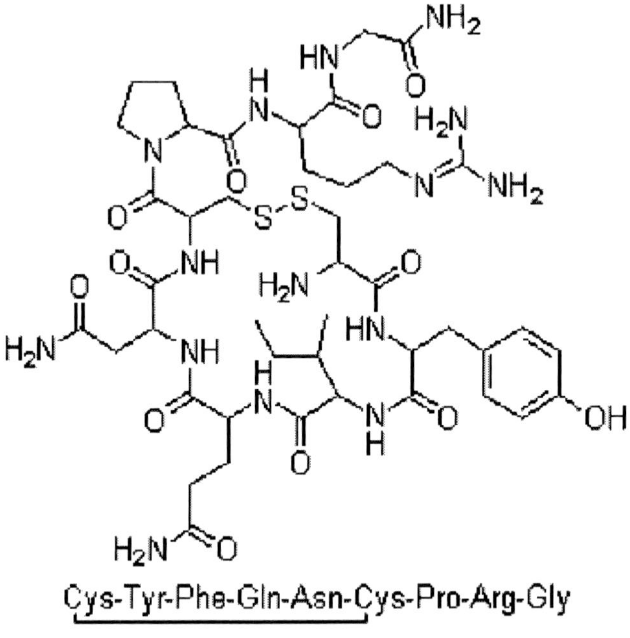

Cys-Tyr-Phe-Gln-Asn-Cys-Pro-Arg-Gly

Figure 3.3. Molecular formula of vasopressin. One can see the sequential series of amino-acids that form the chemical product. Reproduced with the permission of Online Informational Database of China [45].

Increased concentrations of vasopressin produce coronary vasoconstriction throughout a direct mechanism [42, 46]. However, myocardial perfusion may be affected also indirectly by the effects of vasopressin on the aortic pressure and cardiac output. Additionally, the significant interaction that exists between vasopressin and catecholamines potentiates vasoconstrictor properties of the hormone [47].

Different pathological states, particularly shock accompanied by a significant dehydration, hemorrhage and heart failure, induce changes in vasopressin release. However, a significant increase in vasopressin blood levels needs to induce a direct vasoconstrictor effect on coronary circulation [42, 48].

Adenosine

Adenosine is, probably, the most potent known vasodilator in normal arteries. Coronary tone is strongly influenced by the action of this chemical.

Different responses, however, may be obtained with regard to the functional stimulation of coronary vessels and possible compensatory mechanisms that follow stimulation itself [49–53].

Adenosine originates from the energetic metabolism that involves phospathe chains. The result of the metabolic pathways is to provide aerobic constituents for heart and vessel function.

Chemically, adenosine is a nucleoside that is composed by adenine and d-ribose with a chemical formula of C10H13N5O4, and a chemical name of 2-(6-aminopurin-9-yl)-5-(hydroxymethyl)oxolane-3,4-diol. Spatial formula (figure 3.4.) may be reproduced as follows:

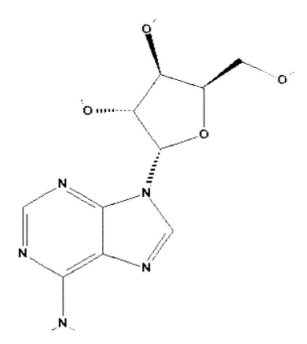

Figure 3.4. Adenosine, a chemical compound formed by adenine and d-ribose.

In the coronary circulation, adenosine can produce maximal coronary dilation with a degree that varies for the different layers of the heart. Thus, intermediate doses of the substance produce higher vasodilator effects on subendocardial coronary vessels than subepicardial coronary arteries of the left ventricle [50]. On the contrary, maximal doses of the drug induce effects that are the result of direct vasodilator action on coronary wall and combined effects on cardiac output, blood pressure and degree of compressive extravascular forces.

In conclusion, adenosine relaxes primarily the small coronary vessels [54–55] more than subepicardial conduit coronary arteries where vasodilator effects of the substance may be identified although with a different degree. Moreover, collateral coronary circulation that is, usually, developed when coronary stenoses exist responds to adenosine effects with a vessel dilation.

Other Chemicals

A large group of other chemicals may influence metabolically and humorally the vascular tone of the coronary arteries, although they can produce responses that can vary with regard to blood concentrations of themselves, myocardial function, and coronary vessel tone and anatomy.

Among these substances, there are some with dilator effects even if, sometimes, with paradoxical vasoconstrictor responses, like acetylcholine [56–59], histamine, which produces its vasodilator effects both directly on coronary tone and indirectly by changes in inotropic and chronotropic responses of the heart [60–63], and serotonin, that produces a mild coronary vasodilation. Vasodilator responses determined by Calcium and Magnesium ions on coronary tone are often of not significant levels, whereas the K-ion stimulation can determine either vasodilator or vasoconstrictor responses which depend on ion concentration [64–67].

Among vasoconstrictor chemicals, it is worthwhile to mention the effects of thyroid hormone that, at the end, produces coronary vasodilation as a consequence of its complex effects that increase heart rate, myocardial oxygen consumption, and myocardial contractility and, then, activate the vasodilator compensatory coronary response [68]. Also glucagon, potentially a vasoconstrictor agent of isolated coronary segments, causes coronary vasodilation as a consequence of its stimulating effects on inotropism and chronotropism of the heart [69].

A more detailed description needs to clarify the role of prostaglandins on coronary tone since these substances play complex effects either directly on the coronary wall or indirectly causing changes in platelet functions and pathological alterations of both heart and vessels.

Prostaglandins

Prostaglandins are a group of substances which may be synthesized by all tissues in the body as products of polyunsaturated acid metabolism, particularly arachidonic acid released from membrane phospholipids by the action of the enzyme phospholipase A2 in response to a large series of physical, chemical, biological and neurohormonal factors.

The precursor, arachidonic acid, chemically originates from 20-carbon essential fatty acids. Then, it is converted into two classes of substances which are respectively primary prostaglandins and leukotrienes by the action of two enzymatic chains respectively cyclooxygenases and lipoxygenases (figure 3.5.) [70-72].

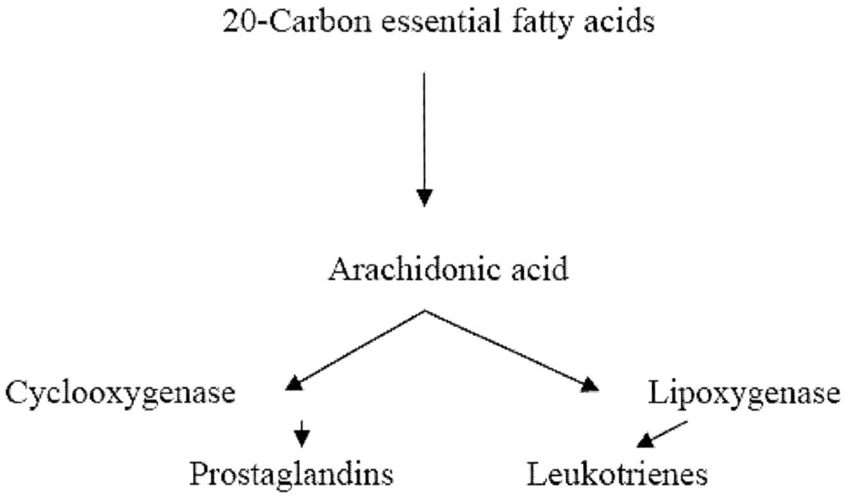

20-Carbon essential fatty acids

Arachidonic acid

Cyclooxygenase   Lipoxygenase

Prostaglandins   Leukotrienes

Figure 3.5. Main metabolic pathways of arachidonic acid.

Prostaglandins exhibit a broad spectrum of effects.

Those substances belonging to E group and PGI2 originate from endothelium and vessel wall and have significant circulatory properties that contribute to maintain primarily the microcirculation and counterbalance the vasoconstrictive and proaggregatory properties of Thromboxane A2. These prostaglandins are potent vasodilators in various vascular beds and have also, primarily PGI2, antithrombotic effects [73-76]. Coronary tone strongly feels vasodilator effects of PGE and PGI2 since they strongly counteract the effects of Thromboxane A2, released by platelets, that increases platelet aggregation and simultaneously induces vasoconstriction [77].

Vasodilator effects of PGE and PGI2 may be seen primarily "in vivo" in animal studies, since a balance in their vasodilator effects when these prostaglandins are circulating may be observed as a consequence of their instability or pulmonary uptake.

Cigarette smoking is one of the most potent factors that determines changes in coronary tone since smoking, either as active smoking or passive smoking [78–85], influences heavily the system prostaglandin-thromboxane by blood platelet activation and, consequently, thromboxane A2 production. Moreover, complex enzymatic mechanisms that stimulate an abnormal platelet response potentiate cardiovascular damage.

In conclusion, coronary tone [86], and consequently possible coronary spasm, particularly when ischemic areas exist into the myocardium, may be influenced by interplay between prostaglandins, thromboxane formed by platelets, and also endoperoxides, which are active precursors in the biosynthesis of both prostaglandins and thromboxanes from arachidonic acid. Thus, in this way, chemical compounds of smoking can negatively involve coronary vessel function and determine, in the long run, the appearance of those structural lesions that may be the basis of ischemic heart disease and nonfatal or fatal cardiac events.

References

[1] Axelrod J. The metabolism, storage and release of catecholamines. *Recent Prog. Hormone Research.* 1965; 21: 597 – 622.

[2] Chalmers JP, West MJ. The nervous system in the pathogenesis of hypertension. In: Robertson JIS ed, *Handbook of hypertension. Clinical Aspects of Essential Hypertension.* Elsevier, Amsterdam, Netherlands, 1983; Vol 1: 64 – 96.

[3] Calaresu FR, Yardley CP. Medullary basal sympathetic tone. *Ann. Rev. Physiol.* 1988; 50: 511 – 24.

[4] Markwalder J, Starling EH. Note on some factors which determine blood flow through coronary circulation. *J. Physiol.* 1914; 47: 275 – 85.

[5] Berne RM. Effect of epinephrine and norepinephrine on coronary circulation. *Circ. Res.* 1958; 6: 644 – 55.

[6] Vatner SF, Higgins CB, Braunwald E. Effects of norepinephrine on coronary circulation and left ventricular dynamics in the conscious dog. *Circ. Res.* 1974; 34: 812 – 23.

[7] Breuer HW, Skyschally A, Schulz R, Martin C, Wehr M, Heusch G. Heart rate variability and circulating catecholamine concentrations during steady state exercise in healthy volunteers. *Br. Heart J.* 1993; 70: 144 – 9.

[8] Anton AH, Sayre DF. A study of the factors affecting the aluminum oxide-trihydroxyindole procedure for the analysis of catecholamines. *J. Pharmacol. Exp. Ther.* 1966; 138: 360 – 74.

[9] Hasking GJ, Esler MD, Jennings JL, Dewar E, Lambert J. Norepinephrine spillover to plasma during steady-state supine bicycle exercise. *Circulation.* 1988; 78: 516 – 21.

[10] Riegger AJG, Liebau G. The renin-angiotensin-aldosterone system, antidiuretic hormone and sympathetic nerve activity in an experimental model of congestive heart failure in the dog. *Clin. Sci.* 1982; 62: 465 – 9.

[11] Schievelbein H, Richter F. The influence of passive smoking in the cardiovascular system. *Prev. Med.* 1984; 13: 626 – 44.

[12] Glantz SA. Air pollution as a cause of heart disease: Time for action. *J. Am. Coll. Cardiol.* 2002; 39: 943 – 5.

[13] Pope CA 3rd, Eatough DJ, Gold DR, Pang Y, Nielsen KR, Nath P, Verrier RL, Kanner RE. Acute exposure to environmental tobacco smoke and heart rate variability. *Environ. Health Perspect.* 2001; 109: 711 – 6.

[14] Leone A. Relationship between cigarette smoking and other coronary risk factors in atherosclerosis: Risk of cardiovascular disease and preventive measures. *Curr. Pharm. Design.* 2003; 9: 2417 – 23.

[15] Akhtar N, Mikulic E, Cohn JN, Chaudhry MH. Hemodynamic effect of dobutamine in patients with severe heart failure. *Am. J. Cardiol.* 1975; 36: 202 – 5.

[16] Braunwald E. Control of myocardial oxygen consumption: physiologic and clinical considerations. *Am. J. Cardiol.* 1971; 27: 416 – 32.

[17] Gaal PG, Kattus AA, Kolin A, Ross G. Effects of adrenaline and noradrenaline on coronary blood flow before and after beta-adrenergic blockade. *Br. J. Pharmacol. Chemother.* 1966; 26: 713 – 22.

[18] Goldberg LI. Cardiovascular and renal actions of dopamine: potential clinical applications. *Pharmacol. Rev.* 1972; 24: 1 – 29.

[19] Lewis FB, Coffman JD, Gregg DE. Effect of heart rate and intracoronary isoproterenol, levarterenol, and epinephrine on coronary flow and resistance. *Circ. Res.* 1961; 9: 89 – 95.

[20] Maroko PR, Kjekshus JK, Sobel BE, Watanabe T, Covell JW, Ross J Jr, Braunwald E. Factors influencing infarct size following experimental coronary artery occlusions. *Circulation.* 1971; 43: 67 – 82.

[21] Mueller H, Ayres SM, Giannelli S Jr, Conklin EF, Mazzara JT, Grace WJ. Effect of isoproterenol, l-norepinephrine, and intra-aortic counterpulsation on hemodynamics and myocardial metabolism in shock following acute myocardial infarction. *Circulation.* 1972; 45: 335 – 51.

[22] Stephens J, Hayward R, Ead H, Adams L, Hamer J, Spurrel R. Effects of selective and non-selective beta-adrenergic blockade on coronary dynamics in man assessed by rapid atrial pacing. *Br. Heart J.* 1978; 40: 856 – 63.

[23] Drake-Holland AJ, Laird JD, Noble MI, Spaan JA, Vergroesen I. Oxygen and coronary vascular resistance during autoregulation and metabolic vasodilation in the dog. *J. Physiol.* 1984; 348: 285 –99.

[24] Samuels MA. Neurally induced cardiac damage : definition of the problem. *Neurol. Clin.* 1993; 11: 273 – 92.

[25] Carrel R, Travis J. A1-antitrypsin and serpins: variation and countervariation. *Trends Biochem. Sci.* 1985; 10: 20 – 4.

[26] Regoli D, Park WK, Rioux F. Pharmacology of angiotensin. *Pharmacol. Rev.* 1974; 26: 69 – 123.

[27] Davis JO, Freeman RH. Mechanisms regulating renin release. *Physiol. Rev.* 1976; 56: 1 – 56.

[28] Ferrario CM, Gildenberg PL, McCubbin JW. Cardiovascular effects of angiotensin mediated by the central nervous system. *Circ. Res.* 1972; 30: 257 – 62.

[29] Fowler NO, Holmes JC. Coronary and myocardial actions of angiotensin. *Circ. Res.* 1964; 14: 191 – 201.

[30] Lorber V. The action of angiotensin on the completely isolated mammalian heart. *Am. Heart J.* 1942; 23: 37.

[31] Britton S, DiSalvo J. Effects of angiotensin I and angiotensin II on hindlimb and coronary vascular resistance. *Am. J. Physiol.* 1973; 225: 1226 – 31.

[32] Saino A, Pomidossi G, Perondi R, Valentini R, Rimini A, Di Francesco L, Mancia G. Intracoronary angiotensin II potentiates coronary sympathetic vasoconstriction in humans. *Circulation.* 1997; 96: 148 – 53.

[33] Zimmerman BG, Sybertz EG, Wong PC. Interaction between sympathetic and renin-angiotensin system. *J. Hypertens.* 1984; 2: 581 – 8.

[34] Lanier SM, Malik KU. Facilitation of adrenergic transmission in the canine heart by intracoronary infusion of angiotensin II: effect of prostaglandin synthesis inhibition. *J. Pharmacol. Exp. Ther.* 1983; 227: 676 – 82.

[35] Hatton R, Clough DP, Adigun SA, Conway J. Functional interaction between angiotensin and sympathetic reflexes in cats. *Clin. Sci.* 1982; 62: 51 – 6.

[36] Drimal J, Pavek K, Selecky FV. Primary and secondary effects of angiotensin on the coronary circulation. *Cardiologia.* 1969; 54: 1 – 15.

[37] Cohen MV, Kirk ES. Differential response of large and small coronary arteries to nitroglycerin and angiotensin. *Circ. Res.* 1973; 33: 445 – 53.

[38] Zimmerman BG, Gomer SK, Chia Liao J. Action of angiotensin on vascular adrenergic nerve endings: facilitation of norepinephrine release. *Fed. Proc.* 1972; 31: 1344 – 50.

[39] Blumberg AL, Denny SE, Marshall GR, Needleman P. Blood vessel hormone interactions: angiotensin, bradykinin and prostaglandins. *Am. J. Physiol.* 1977; 232: H305 – 10.

[40] Urata H, Healy B, Stewart RW, Pumpus FM, Husain A. Angiotensin II receptors in normal and failing human hearts. *J. Clin. Endocrinol. Metab.* 1989; 69: 54 – 66.

[41] Gunther S, Cannon PJ. Modulation of angiotensin II coronary vasoconstriction by cardiac prostaglandin synthesis. *Am. J. Physiol.* 1980; 238: H895 – 901.

[42] Nakano J.Cardiovascular actions of vasopressin. *Jpn. Circ. J.* 1973; 37: 363 – 81.

[43] de Aguilera EM, Vila JM, Irurzun A, Martinez MC, Martinez-Cuesta MA, Lluch S. Endothelium-independent contractions of human cerebral arteries in response to vasopressin. *Stroke.* 1990; 21: 1689 – 93.

[44] Tallarida G, Ceccamea A, Leone A, Semprini A, Parrinello A, Condorelli M. Effetti indotti dal salasso parziale e totale sulla struttura istologica post-ipofisaria. *Ric. Sci.* 1967; 37: 785 – 93.

[45] Chemical-Blink: Online Informational Database from China.

[46] Khayyal MA, Heng C, Franzen D, Breall JA, Kirk ES. Effects of vasopressin on the coronary circulation reserve and during ischemia. *Am. J. Physiol.* 1985; 248: H516 – 22.

[47] Vanhoutte PM, Verbeuren TJ, Webb RC. Local modulation of adrenergic neuroeffector interaction in the blood vessel wall. *Physiol. Rev.* 1981; 61: 151 – 247.

[48] Pullan PT, Johnston WP, Anderson WP, Korner PI. Plasma vasopressin in blood pressure homeostasis and in experimental renal hypertension. *Am. J. Physiol.* 1980; 239: H81 – 7.

[49] Berne RM. The role of adenosine in the regulation of coronary blood flow. *Circ. Res.* 1980; 47: 807 – 13.

[50] Rembert JC, Boyd LM, Watkinson WP, Greenfield JC Jr. Effect of adenosine on transmural myocardial blood flow distribution in the awake dog. *Am. J. Physiol.* 1980; 239: H7 – 13.

[51] Vanhoutte PM, Mombouli JV. Vascular endothelium: Vasoactive mediators. *Prog. Cardiovasc. Dis.* 1996; 39: 229 – 38.

[52] Wusten B, Buss DD, Deist H, Schaper W. Dilatory capacity of the coronary circulation and its correlation to the arterial vasculature in the canine left ventricle. *Basic Res. Cardiol.* 1977; 72: 636 – 50.

[53] Hori M, Kitakaze M. Adenosine, the heart, and coronary circulation. *Hypertension.* 1991; 18: 565 – 74.

[54] Harder DR, Belardinelli L, Sperelakis N, Rubio R, Berne RM. Differential effects of adenosine and nitroglycerin on the action potentials of large and small coronary arteries. *Circ. Res.* 1979; 44: 176 – 82.

[55] Patterson RE, Kirk ES. Apparent improvement in canine collateral myocardial blood flow during vasodilation depends on criteria used to identify ischemic myocardium. *Circ. Res.* 1980; 47: 108 – 116.

[56] Yasue H, Horio Y, Nakamura N, Fujii H, Himoto N, Sonoda R, Kugiyama K, Obata K, Morikami Y, Kimura T. Induction of coronary artery spasm by acetylcholine in patients with variant angina: Possible role of the parasympathetic nerve system in the pathogenesis of coronary artery spasm. *Circulation.* 1986; 74: 955 – 63.

[57] Okumura K, Yasue H, Horio Y, Takaoka K, Matsuyama K, Fujii H, Morikami Y. Multivessel coronary spasm in patients with variant angina: A study with intracoronary injection of acetylcholine. *Circulation.* 1988; 77: 535 – 42.

[58] Ludmer PL, Selwyn AP, Shook TL, Wayne R, Mudge GH, Alexander RW, Ganz P. Paradoxical vasoconstriction induced by acetylcholine in atherosclerotic coronary arteries. *N. Engl. J. Med.* 1986; 315: 1046 – 51.

[59] Yamamoto H, Bossaller C, Cartwright J Jr, Henry PD. Videomicroscopic demonstration of defective cholinergic arteriolar vasodilation in atherosclerotic rabbit. *J. Clin. Invest.* 1988; 81: 1752 – 8.

[60] Owen DAA. Histamine receptors in the cardiovascular system. *Gen. Pharmac.* 1977; 8: 141 – 56.

[61] Black JW, Duncan WAM, Durant CJ, Ganellin CR, Pearsons EM. Definition and antagonism of histamine-H2-receptors. *Nature.* 1972; 236: 385 – 90.

[62] Carrol GJ, Clark DWJ. Peripheral cardiovascular effects in rats after central administration of histamine and antihistamines. *Clin. Exper. Pharmacol. and Physiol.* 1979; 6: 393 – 402.

[63] Brashear RE, Ross JC, Martin RR. Plasma histamine levels and cardiovascular effects after compound 48-80. *J. Appl. Physiol.* 1969; 27: 170 – 3.

[64] Teragawa H, Kato M, Yamagata T, Matsuura H, Kajiyama G. The preventive effect of magnesium on coronary spasm in patients with vasospastic angina. *Chest.* 2000,118:1690 –5.

[65] Kafka H, Langevin R, Armstrong PW. Serum magnesium and potassium in acute myocardial infarction. *Arch. Intern. Med.* 1987; 147: 465 – 9.

[66] Sasaguri T, Itoh T, Hirata M, Kitamura K, Kuriyama K. Regulation of coronary artery tone in relation to the activation of signal transductors that regulate calcium homeostasis. *J. Am. Coll. Cardiol.* 1987; 9: 1167 – 75.

[67] Brayden JE, Nelson MT. Regulation of arterial tone by activation of calcium-dependent potassium channels. *Science.* 1992; 256: 532 – 5.

[68] Buccino RA, Spann JF Jr, Pool PE, Sonnenblick EH, Braunwald E. Influence of thyroid state on the intrinsic contractile properties and energy stores of the myocardium. *J. Clin. Invest.* 1967; 46: 1669 – 82.

[69] Farah A, Tuttle R. Studies on the pharmacology of glucagon. *J. Pharmacol. Exp. Ther.* 1960; 129: 49 – 55.

[70] Fitzgerald GA, Patrono C. The coxibs, selective inhibitors of cyclooxygenase-2. *N. Engl. J. Med.* 2001; 345: 433 – 42.

[71] Vane JR, Bakhle YS, Botting RM. Cyclooxygenases 1 and 2. *Annu. Rev. Pharmacol. Toxicol.* 1998; 38: 97 – 120.

[72] Fitzgerald GA, Austin S, Egan K, Cheng Y, Pratico D. Cyclooxygenase products and atherothrombosis. *Ann. Med.* 2000; 32S: 21 – 6.

[73] Linton MF, Fazio S. Cyclooxygenase-2 and atherosclerosis. *Curr. Opin. Lipidol.* 2002; 13: 497 – 504.

[74] Needleman P, Kaley S. Cardiac and coronary prostaglandin synthesis and function. *N. Engl. J. Med.* 1978; 298: 1122 – 8.

[75] Sivakoff M, Pure E, Hsueh W, Needleman P. Prostaglandins and the heart. *Fed. Proc.* 1979; 38: 78 – 82.

[76] Dusting GJ, Moncada S, Vane JR. Prostaglandins, their intermediates and precursors : Cardiovascular actions and regulatory roles in normal and abnormal circulatory systems. *Prog. Cardiovasc. Dis.* 1979; 21: 405 – 30.

[77] Robertson RM, Robertson D, Roberts LJ, Maas RL, Fitzgerald GA, Friesinger GC, Oates JA. Thromboxane A2 in vasotonic angina pectoris. *N. Engl. J. Med.* 1981; 304: 998 – 1003.

[78] Pittilo RM, Mackie IJ, Rowles PM, Machine SJ, Woolf N. Effects of cigarette smoking on the ultrastructure of rat thoracic aorta and its ability to produce prostacyclin. *Thromb. Haemost.* 1982; 48: 173 –6.

[79] Davis J, Shelton L, Watanabe I, Arnold J. Passive smoking affects endothelium and platelets. *Arch. Intern. Med.* 1989; 149: 386 – 9.

[80] Sinzinger H, Kefalides A. Passive smoking severely decreases platelet sensitivity to antiaggregatory prostaglandins. *Lancet.* 1982; 2: 392 – 3.

[81] Burghuber O, Punzengruber C, Sinzinger H, Haber P, Silberbauer K. Platelet sensitivity to prostacyclin in smokers and non-smokers. *Chest.* 1986; 90: 34 – 8 .

[82] Sinzinger H, Virgolini I. Are passive smokers at greater risk of thrombosis? *Wien Klin. Wochenschr.* 1989; 20: 694- 8.

[83] Leone A, Giannini D, Bellotto C, Balbarini A. Passive smoking and coronary heart disease. *Current Vascular Pharmacology.* 2004; 2: 175 – 82.

[84] Steinberg D, Parthasarathy S, Carew TE, Khoo JC, Witztum JL. Beyond cholesterol: modifications of low-density lipoprotein that increase its atherogenicity. *N. Engl. J. Med.* 1989; 320: 915 – 24.

[85] Glantz SA, Parmley WW. Passive smoking and heart disease. Mechanisms and risk. *JAMA.* 1995; 273: 1047 – 53.

[86] Needleman P, Kulkarni PS, Raz A. Coronary tone modulation: formation and actions of prostaglandins, endoperoxides,and thromboxanes. *Science.* 1977; 195: 409 – 12.

Chapter IV

Coronary Vascular Endothelium

Abstract

The vascular endothelium has been long viewed as simply a physical separation between the blood and contiguous tissues. Nowadays, there is evidence that endothelial cells exert a rich "mosaic" of functions and, among these, primarily the regulation of vascular tone, particularly coronary vasomotor tone. When endothelium is intact, a balanced control of vessel response is a consequence of the action between vasodilator and vasoconstrictor substances produced by the endothelium itself.

Endothelium-derived NO is not only a potent vasodilator, but also inhibits platelet aggregation, vascular smooth muscle cell migration and proliferation, monocyte adhesion, which trigger those pathogenetic mechanisms that lead to atherosclerotic plaque formation.

When endothelial surface is altered by stimuli of different types, primarily the negative effects of major coronary risk factors including cigarette smoking, vasodilator capacity is impaired up to a level that depends on the power of applied stimulus and, therefore, endothelial dysfunction appears.

Endothelial dysfunction may be followed by endothelial activation characterized by a series of inflammatory and infiltrating processes that are considered "the sliding door of atherosclerosis".

Among major coronary risk factors, the main chemical compounds that characterize cigarette smoking such as nicotine and carbon monoxide exert a significantly negative action, either early or late, on the endothelium that heavily involves coronary function and structure.

Keywords: Endothelium, endothelial function, endothelial dysfunction, endothelial activation, vasodilator effect, vasoconstrictor effect, NO (nitric oxide), endothelium-derived relaxing factor(s), biopterin, l-arginine, NOS, cyclooxygenase-dependent contracting factor(s), endothelin-1, carbon monoxide, nicotine, preventive measures, coronary risk factors, prostacyclin, catecholamine, adrenergic response.

Following the excellent paper of Furchgott and Zawadzki [1], there is evidence that vascular endothelium plays a primary autocrine and paracrine regulatory role of the vascular tone at any artery level by producing a large series of chemical substances that control both arterial function and structure.

The vascular endothelium is a cellular monolayer that lines the entire vascular bed at the interface between both plasma and cellular blood and the vessel wall. As mentioned previously, endothelial cells are contiguous elements linked among themselves by interdigitations that contribute to form, however, a continuous structure which is capable of influencing and interacting with both the blood surface and subendothelial layer. In so doing, the endothelium is intimately linked to controlling vasomotor tone and preventing atherosclerotic plaque formation [2].

Studies [3–4] would seem to demonstrate that a close relationship exists between brachial, carotid and coronary endothelial changes that would be similar in type when arterial pathology may be seen by ultrasonography techniques. Moreover, a smoking habit plays a strongly negative effect on the vascular endothelium either as active smoking or passive smoking. Yet, passive smoking exposure increases more and more our knowledge of endothelial damage as one can easily observe by the analysis of both clinical and experimental findings on the subject [5–8].

From these preliminary concepts, there is evidence that a clear knowledge of endothelial properties is worthwhile to keep in mind to better understand the coronary pathology related to cigarette smoking, since accumulating results indicate that a dysfunctional endothelium, which, usually, is associated with the other major coronary risk factors, is one of the major determinants of atherothrombosis and, consequently, cardiovascular non-fatal and fatal attacks.

At first, endothelial function of the coronary arteries could be assessed by invasive techniques by using intracoronary injection of acetylcholine [9]. The use of brachial artery ultrasonography permitted a non-invasive study of endothelial function and, consequently, coronary endothelium properties since there was a demonstration of a clear correspondence between systemic and coronary artery responses [3–4].

In this chapter, those responses that characterize or interfere with endothelial function will be analyzed in regard to their main effects on the cardiovascular system.

Endothelium Metabolites

The endothelium produces several chemicals which determine primarily relaxing effects but also there are chemicals which act as contracting factors (table 4.1.).

Table 4.1. Main metabolites produced by endothelial cells

Relaxing factors	Contracting factors
Nitric Oxide (NO)	Cyclooxygenase-dependent contracting factor
Prostacyclin (PG)	Endothelin-1 (ET-1)
Hyperpolarizing relaxing factor (EDHF)	

By these substances, when there is a balanced endothelial function, the structure regulates the cardiovascular system [10] and coronary vessel vasomotor tone .

Endothelium-Derived Relaxing Factors

NO (Nitric Oxide)

NO plays a basic role in the regulation of vascular tone. It has been well demonstrated that impaired NO availability has been often associated with other coronary risk factors [11–20] and it must be identified as the triggering key for development of atherosclerotic lesions.

The metabolic pathways that lead to endothelial NO biosynthesis consist of a complex series of chemical reactions. The main ones are listed in figure 4.1.

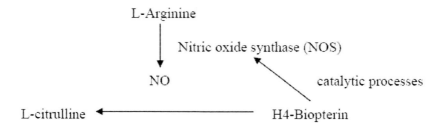

Figure 4.1. Biosynthesis of endothelial NO from L-arginine. All a series of complex processes that will be described in the text characterize NO synthesis.

Five processes of electronic oxidation that utilize three different NOS enzymatic isoforms lead to NO production [21]. Two of these substrates are constituents of vascular endothelial cells and are activated by increased levels of intracellular calcium.

In vivo, the activity of L-arginine-NO pathway is a balance between NO synthesis and breakdown. NO synthesis may meet changes in its amount [22], but the main factor that is capable to induce endothelial alterations seems to be enhanced catabolic pathways that concern NO with consequent impairment in NO availability.

These observations would seem to indicate that catabolic reactions that involve NO metabolism would be one of the major factors responsible for NO impairment and, consequently, a mechanism that could trigger the appearance of endothelial dysfunction.

NO has a very short half-life once released from endothelial cells since it rapidly interacts with free radicals, primarily superoxides, and it is destroyed after entering red blood cells to react with oxyhemoglobin. In coronary subepicardial arteries, endothelium-dependent vasodilation due to NO may be actively inhibited by substances blocking NO synthesis like N-monomethyl-L –arginine in both humans and experimental animals [23].

NO increases blood flow in response to metabolic stimuli when there is an intact endothelium. Inhibited NO production determines a reduced degree of metabolic dilation of coronary and systemic arteries in both humans and animals [24].

Two main mechanisms induce NO production and, then, regulation under the effects of metabolic stimuli: hypoxia, that stimulates endothelial cells to release NO, and coronary flow-mediated vasodilation produced also as an effect of hypoxia. Primarily, hypoxia promotes vascular hyperemia and coronary flow-mediated vasodilation increases and maintains hyperemic response. However, increased concentrations of peroxides may be seen in a dysfunctional endothelium where increased oxygen availability originates from the action of a series of oxidizing compounds and possible decrease in availability of H4 Biopterin [25–28].

Studies [29–32] investigated also the relationship between H4 Biopterin and NO synthesis since the role that this cofactor plays in regulation of NOS catalytic activity is not yet well identified.

Inhibition of H4 Biopterin synthesis reduces the production and availability of NO throughout the influence of Calcium ions and bradykinin. Thus, an optimal concentration of H4 Biopterin would seem to need adequate calcium-dependent production of NO.

From these explanations, there is evidence that NO synthesis and production is regulated by a series of different factors, the main of which may be seen in table 4.2.

Table 4.2. Main factors that regulate biosynthesis and degree in availability of NO

Hypoxia
Hyperemia (flow-mediated vasodilation)
NOS
Calcium ions
Peroxides (oxygen free radicals)
Oxyhemoglobin
H4 Biopterin

In conclusion, NO has basic vasodilator effects on the arterial wall that, however, require the presence of an intact endothelium. Coronary tone regulation due to NO production and availability has been demonstrated to be completely similar to vasodilator responses observed on the systemic arteries, primarily carotid and brachial arteries where endothelial function may be carefully assessed by non-invasive techniques like ultrasonography.

EDHF

Endothelial cells may release a relaxing factor [33] that differs from either NO or prostacyclin as it has been shown in studies on porcine coronary circulation [34].

Really, the block of NO action or prostacyclin by specific inhibitors [34, 35–39] does not totally remove possible endothelial vasodilation. Endothelium-derived hyperpolarizing factors (EDHF) have been identified as those factors which have these properties, at least under some circumstances [39, 40].

The EDHF activate adenosine triphosphate-sensitive K-channels as well as Na or K-adenosine triphosphate in smooth cells.

The role of these substances has yet to be completely clarified. There would be a series of substances belonging to different chemical families. Among these, other similar property substances would exist like a hyperpolarizing factor derived from lipoxygenase and cytochrome P450.

Hyperpolarization of endothelial cells, determined by these substances, causes an efflux of potassium from the intracellular zone that lead to intercellular accumulation of K ions between endothelial and smooth muscle cells [41].

A large series of findings that demonstrated the EDHF properties has been conducted either clinically or experimentally, and many of these involved coronary circulation.

PG (Prostacyclin)

PG is the major product of vascular cyclooxygenase metabolism and may originate on various places of the arterial wall. Endothelial cells, but particularly intima coat, media and adventitia, metabolize and release this substance under the effects of physical or biochemical stimuli which may also induce NO production [10]. Moreover, data would support that an action of nitroglycerin and its derivatives potentiate prostacyclin production [42–44]. However, some reports [45–47] would suggest that further observations need to validate the hypothesis that nitrates stimulate prostacyclin synthesis.

The stimulation by endothelial prostacyclin to induce endothelium-dependent relaxation in most blood vessels has been identified to be of weak significance [34, 48–49].

The mechanism of relaxation induced by prostacyclin is due to an increased production of cyclic 3',5'-adenosine monophosphate (cAMP) in smooth muscle cells and platelets which reduce also their aggregation properties [50].

Endothelium-Derived Contracting Factors (EDCFs)

Cyclooxygenase-Dependent Endothelium-Derived Contracting Factor

The different pathways that may lead to endothelium-dependent contraction involve the role of cyclooxygenase that plays a leading action.

Cyclooxygenase-dependent endothelium-derived contracting factor activity has been documented by the fact that cyclooxygenase blockers inhibited endothelium-dependent contraction which could be induced by arachidonic acid [51–52]. Moreover, cyclooxygenase-dependent endothelium-derived contracting factors could be also induced by acetylcholine in different vessels of experimental models of hypertension and diabetes mellitus [53–54].

Two kinds of mediators of cyclooxygenase-dependent endothelium-derived contracting factor have been identified according to their response respectively to acetylcholine or histamine [49]. These mediators belong to the family of prostanoids, particularly thromboxane A2, in case of response to acetylcholine, whereas endoperoxides are related to histamine response.

Usually, prostanoids are direct vasoconstrictors, while endoperoxides may act either as direct vasoconstrictors of vascular smooth muscle cells by acting on prostaglandin H2, or indirectly by inducing NO impairment [55–56]. Increased platelet aggregation induced by this group of substances plays a significant role to potentiate the action of endothelium-derived contracting factors.

Finally, there is evidence that metabolic pathways of cyclooxygenase produce contracting effects primarily on vascular endothelium of cerebral and ophthalmic arteries as well as veins [10].

Endothelin-1

Endothelin-1 (ET-1) is the main EDCF produced by the endothelial cells. There are three types of endothelins: endothelin-1, endothelin-2, and endothelin-3. Among these, only ET-1 is almost completely produced by endothelial cells.

Chemically, ET-1 is a 21 amino acid peptide, the chemical characteristics of which [57–59] are listed in table 4.3.

Table 4.3. Chemical characteristics of ET-1

Molecular formula	$C109H163N25O32S$
Amino acid sequence	Ala-Ser-Ala-Ser-Ser-Leu-Met-Asp-Lys-Glu-Ala-Val-Tyr-Phe-Ala-His-Leu-Asp-Ile-Ile-Trp.
Enzymatic conversion	
Molecular Weight	2367.67
Biochemical action	Selective agonist for ET- endothelin receptors

ET-1 acts by specific receptors called ETA and ETB [60–63]. ETA receptors are located only on smooth muscle cells and function inducing growth and mediating contractions. On the contrary, ETB receptors are located on both endothelial cells and smooth muscle cells where they have different effects. Smooth muscle cell ETB receptors stimulate contraction, whereas endothelial cell ETB receptors cause relaxation throughout the production of endothelium-derived relaxing factors including NO and prostacyclin [64–65].

ET-1 is a potent vasoconstrictor although it may exert a multiphasic action according to its blood concentrations. Usually, lowest concentrations of substance circulate, physiologically, into the blood. However, lower ET-1 concentrations exert a vasodilator effect on coronary and systemic arteries, whereas high substance concentrations vasoconstrict arterial vessels, and they can cause myocardial ischemia, arrhythmias and sudden cardiac death [66–68]. Vasoconstrictor effects of high ET-1 concentrations have been identified also in arterial and venous coronary bypass [69].

ET -1 can also release NO and prostacyclin via ETB receptors by a negative feedback mechanism [70].

In conclusion, the metabolic effect of ET-1 on coronary vascular tone is a consequence of the balance that exists between the direct effect on smooth muscle cells regulated by ETA and ETB receptors and NO or prostacyclin stimulation mediated by ETB receptors [71].

Breakdown of this balance, primarily due to coronary risk factors, increases vasoconstrictor effects of ET-1, which, under these circumstances, plays a pathological role in inducing coronary pathology.

From these biochemical and physiological characteristics that regulate endothelium-derived factors, there is clear evidence that a series of complex responses may be evoked with regard to the type of endothelial stimulation, and endothelium response depends on the structural characteristics of this anatomical layer.

Endothelial Dysfunction

When endothelium is intact, physiological stimulation causes vasodilation and there is also a protective effect against the development of atherosclerotic lesions. The benchmark of endothelium response is certainly NO availability.

Impaired NO availability or enhanced vasoconstrictor activity affect negatively vasodilation of the blood vessels causing altered endothelium response that may be, primarily, of two types: transient alterations, potentially reversible, or chronically irreversible alterations, which lead to atherosclerotic pathology throughout various steps [72]. Really, there is an impaired endothelial integrity triggered, usually, by the major coronary risk factors to initiate endothelial function changes.

The reduction or loss of endothelial vasodilator response characterize endothelial dysfunction, which is the first step of a series of active processes involving mechanisms like inflammation, proliferation or apoptosis, that determine endothelial activation..

Thus, endothelial activation initiates a large series of reactions that lead to formation of an atherosclerotic plaque, as a final step. The progression of endothelial activation phenomena extends the other artery coats with progressive reduction in their function as well as changes in their anatomical structure (table 4.4.).

Table 4.4. Main steps of endothelial alterations that lead to atherosclerosis

Endothelial dysfunction (loss of vasodilator capacity)	Impaired NO availability
	Enhanced vasoconstrictor activity
Endothelial activation	Inflammation
	Proliferation
	Apoptosis
Intermediated phase	Infiltration
	Artery coat alterations
Final phase	Atherosclerotic plaque

Endothelial activation usually leads to vessel inflammation and proliferation. As a consequence of endothelial dysfunction, there is a production of pro-inflammatory metabolites like cytochines, primarily interleukins, that interfere with leukocyte migration and adhesion by an active process that involves both endothelial cells and leukocytes [73–74]. Furthermore, C-reactive protein – an aspecific marker of inflammatory processes – undergoes an increased production in the liver through an interleukin mediated action [75].

Leukocyte adhesion to endothelial cells is followed by leukocyte transmigration into the subendothelial layer in response to stimuli mediated by different chemokines [76–78]. On this step, also monocyte migration and entry into macrophages have been identified at the level of subintimal layer. Therefore, the initial endothelial dysfunction, when it is not transient, triggers a series of pathologic phenomena locally at the arterial wall level as well as at a systemic level, which promote the progression of a vascular event such as atherosclerosis that affects both coronary and systemic arteries.

The steps that lead to atherosclerosis as well as atherosclerotic plaque complications that influence both coronary and cardiac pathology will be described with major details in a later chapter of this book.

Thus, coronary vessel bed alterations [79] have been primarily identified in changes of endothelial properties, although vascular media and adventitia with vasa vasorum are also structures characterized by the appearance of patterns that contribute actively to those complex phenomena that affect the artery tree under the action of stimuli, particularly cardiovascular risk factors, which may induce different types of alterations. Among these stimuli, there is, undoubtedly, cigarette smoking.

As just mentioned, endothelial dysfunction may be a phenomenon in progress but also transient followed by endothelial function restoration. Really, endothelial progenitor cells seem to participate actively in endothelium restoration [80].

Endothelial progenitor cells are primitive cells which originate from bone marrow, may enter into the bloodstream and, then, reach injured vessels where they contribute to injury repair.

The role and mechanism of action of endothelial progenitor cells are yet far from being completely clarified.

In the past, restoration of a damaged endothelium was attributed to migration of endothelial progenitor cells to the site of vessel alteration and consequent replacement and regeneration of those endothelial cells damaged by an injured stimulus. However, other studies [81–85] identified that additional factors, and not only endothelial progenitor cells, contributed actively to repair the injured endothelium. Therefore, the role of endothelial progenitor cells would be of lower importance according to what the findings would demonstrate.

Two types of endothelial progenitor cells would act specifically to repair the injured endothelium: cells coming from bone marrow and non-bone marrow cells arising from extra bone-marrow sources like tissue cells and vessel wall-derived endothelial cells.

Factors, including nicotine, influence both number and activity of endothelial progenitor cells determining enhanced functional activity of these cells at a relatively low concentration.In contrast, high concentrations of nicotine would have a toxic effect [86].

In conclusion, endothelial dysfunction not only may impair transiently endothelium-dependent vasodilation, but when dysfunction itself is prolonged or triggers inflammatory-proliferative mechanisms, becomes the promoter of those changes which lead to atherosclerotic plaque formation although a lot of factors, including primarily smoking, may interact among themselves to cause alterations, the degree of which may widely vary in different individuals.

Endothelial Dysfunction and Cigarette Smoking

As previously mentioned, several smoking compounds act negatively on endothelial cells. They can induce endothelial dysfunction of different type and degree, sometimes earlier than that due to other major coronary risk factors which, usually, need a chronic damaging activity.

Really, functional disorders of endothelial cells due to cigarette smoking develop as early as when smoking exposure begins. However, endothelial changes are, initially, transient and followed by endothelium restoration after smoking cessation.

It has been well established that functional disorders due to cigarette smoking are the result of either adrenergic stimulation or endothelial dysfunction [6–8, 87–90], and both these mechanisms interact actively among themselves since the main compounds of tobacco smoke such as nicotine and carbon monoxide are capable of causing changes in both parameters, adrenergic system and endothelial cells [91].

Nicotine interferes primarily with adrenergic responses, whereas carbon monoxide, by a direct action, induces a series of changes, including endothelial dysfunction, which recognize either a functional mechanism or later structural changes related to atherosclerosis development [89, 92–93]. Findings on selected populations [92] would show that carbon monoxide acted as a stress factor that potentiated other major coronary risk factors through its binding with hemoglobin. Increased carboxyhemoglobin concentrations induce hypoxia which is a potent promotor in endothelial cell changes, as seen in table 4.2.

Smoking is a strong factor of endothelial dysfunction even after transient acute exposure [5–7, 90]. Findings [94] compared endothelial function in the artery vessels of three different groups of healthy individuals. The first group enrolled active smokers, the second group lifelong nonsmokers who, however, were exposed to environmental tobacco smoke, and, finally, the third group consisted of individuals who were exposed inconstantly and irregularly to passive smoking. Endothelial function was assessed by using ultrasonography that estimated vascular reactivity of brachial artery. Results identified that either active or also passive smokers had significantly impaired endothelial function, although of a different degree, because of reduced NO production and release.

As far as here, functional damage caused by smoking exposure has been interpreted to be an isolated effect of an alterated adrenergic response or isolated endothelial dysfunction.

Indeed, there is evidence that smoking acts simultaneously on both parameters by a synergy of mechanisms which potentiates the final result.

Smoking stimulates a major release of epinephrine that determines production of endothelin with consequent increased level of vasoconstriction which is followed by endothelial dysfunction [95]. Moreover, both nicotine and carbon monoxide can directly cause endothelial dysfunction impairing endothelium-vasodilator responses.

There is evidence that endothelial dysfunction in smokers is due to three factors (figure 4.2.): smoking compounds, adrenergic stimulation, catecholamine action. However, the last two mechanisms may be joined together since they depend strictly on each other.

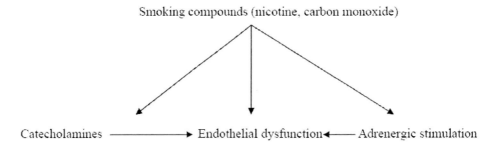

Figure 4.2. Factors that cause endothelial dysfunction in smokers. There is evidence of a direct action of the main smoking compounds associated with an indirect stimulation due to adrenergic stimulation via sympathetic system and catecholamine release.

Thus, endothelial dysfunction in smokers recognizes a multifactorial mechanism where, however, smoking compounds exert a direct action on every phase of the process. Indirect stimulation by catecholamines and sympathetic adrenergic system potentiates the degree of dysfunction. Such an occurrence may explain the early alterations, firstly functional but later structural, that affect coronary arteries of smokers which, as will be described in a new chapter, show a heavier damage than those of nonsmokers even when cardiac pathology is similar. Therefore, it could be very suitable to begin all those preventive measures which may reduce endothelial dysfunction. Among those measures which can fight endothelial dysfunction, there are some linked to individuals' lifestyle such as physical activity and antioxidant dietary supplementation with vitamin C and E, folates, fish oil or red wine, some addressed to reduce the incidence and negative effects of major coronary risk factors, and, finally, some others that require specifically a therapeutic approach when non-pharmacological prevention is unable to obtain the settled result.

Really, a large series of longitudinal studies identified endothelial dysfunction as an independent prognostic marker for cardiovascular disease. Moreover, some of these studies [18, 96–99] demonstrated endothelial dysfunction associated with coronary pathology. Totally, there were 964 patients for a mean-month follow-up of a total of 53.4 months in examined studies. Epicardial coronary arteries as well as brachial arteries in some cases showed a clear evidence of endothelial function disorders primarily linked to an impaired flow-mediated vasodilation. Moreover, endothelial dysfunction could be associated also with an increased occurrence of fatal and non-fatal cardiovascular events. It is worthy noting that impaired endothelium-dependent vasodilation can predict clinical events independent of whatever vascular district and type of vessel affected.

In conclusion, there is evidence that different endothelium-derived factor changes play a crucial role in originating atherosclerotic vessel alterations [72, 100–101] because of local blood changes, platelet function alterations, cell migration and proliferation. Among affected vessels, there is no doubt that vascular coronary arteries feel particularly the negative effects of endothelial dysfunction triggered by cigarette smoking, and such an occurrence explains the more evident impairment of coronary circulation in smokers when they are compared with nonsmokers.

References

[1]   Furchgott RF, Zawadzki JV. The obligatory role of endothelial cells in the relaxation of arterial smooth muscle by acetylcholine. *Nature.* 1980; 288: 373 –6.

[2]   Vane JR, Anggard EE, Botting RM. Regulatory functions of the vascular endothelium. *N. Engl. J. Med.* 1990; 323: 27 – 36.

[3]   Anderson TJ, Uehata A, Gerhard MD, Meredith IT, Knab S, Delagrange D, Lieberman EH, Ganz P, Creager MA, Yeung AC, Selwyn AP. Close relation of endothelial function in the human coronary and peripheral circulations. *J. Am. Coll. Cardiol.* 1995; 26: 1235 – 41.

[4]   Kallikazaros I, Tsioufis C, Sideris S, Stefanidis C, Toutouzas P. Carotid artery disease as a marker for the presence of severe artery coronary disease in patients evaluated for chest pain. *Stroke.* 1999; 30: 1002 – 7.

[5]   Davis J, Shelton L, Watanabe I, Arnold J. Passive smoking affects endothelium and platelets. *Arch. Intern. Med.* 1989; 149: 386 – 9.

[6]   Celermajer DS, Sorensen KE, Gooch VM, Spiegelhalter DJ, Miller OL, Sullivan ID, Lloyd JK, Deanfield JE. Non-invasive detection of endothelial dysfunction in children and adults at risk of atherosclerosis. *Lancet.* 1992; 340: 1111 – 5.

[7]   Celermajer DS, Sorensen KE, Georgakopoulos D. Cigarette smoking is associated with dose-related and potentially reversible impairment of endothelium-dependent dilation in healthy young adults. *Circulation.* 1993; 88: 2149 – 55.

[8]   Leone A, Giannini D, Bellotto C, Balbarini A. Passive smoking and coronary heart disease. *Current Vascular Pharmacology.* 2004; 2: 175 – 82.

[9]   Ludmer PL, Selwyn AP, Shook TL, Wayne RR, Mudge GH, Alexander RW, Ganz P. Paradoxical vasoconstriction induced by acetylcholine in atherosclerotic coronary arteries. *N. Engl. J. Med.* 1986;315: 1046 – 51.

[10]   Luscher TF,Vanhoutte PM. *The endothelium: modulator of cardiovascular function.* CRC Press, Boca Raton, USA,1990.

[11]   Creager MA, Cooke JP, Mendelsohn ME, Gallagher SJ, Coleman SM, Loscalzo J, Dzau VJ. Impaired vasodilation of forearm resistance vessels in hypercholesterolemic humans. *J. Clin. Invest.* 1990: 86: 228 – 34.

[12]   Ghiadoni L, Taddei S, Virdis A, Sudano I, Di Legge V, Meola M, Di Venanzio L, Salvetti A. Endothelial function and common carotid artery wall thickening in patients with essential hypertension. *Hypertension.* 1998; 32: 25 – 32.

[13]   Stroes ES, Koomans HA, deBruin TW, Rabelink TJ. Vascular function in the forearm of hypercholesterolaemic patients off and on lipid-lowering medication. *Lancet.* 1995; 346: 467 – 71.

[14]   Taddei S, Ghiadoni L, Virdis A, Versari D, Salvetti A. Mechanisms of endothelial dysfunction: clinical significance and preventive non-pharmacological therapeutic strategies. *Curr. Pharm. Design.* 2003; 9: 2385 – 402.

[15]   Barenbrock M, Hausberg M, Kosch M, Golubev SA, Kisters K, Rahn KH. Flow-mediated vasodilation and distensibility in relation to intima-media thickness of large arteries in mild essential hypertension. *Am. J. Hypertension.* 1999; 12: 973 – 9.

[16] Panza JA, Garcia CE, Kilcoyne CM, Quyyumi AA, Cannon RO. Impaired endothelium-dependent vasodilation in patients with essential hypertension. Evidence that nitric oxide abnormality is not localized to a single signal transduction pathway. *Circulation.* 1995; 91: 1732 – 8.

[17] Johnstone MT, Creager SJ, Scales KM, Cusco JA, Lee BK, Creager MA. Impaired endothelium-dependent vasodilation in patients with non-insulin-dependent diabetes mellitus. *Circulation.* 1993; 88: 2510 – 6.

[18] Schachinger V, Britten MB, Zeiher AM. Prognostic impact of coronary vasodilator dysfunction on adverse long-term outcome of coronary heart disease. *Circulation.* 2000; 101: 1899 – 906.

[19] Egashira K, Inou T, Hirooka Y, Kai H, Sugimaki M, Suzuki S, Kuga T, Urabe Y, Takeshita A. Effects of age on endothelium-dependent vasodilation of resistance coronary artery by acetylcholine in humans. *Circulation.* 1993; 88: 77 – 81.

[20] Reddy KG, Nair RN, Sheehan HM, Hodgson JM. Evidence that selective endothelial dysfunction may occur in the absence of angiographic or ultrasound atherosclerosis in patients with risk factors for atherosclerosis. *J. Am. Coll. Cardiol.* 1994; 23: 833 – 43.

[21] Knowles RG, Moncada S. Nitric oxide synthases in mammals. *Biochem. J.* 1994; 298: 249 – 58.

[22] Cooke JP, Tsao PS. Arginine: a new therapy for atherosclerosis? *Circulation.* 1997; 95: 311 – 2.

[23] Ignarro LJ, Cirino G, Casini A, Napoli C. Nitric oxide as a signaling molecule in the vascular system. *J. Cardiovasc. Pharmacol.* 1999; 34: 879 – 86.

[24] Yada T, Richmond KN, Van Bibber R, Kroll K, Feigl EO. Role of adenosine in local metabolic coronary vasodilation. *Am. J. Physiol.* 1999; 276: H1425 – 33.

[25] Cosentino F, Sill JC, Katusik ZS. Role of superoxide anions in the mediation of endothelium-dependent contractions. *Hypertension.* 1994; 23: 229 – 35.

[26] Kontos HA, George E. Oxygen radicals in cerebral vascular injury. *Circ. Res.* 1985; 57: 508 – 16.

[27] Mohazzab KM, Kaminski PM, , Wolin MS. NADH oxidoreductase is a major source of superoxide anion in bovine coronary artery endothelium. *Am. J. Physiol.* 1994; 266: H2568 – 72.

[28] Schmidt K, Werner ER, Mayer B, Wachter H, Kukovetz WR. Tetrahydrobiopterin-dependent formation of endothelium-derived relaxing factor (nitric oxide) in aortic endothelial cells. *Biochem. J.* 1992; 281: 297 – 300.

[29] Mayer B, Werner ER. In search of a function for tetrahydrobiopterin in the biosynthesis of nitric oxide. *Naunyn. Schmiedebergs. Arch. Pharmacol.* 1995;351: 453 – 63.

[30] Nagao K, Takenaka S, Yamaji R, Inui H, Nakano Y. Nitric oxide synthase induction, cGMP elevation, and biopterin synthesis in vascular smooth muscle cells stimulated with interleukin-1β in hypoxia. *J. Biochem.* 2003; 133: 501 – 5.

[31] Riethmuller C, Gorren ACF, Pitters E, Hemmens B, Habisch HJ, Heales SJR, Schmidt K, Werner ER. Activation of neuronal nitric-oxide synthase by the 5-methyl analog of tetrahydrobiopterin. Functional evidence against reductive oxygen activation by the pterin cofactor. *J. Biol. Chem.* 1999; 274: 16047 – 51.

[32] Werner-Felmayer G, Werner ER, Fuchs D, Hausen A, Reibnegger G, Schmidt K, Weiss G, Wachter H. Pteridine biosynthesis in human endothelial cells. Impact on nitric oxide-mediated formation of cyclic GMP. *J. Biol. Chem.* 1993; 268: 1842 – 6.

[33] Vanhoutte PM. The end of the quest? *Nature.* 1987; 327: 459 – 60.

[34] Richard V, Tschudi MR, Luscher TF. Differential activation of the endothelial L-arginine pathway by bradykinin, serotonin and clonidine in porcine coronary arteries. *Am. J. Physiol.* 1990; 259: H1433 – 9.

[35] Feletou M, Vanhoutte PM. Endothelium-dependent hyperpolarization of canine coronary smooth muscle. *Br. J. Pharmacol.* 1988; 93: 515 – 24.

[36] Tare M, Parkington HC, Coleman HA, Neild TO, Dusting GJ. Hyperpolarization and relaxation of arterial smooth muscle caused by NO derived from the endothelium. *Nature.* 1990; 346: 69 – 71.

[37] Nelson MT, Patlak JB, Worley JF, Standen NB. Calcium channels, potassium channels, and voltage dependence of arterial smooth muscle tone. *Am. J. Physiol.* 1990; 259: C3 – 18.

[38] Parkington HC, Tare M, Tonta MA, Coleman HA. Stretch revealed three components in the hyperpolarization of guinea-pig coronary artery in response to acetylcholine. *J. Physiol.* 1993; 465: 459 – 76.

[39] Murphy ME, Brayden JE. Nitric oxide hyperpolarizes rabbit mesenteric arteries via ATP-sensitive potassium channels. *J. Physiol.* 1995; 486: 47 – 58.

[40] Standen NB, Quayle JM, Davies NW, Brayden JE, Huang Y, Nelson MT. Hyperpolarizing vasodilators activate ATP-sensitive K-channels in arterial smooth muscle. *Science.* 1989; 245: 177 – 80.

[41] Edwards G, Dora KA, Gardener MJ, Garland CJ, Weston AH. K is an endothelium-derived hyperpolarizing factor in rat arteries. *Nature.* 1998; 396: 269 – 72.

[42] Levin RI, Jaffe EA, Weksler BB, Tack-Goldman K. Nitroglycerin stimulates synthesis of prostacyclin by human endothelial cells. *J. Clin. Invest.* 1981; 67: 762 - 9.

[43] Schror K, Grozinska L, Darius H. Stimulation of coronary vascular prostacyclin and inhibition of human platelet thromboxane A2 after low-dose nitroglycerin. *Thromb. Res.* 1981; 23: 59 – 67.

[44] Mehta J, Mehta P, Roberts A, Faro R, Ostrowski N, Brigmon L. Comparative effects of nitroglycerin and nitroprusside on prostacyclin generation in adult human vessel wall. *J. Am. Coll. Cardiol.* 1983; 6: 625 – 30.

[45] De Caterina R, Dorso CR, Tack-Goldman K, Weksler BB. Nitrates and endothelial prostacyclin production: studies in vitro. *Circulation.* 1985; 71: 176 – 82.

[46] Forster W. Significance of prostaglandins and thromboxane A2 for the mode of action of cardiovascular drugs. *Adv. Prostaglandins Thromboxane Res.* 1980; 7: 609 – 18.

[47] Neichi T, Tomisawa S, Kubodera N, Uchida Y. Enhancement of PGI2 formation by a new vasodilator, 2-nicotinamido-ethyl-nitrate in the coupled system of platelets and aortic microsomes. *Prostaglandins.* 1980; 19: 577 - 86.

[48] Tschudi M, Richard V, Bulher FR, Luscher TF. Importance of endothelium- derived nitric oxide in intramyocardial porcine coronary arteries. *Am. J. Physiol.* 1990; 260: H13 – 20.

[49] Yang Z, von Segesser L, Bauer E, Stulz P, Tschudi M, Luscher TF. Differential activation of the endothelial L-arginine and cyclooxygenase pathway in the human internal mammary artery and saphenous vein. *Circ. Res.* 1991; 68: 52 – 60.

[50] Moncada S, Vane JR. Pharmacology and endogenous roles of prostaglandin endoperoxides, thromboxane A2, and prostacyclin. *Pharmacol. Rev.* 1979; 30: 293 – 331.

[51] Miller VM, Vanhoutte PM. Endothelium-dependent contractions to arachidonic acid are mediated by products of cyclooxygenase. *Am. J. Physiol.* 1985; 248: H432 – 7.

[52] Katusic ZS, Shepherd JT. Endothelium-derived vasoactive factors: II. Endothelium-dependent contraction. *Hypertension.* 1991; 18: 86 – 92.

[53] Konishi M, Su C. Role of endothelium in dilator responses of spontaneously hypertensive rat arteries. *Hypertension.* 1983; 5: 881 – 6.

[54] Tesfamariam B, Jakubowski JA, Cohen RA. Contraction of diabetic rabbit aorta caused by endothelium-derived PGH2-TxA2. *Am. J. Physiol.* 1989; 257: H1327 – 33.

[55] Vanhoutte PM, Katusic ZS. Endothelium-derived contracting factor: endothelin and/or superoxide anion? *Trends Pharmacol. Sci.* 1988; 9: 229 – 30.

[56] Katusic ZS, Vanhoutte PM. Superoxide anion is an endothelium-derived contracting factor. *Am. J. Physiol.* 1989; 257: H33 – 7.

[57] Bigand M, Pelton JT. Discrimination between ETA-and ETB-receptor-mediated effects of endothelin-1 and (Ala131115)endothelin-1 by BQ-123 in the anaesthetized rat. *Br. J. Pharmacol.* 1992; 107: 912 – 8.

[58] Widdowson PS, Kirk CN. Characterization of (125)-endothelin-1 and (125l)-BQ3020 binding to rat cerebellar endothelin receptors. *Br. J. Pharmacol.* 1996; 118: 2126 – 30.

[59] Nakamichi K, Ihara M, Kobayashi M, Saeki T, Ishikawa K, Yano M. Different distribution of endothelin receptor subtypes in pulmonary tissues revealed by the novel selective ligands BQ-123 and (Ala1,3,11,15)ET-1. *Biochem. Biophys. Res. Commun.* 1992; 182: 144 – 50.

[60] Arai H, Hori S, Aramori I, Ohkubo H, Nakanishi S. Cloning and expression of a cDNA encoding an endothelin receptor. *Nature.* 1990; 348: 730 – 2.

[61] Vane J. Endothelins come home to roost. *Nature.* 1990; 348: 673 – 5.

[62] Seo B, Oemar BS, Siebenmann R, von Segesser L, Luscher TF. Both ETA and ETB receptors mediate contraction to endothelin-1 in human blood vessels. *Circulation.* 1994; 89: 1203 – 8.

[63] Sakurai T, Yanagisawa M, Takuwat Y, Miyazakit H, Kimura S, Goto K, Masaki T. Cloning of a cDNA encoding a non-isopeptide-selective subtype of the endothelin receptor. *Nature.* 1990; 348: 732 – 5.

[64] Tsukahara H, Ende H, Magazine HI, Bahou WF, Goligorsky MS. Molecular and functional characterization of the non-isopeptide-selective ETB receptor in endothelial cells. Receptor coupling to nitric oxide synthase. *J. Biol. Chem.* 1994; 269: 21778 – 85.

[65] de Nucci G, Thomas R, D'Orleans-Juste P, Antunes E, Walder C, Warner TD, Vane JR. Pressor effects of circulating endothelin are limited by its removal in the pulmonary circulation and by the release of prostacyclin and endothelium-derived relaxing factor. *Proc. Natl. Acad. Sci. USA.* 1988; 85: 9797 – 800.

[66] Meyer P, Flammer J, Luscher TF. Endothelium-dependent regulation of the ophthalmic microcirculation in the perfused porcine eye. Role of nitric oxide and endothelins. *Invest. Ophthalmol. Vis. Sci.* 1993; 34: 3614 – 21.

[67] Kiowski W, Luscher TF, Linder L, Buhler FR. Endothelin-1-induced vasoconstriction in man: reversal by calcium channel blockade but not by nitrovasodilators or endothelium-derived relaxing factor. *Circulation.* 1991; 83: 469 – 75.

[68] Neubauer S, Ertl G, Haas U, Pulzer F, Kochsiek K. Effects of endothelin-1 in isolated perfused rat heart. *J. Cardiovasc. Pharmacol.* 1990; 16: 1 – 8.

[69] Luscher TF, Yang Z, Tschudi M, von Segesser L, Stulz P, Boulanger C, Siebenmann R, Turina M, Buhler FR. Interaction between endothelin-1 and endothelium-derived relaxing factor in human arteries and veins. *Circ. Res.* 1990; 66: 1088 – 94.

[70] Warner TD, Mitchell JA, de Nucci G, Vane JR. Endothelin-1 and endothelin-3 release EDRF from isolated perfused arterial vessels of the rat and rabbit. *J. Cardiovasc. Pharmacol.* 1989; 13 (Suppl 5): 85 – 8.

[71] Haynes WG, Webb DJ. Endothelin as a regulator of cardiovascular function in health and disease. *J. Hypertens.* 1998; 16: 1081 – 98.

[72] Ross R. Atherosclerosis – An inflammatory disease. *N. Engl. J. Med.* 1999; 340: 115 – 26.

[73] Adams DH, Shaw S. Leukocyte endothelial interactions and regulation of leukocyte migration. *Lancet.* 1994; 343: 831 – 6.

[74] Springer TA. Traffic signals for lymphocyte recirculation and leukocyte emigration: the multistep paradigm. *Cell.* 1994; 76: 301 – 4.

[75] Pasceri V, Willerson JT, Yeh ET. Direct proinflammatory effect of C-reactive protein on human endothelial cells. *Circulation.* 2000; 102: 2165 – 8.

[76] Libby P. Inflammation in atherosclerosis. *Nature.* 2002; 420: 868 – 74.

[77] Libby P, Ridker PM, Maseri A. Inflammation and atherosclerosis. *Circulation.* 2002; 105: 1135 – 43.

[78] Desideri G, Ferri F. Endothelial activation. Sliding door to atherosclerosis. *Curr. Pharm. Design.* 2005; 11: 2163 – 75.

[79] Herrman J, Lerman LO, Rodriguez-Porcel M, Holmes DR, Richardson DM, Ritman EL, Lerman A. Coronary vasa vasorum neovascularization precedes epicardial endothelial dysfunction in experimental hypercholesterolemia. *Cardiovasc. Res.* 2001; 51: 762 – 6.

[80] Rafii S, Lyden D. Therapeutic stem and progenitor cell transplantation for organ vascularization and regeneration. *Nat. Med.* 2003; 9: 702 – 12.

[81] Shi Q, Rafii S, Wu MH, Wijelath ES, Yu C, Ishida A, Fujita Y, Kothary S, Mohle R, Sauvage LR, Moore MA, Storb RF, Hammond WP. Evidence for circulating bone marrow-derived endothelial cells. *Blood.* 1998; 92: 362 – 7.

[82] Hillebrands JL, Klatter FA, van Dijk WD, Rozing J. Bone marrow does not contribute substantially to endothelial-cell replacement in transplant atherosclerosis. *Nat. Med.* 2002; 8: 194 – 5.

[83] Walter DK, Rittig K, Bahlmann FH, Kirchmair R, Silver M, Murayama T, Nishimura H, Losordo DW, Asahara T, Isner JM. Statin therapy accelerates reendothelization: a

novel effect involving mobilization and incorporation of bone marrow-derived endothelial progenitor cells. *Circulation.* 2002; 105: 3017 – 24.

[84] Werner N, Junk S, Laufs U, Link A, Walenta K, Bohm M, Nickering G. Intravenous transfusion of endothelial progenitor cells reduces neointima formation after vascular injury. *Circ. Res.* 2003; 93: E17 – 24.

[85] Kaushal S, Amiel GE, Guleserian KJ, Shapira OM, Perry T, Sutherland FW, Rabkin E, Moran AM, Schoen FJ, Atala A, Soker S, Bischoff J, Mayer JE Jr. Functional small-diameter neovessels created using endothelial progenitor cells expanded ex vivo. *Nat. Med.* 2001; 7: 1035 – 40.

[86] Wang XX, Zhu JH, Chen JZ, Shang YP. Effects of nicotine on the number and activity of circulating endothelial progenitor cells. *J. Clin. Pharmacol.* 2004; 44: 881 - 9.

[87] Koch A, Hoffmann K, Steck W, Horsch A, Hengen N, Morl H, Harenberg J, Spohr U, Weber E. Acute cardiovascular reactions after cigarette smoking. *Atherosclerosis.* 1980; 35: 67 – 75.

[88] Pachinger O, Hellberg KD, Bing JR. The effect of nicotine, propranolol, phentolamine and hexamethonium on the coronary microcirculation of the cat. *J. Clin. Pharmacol.* 1972; 12: 432 – 9.

[89] Spohr U, Harenberg J, Walter E, Augustin J, Morl H, Koch A, Weber E. Smoking-induced effects on circulatory and metabolic variables with respect to plasma nicotine and COHb levels. In: Greenhalgh RM ed., *Smoking and Arterial Disease.* Pitman Medical, London, UK, 1981; 98 – 106.

[90] Giannini D, Leone A, Di Bisceglie D, Nuti M, Strata G, Buttitta F, Masserini L, Balbarini A. The effects of acute passive smoke exposure on endothelium-dependent brachial artery dilation in healthy individuals. *Angiology.* 2007; 58: 211 – 7.

[91] Glantz S, Parmley WW. Even a little secondhand smoke is dangerous. *JAMA.* 2001; 286: 462 – 3.

[92] Turino GM. Effect of carbon monoxide on the cardiorespiratory system. Carbon monoxide toxicity: Physiology and biochemistry. *Circulation.* 1981; 63: A253 – 9.

[93] Anderson EW, Andelman RJ, Strauch JM, Fortuin NJ, Knelson JK. Effect of low-level carbon monoxide exposure on onset and duration of angina pectoris. *Ann. Intern. Med.* 1973; 79: 46 – 50.

[94] Celermajer DS, Adams MR, Clarkson P, Robinson J, McCredie R, Donald A, Deanfield JE. Passive smoking and impaired endothelium-dependent arterial dilatation in healthy young adults. *N. Engl. J. Med.* 1996; 334: 150 – 4.

[95] Barnoya J, Glantz SA. Cardiovascular effects of secondhand smoke. Nearly as large as smoking. *Circulation.* 2005; 111: 2684 – 98.

[96] Suwaidi JA, Hamasaki S, Higano ST, Nishimura RA, Holmes DR Jr, Lerman A. Long-term follow-up of patients with mild coronary artery disease and endothelial dysfunction. *Circulation.* 2000; 101: 948 – 54.

[97] Neunteufl T, Heher S, Katzenschlager R, Wolfl G, Kostner K, Maurer G, Weidinger F. Late prognostic value of flow-mediated dilation in the brachial artery of patients with chest pain. *Am. J. Cardiol.* 2000; 86: 207 – 10.

[98] Heitzer T, Schlinzig T, Krohn K, Meinertz T, Munzel T. Endothelial dysfunction, oxidative stress, and risk of cardiovascular events in patients with coronary artery disease. *Circulation.* 2001; 104: 2673 – 8.

[99] Halcox JP, Schenke WH, Zalos G, Mincemoyer R, Prasad A, Waclawiw MA, Prognostic value of coronary vascular endothelial dysfunction. *Circulation.* 2002; 106: 653 – 8.

[100] Hansson GK, Libby P, Schonbeck U, Yan ZQ. Innate and adaptive immunity in the pathogenesis of atherosclerosis. *Circ. Res.* 2002; 91: 281 – 91.

[101] Casscells W. Migration of smooth muscle and endothelial cells: critical events in restenosis. *Circulation.* 1992; 86: 723 – 9.

Chapter V

Biochemistry of Smoking Compounds

Abstract

Growing evidence that several biochemical compounds of cigarette smoke play a significant role in the development, maintainance, and progression of heart and coronary vessel damage exists.

Some of these substance may be interpreted as biomarkers and may be dosed in blood samples, urine and saliva providing data about smoking exposure and type of cardiovascular and coronary damage.

Among the thousands of chemical compounds in tobacco smoke, usually nicotine, cotinine, carbon monoxide and thiocyanate have been, time to time, dosed, although obtained measures could not be conducted on a large-scale sample since there is not a large number of laboratories equipped for that. Actually, cotinine concentrations particularly in urine, but also in blood and/or saliva, are measured since cotinine dosage in urine is easier to determine than that of other metabolites to assess a smoking habit. Also carboxyhemoglobin levels may provide qualitative but not quantitative data, unless in experimental studies, to estimate either the degree of cardiovascular damage or the level and duration of exposure to smoking.

Some hematologic markers may also be assessed to estimate a cigarette smoking habit, although with results worthwhile to be evaluated with prudence. Increased white blood cells, platelet aggregation and adhesiveness, fibrinogen level, and changes in serum lipids characterize chronic and prolonged smoking use with evidence of significantly heavy damage on heart and coronary vessels.

Finally, smoking biomarkers structured usually with chemically open chains can cause possible chemical reactions in the tissues and organs of the body. That can potentiate the harmful effects of smoking compounds, triggering, usually, a hypoxic mechanism that is further increased by a direct action of smoking components on the cardiovascular system.

Keywords: Smoking Biomarkers, Nicotine, Cotinine, Carbon Monoxide, Thiocyanate, Chemistry, Toxicity, Measuring Method, Gas Chromatography, HPLC, HPLC coupled with Mass Spectrophotometry, Spectrophotometry, RIA, ELISA, Polycyclic aromatic hydrocarbons, Benzene, Benzopyrene, Toluene.

Tobacco smoke has a different chemical composition with regard to its phase of harvesting or manufacturing: fresh leaves of tobacco and leaves prepared for cigarette or similar products.

As it can be deduced from the previous chapters concerning the structural, physiological, and bio-humoral characteristics of coronary circulation, there are several factors which may cause coronary changes, and among these, chemical compounds of tobacco smoke play a crucial role in inducing coronary pathology. It depends on the type and form of the tobacco products, characteristics of burned tobacco, environment, health and lifestyle of individuals.

Among the thousands of components of smoking, those which lead particularly to coronary damage are nicotine and its metabolites, carbon monoxide and thiocyanate. All together, these chemicals can cause a large majority of the cardiovascular alterations observed, although almost each or other compound of cigarette smoking has primarily a tropism for some structures rather than others, and, consequently, functional responses of heart and coronary vessels as well as type of pathology depend on the prevalence of action of the involved chemical. Indeed, experimental study material may be exposed to a selected smoking compound.

This chapter aims to focus on chemistry and the main properties of those tobacco compounds which usually have negative effects on the cardiovascular system, analyzing their metabolic characteristics, pharmacological effects, biochemical significance as markers of exposure to tobacco smoke, dosage in biologic liquids, and, finally, their involvement as markers of coronary or systemic artery damage.

Nicotine and Its Metabolites

Nicotine [1] is a natural alkaloid with a basic charge obtained from the dried leaves and stems of the Nicotiana tabacum and Nicotiana rustica of Solanaceae family where this compound varies in concentration from 0.5 percent to 8 percent.

Nicotine has been always identified as the most powerful toxic of cigarette smoking since its harmful action, either functionally or structurally, could be largely demonstrated at a relative low blood concentration in both clinical and experimental studies that involved almost all organs of the body. However, target organs were particularly the cardiovascular district, lung, and some structures of the endocrine system. The first two structures are usually involved functionally and anatomically on the same degree. On the contrary, the endocrine system feels a direct action which stimulates some hormone production and release, but also an indirect functional stimulation mediated by the sympathetic system. However, both these stimulations are very closely dependent on themselves.

Nicotine biosynthesis takes place in the roots of Nicotiana tabacum or Nicotiana rustica. Then, it accumulates in the leaves, the particular shape and composition of which, described as a "cupola", is a basic factor for harvesting and extraction of the alkaloid. Each cigarette, depending on its preparation, may reach nicotine concentration from 1.5 mg to 2.5 mg, but not the whole amount of burned substance enters the blood, which, however, is affected negatively by the amount of nicotine released by smoked cigarettes.

Chemistry

Chemically, nicotine is 3(1-Methyl-2-pyrrolidinyl)pyridine, with a chemical formula $C_{10}H_{14}N_2$, and a molecular mass of 162.23 g/mol. Nicotine stechiometry, that characterizes spatially nicotine structural formula, is like figure 5.1.

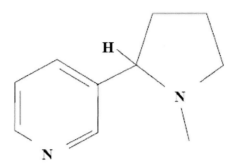

Figure 5.1. Chemical structure of nicotine. Stechiometry identifies the type of spatial aggregation of those elements that take part in nicotine composition. Evidence indicates that nicotine S(-) isomer is the main nicotine isomer [74]. Different isomers would also have a different taste sensation: S(-)isomer would be pleasant for smokers but not for non-smokers, whereas S(+)isomer would be generally unpleasant.

Different isomers characterize spatially the nicotine structure. The main isomer, S(-), gives a pleasant taste to cigarette smoke only for regular smokers but not for non-smokers. That explains clearly the reasons which determine a disgusting taste following, usually, the first cigarette smoked. Then, disgusting taste is followed by a pleasant habit when a smoker becomes a regular smoker.

Table 5.1. summarizes the main physico-chemical characteristics and use of the alkaloid.

Table 5.1. Physico-chemical characteristics and use of Nicotine

Form	Liquid oil
Mixture	Water soluble
Chemical name	3-(1-Methyl-2-pyrrolidinyl)pyridine
Chemical nature	Alkaloid with a basic charge
Isomeric structure	S(-)isomer – main isomer-, S(+)isomer
Chemical formula	C10H14N2
Molecular mass	162.23 g/mol
Density	1.01 g/ml
Boiling point	247°C (degree of decomposition)
Melting point	-79°C
Autoignition temperature	240°C
Half life	2 h
Habit-bound use	Smoked (tobacco)
	Insufflated (snuff)
	Chewed

Nicotine is a hygroscopic liquid that is miscible with water in its form as base. Such a chemical characteristic makes the alkaloid diffusible on the whole tobacco leaf so that harvesting tobacco leaves fills up the greatest amount of nicotine. As a nitrogenous base, nicotine interacts with acid compounds forming salts usually soluble in water.

Physico-chemical properties of nicotine have been identified throughout studies which used different methodologies, although those methods with radioactive isotope provided more valid data particularly for what involved tobacco which is the most popular worldwide producer of nicotine.

A study conducted using C14-labeled nicotine showed that about 15 percent of it was entering the mainstream smoke, while as much as 37 percent characterized sidestream smoke with 18 percent contained in the butt, and the remainder formed pyrolysis products [2]. As shown by table 5.1, free base nicotine burns at a temperature of 240°C. Therefore, there is evidence that burning temperature is below the boiling point (247°C) of the alkaloid. That means that nicotine is burned particularly when cigarette is still smoked and boiling point has not yet been reached. Thus, a smoker inhales the alkaloid before its decomposition, and the result of this consists of a potentiate effect due to nicotine itself together with other burned products of tobacco smoking. Therefore, nicotine may play almost entirely its adverse effects, the harmful of which is the addiction [3] that makes it difficult to stop smoking. Although nicotine has the property of autoignition before its boiling point, a lower amount than the total of the tobacco leaf is dosable in the different types of smoke.

Metabolism

Liver, followed by kidney, lung and oral cavity are particularly involved in regulating nicotine metabolism, although, as just described, the cardiovascular system and some endocrine glands are the target organs of the substance.

Absorption of nicotine occurs very quickly. In the oral cavity, there is an absorption that usually varies from 4 percent to 45 percent of the total dose [4], whatever introduction method characterizes the nicotine – smoked, chewed or snuffed. However, as nicotine enters the body [5], it reaches the blood and then acts on those sites where its specific receptors are located. Nicotinic acetylcholine receptors are those structures deputed to permit the biochemical action of the alkaloid.

Nicotinic-acetylcholine receptors feel the level of nicotine concentration, which is, therefore, the main factor in regulating receptorial response. When there are small concentrations of nicotine, the activity of the receptors increase, whereas higher concentrations inhibit receptor activity. Thus, that explains the different responses of individuals to nicotine that can induce both stimulant and/or depressant effects according to alkaloid concentrations. Moreover, a complex interaction of factors determines primarily those effects which are related to nicotine action. Nicotine effects are mediated through the interference with the sympathetic system and, then, catecholamine levels. Blood vessels, fat metabolism, carbohydrate metabolism, platelets and coagulation cascade are particularly involved [6–14].

Nicotine exerts a direct and transiently repeated effect on the sympathetic system and similar structures – chromaffin tissue - as well as central nervous system. This effect, which is initially stimulant, changes its characteristics in the long run, and depressant signs will be seen as a consequence of prolonged nicotine stimulation. Similarly, structural changes of those structures which had been involved functionally begin to be identified.

The mechanism by which nicotine could trigger a cardiovascular event is still far from being completely clarified. However, there is evidence that a stimulation of sympathetic nerves and consequent release of intramyocardial catecholamines could be the primary cause [15–16].

Nicotine stimulates the release of norepinephrine from the hypotalamus and antidiuretic hormone from the pituitary gland [17]. Also chemoreceptors in the carotid artery can be stimulated by nicotine [18] triggering different reflexes, which may evoke multiple responses.

As mentioned, several body organs in addition to those which are recognized as target organs of nicotine toxicity may be involved in the metabolic pathway.

Nicotine is metabolized into cotinine principally in the liver. The kidneys and lungs may be involved in the metabolism of the alkaloid, although to a small degree [19–20].

Metabolites of nicotine have interesting properties which may be associated more with the possibility that they provide to follow-up studies on selected populations to estimate smoking habit than with their potential toxicity that is similar to that of nicotine.

Nevertheless, some differences between nicotine and its main metabolites may be identified, primarily the fact that nicotine, usually, acts more rapidly and, therefore, may be dosed earlier in biological liquids. In contrast, chronic toxicity is better estimated by dosing nicotine metabolites in biological liquids.

Table 5.2. lists the pharmacodynamic steps of nicotine.

Table 5.2. Nicotine pharmacodynamic characteristics

Absorption	Skin, oral mucosa, lungs
Type of absorption	Smoking, Snuff, Chewing
Body entry	Blood
Transport	Blood component binding
Site of tissue binding	Receptors (Nicotinic-acetylcholine receptors)
Type of action	Sympathetic effects (mainly)
Type of response	Nicotine blood concentrations
Metabolic steps	Liver (kidney and lung weakly)
Main metabolite	Cotinine
Metabolism organ	Liver (kidney and lung – small amount -)
Excretio	Urine
Target organs	Cardiovascular system, Adrenergic glands

Carbon Monoxide

Strictly speaking, carbon monoxide is not a product of natural tobacco but a product of manufacturated and inhaled burned tobacco similarly to what characterizes the large majority of natural chemicals, which develop carbon monoxide under combustion.

Carbon monoxide is a toxic gas, the formation of which in relation to cigarette smoke is due to decomposition into the burned cone of a cigarette by a chemical reaction between environmental oxygen and burned paper of the cigarette.

Environmental carbon monoxide produced by incomplete combustion of organic substances, comes from automobile exhaust, malfunctioning gas heaters, and tobacco smoke diffused passively from the smoked cigarettes even if, in this case, at a significantly smaller concentration than that of the two previous sources. However, also these smaller environmental concentrations of carbon monoxide could determine carboxyhemoglobin levels into the blood up to four times higher for nonsmokers exposed to passive smoking than those seen in a similar population not exposed [21]. Carboxyhemoglobin blood concentrations in smokers are usually much more elevated and depend on the number of smoked cigarettes, and, therefore, it is hard to establish a mean concentration value among different smokers.

Indeed, the bond between carbon monoxide and hemoglobin is about two hundred times stronger than that of oxygen for hemoglobin. Therefore, carbon monoxide can reduce oxyhemoglobin concentrations very easily and cause clear signs of hypoxia to different organs of the body, particularly cardiovascular system and brain.

Chemistry

Carbon monoxide is a colorless, odorless, tasteless gas which because of these properties and high toxicity is to be considered a potentially silent killer and, therefore, a highly harmful substance for any form of life. With regard to livings, such a property of carbon monoxide is the result of the concentration level reached in the blood. Low concentrations act as a toxic factor, whereas the highest concentrations lead rapidly and acutely to death. In contrast, carboxyhemoglobin concentrations observed in smokers exert their toxic effects primarily chronically and determine structural diseases which are responsible for the prognosis, often negative, of human smokers.

The chemical formula of carbon monoxide is CO, a diatomic molecule with a bond between the two atoms carbon and oxygen as follows:

$$C = O$$

This type of chemical bond is a basic characteristic for the chemical activity of carbon monoxide since it permits an easy dissociation in carbon and oxygen atoms as well as an easy new linking with those substances towards which a major chemical affinity exists like blood hemoglobin. Moreover, carbon monoxide is less dense than air and, therefore, it is capable of spreading out more quickly. It is also slightly soluble in water and burns in air producing carbon dioxide, a metabolite largely diffused in the environment and also an end product of catabolic reactions of intracellular respiratory metabolism.

The chemical characteristics of carbon monoxide are summarized in table 5.3.

Table 5.3. Chemical characteristics of carbon monoxide

Chemical name	Carbon monoxide
Molecular formula	CO
Molar mass	28.01 g/mol
Physical characteristic	Colorless, Odorless gas
Solubility	Water, ethanol, methanol
Melting point	-205°C
Boiling point	-192°C
Structure	Linear molecular shape
Affinity	Hemoglobin
Sites of production	Environment, Body (a very small amount)

Carbon monoxide is also produced spontaneously in the body, in concentrations which are not a hazard for life, by a reaction between heme (a porphyrin to which an iron atom is attached and, in number of four chains, is a component of hemoglobin) and an enzyme called heme-oxygenase.

Toxicity

Carbon monoxide is a very dangerous gas that may be fatal at a concentration as low as 400 parts per million air. Usually, death from carbon monoxide occurs acutely during unconsciously involuntary exposure to the gas, or from "well-informed" suicidal exposure respectively to malfunctioning sources of gas production or normally functioning sources tampered with for specific purposes.

Fatal effects due to acute exposure to relatively high concentrations of carbon monoxide, are the result of a direct action of the gas on the cardiorespiratory and nervous structures of the body with consequent fatal respiratory and cardiac arrest preceded by irreversible coma. Symptoms originate silently since the gas is odorless and, then, progress rapidly leading to death preceded by unconsciousness that impedes exposed individual from avoiding and fighting the harm.

In contrast, carbon monoxide toxicity due to cigarette smoking is the result of some complex reactions that are summarized in table 5.4.

The mechanisms of damage consist of seven main phases, four of which are related to metabolic steps that involve carbon monoxide: oxygen removal from the hemoglobin, its replacement with carbon monoxide and formation of carboxyhemoglobin (these first two steps of removal and replacement have to be kept in mind since they are the chemical factors that trigger the toxic mechanism of carbon monoxide in smokers, past smokers or never smokers exposed passively to cigarette smoke) tissue hypoxia, and, finally, impairment of cellular metabolism due to alterations of intracellular respiratory chains. Furthermore, carbon monoxide potentiates its action damaging directly intracellular structures by inhibiting the function of those cells and intracellular constituents [22–30] which are particularly related to RNA metabolism.

Table 5.4. Steps of carbon monoxide toxicity from smoking

Step 1	Gas enters from smoked cigarette or passively
Step 2	Removing oxygen from oxyhemoglobin
Step 3	Replacement of oxygen with carbon monoxide
Step 4	Circulation of carboxyhemoglobin into the blood
Step 5	Poor oxygen availability
Step 6	Tissue hypoxia
Step 7	Impairment of respiratory cell metabolism

The percentage of carboxyhemoglobin in the body determines, chronically, the type of symptoms, level of damage that may be experienced, and time of development of cardiac and coronary alterations.

As mentioned, structural changes in heart and blood vessels may be seen, experimentally, in different animal models exposed acutely to carbon monoxide derived from cigarette combustion and, then, dosed to pre-fixed concentrations.

Thiocyanate

Thiocyanate [1] is the third chemical of tobacco smoke which causes cardiovascular damage, although results and amount of damage are not yet estimated unanimously.

Thiocyanate is a chemical substance widely distributed in nature, and present in biological liquids such as blood, saliva, and urine. Many plants, particularly of the genus Brassica (cabbages) contain this product.

Thiocyanate interferes with different levels of body metabolism [31–34], particularly with iodine metabolism [32], and causes degrees of tissue alterations that can vary with regard to types of food consumed, characteristics of the living environment, health of the individuals, and possible influence of previous diseases affecting particularly the thyroid gland. Moreover, cigarette smoking exerts its harmful effects particularly in individuals who work in industries manufacturing the chemical by potentiating the stronger toxicity due to work environment.

Thiocyanate develops in the vapor phase of tobacco smoke usually in the form of hydrogen cyanide.

Industrially, it is used in agriculture to prepare insecticides and fungicides, in car industries as a fuel for airbags, and in pharmaceutical industries to prepare antibiotics, thyroid drugs, and chemotherapic drugs.

The effects of the substance on the cardiovascular system may be identified particularly after chronic exposure, and they are added to those of nicotine and carbon monoxide. Totally, there is a potentiating of the toxic effect of tobacco smoke. However, it is very difficult to identify the effects of thiocyanate from tobacco smoke alone on the cardiovascular system since metabolic factors due to diet, lifestyle, and health of humans may hide the appearance of those harms linked to cigarette smoking. Moreover, the coronary district feels the harmful effect of thiocyanate lesser than that of the heart muscle and respiratory system which are strongly influenced by the acute toxicity of the chemical, as it will be described.

Chemistry

Thiocyanate is a colorless, odorless crystalline powder with a chemical formula that changes according to the type of salt linked to the thiocyanate structure, which is: SCN. Among the different salts, potassium and sodium enter more frequently the molecular formula that is KSCN for potassium salt and NaSCN for sodium salt.

Spatially, thiocyanate is structured as shown in figure 5.2.

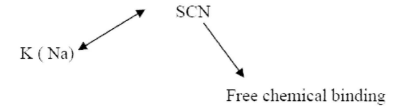

Figure 5.2. Spatial formula of thiocyanate. Sodium or Potassium link chemical structure of SCN group that is the basic nucleus of the molecula. There is evidence, analyzing molecular structure, of those sites of chemical reactions located on the free binding [75].

The chemical characteristics of thiocyanate are listed in table 5.5.

Table 5.5. Chemical characteristics of thiocyanate

Physico-chemical status	Colorless, odorless crystal
Biological status	Natural substance
Solubility	Water (very soluble and depends on salt type)
Density	1.89
Boiling point	500°C
Melting point	173°C
Stability	Slow decomposition under light
Tobacco component	Vapor phase
Decomposition products	Nitrogen oxides, sulfur compounds
Use	Chemical Industries
Toxicity	Hydrogen Cyanide

From the analysis of the thiocyanate characteristics, summarized in table 5.5, evidence emerges that tobacco smoke toxicity is, usually, due to the product in vapor phase

Toxicity

Thiocyanate toxicity has been identified to be due to its metabolic precursors which form in body organs. One of the most toxic substances with potent harmful effects for individuals is the metabolite hydrogen cyanide.

Hydrogen cyanide is metabolized in the liver with production of thiocyanate by a series of chemical reactions that involve enzymatic chains, organic substrates, and shift of metabolic steps. Cyanide is acutely toxic for humans. However, the amount of cyanide inhaled by smokers or individuals who are passively exposed to tobacco smoke, at the most, determines symptoms of chronic intoxication, or, more frequently, inhalation potentiates the harmful effects on the cardiovascular system that nicotine and carbon monoxide usually cause. Thus, coronary arteries may be influenced negatively by the second of damaging mechanisms, namely the total smoking products.

The toxicity of hydrogen cyanide depends particularly on the nature and type of the exposure. The time, dose and manner of exposure are the main parameters to be evaluated to assess the degree of toxicity. However, when cyanide enters the blood, it forms a stable complex with a particular form of cytochrome oxidase, an enzyme usually deputed to permit the synthesis of ATP (adenosine triphosphate). The reduced amount of cytochrome oxidase causes a decrease in ATP synthesis with consequent troubles in mitochondria structure and metabolism, shift of aerobic to anaerobic metabolism, and accumulation of lactate into the blood. The concomitant hypoxia due to carboxyhemoglobin produced as a result of cigarette smoke potentiates the negative effects of cyanide on the cardiovascular system and, particularly on endothelial function.

Figure 5.3. schematizes the main steps of cyanide metabolism.

By observing the main metabolic pathways which involve hydrogen cyanide, evidence emerges that all those factors – physical, humoral and metabolic factors - which have been seen to regulate coronary artery responses and, then, coronary vascular resistance in the previous chapters of this volume, act together to arouse and potentiate their harmful effects.

Cyanide is converted in the body to thiocyanate which interacts with thiosulfates by a chemical reaction catalyzed by sulfur transferase enzymes. Thiocyanate is the compound that can be dosed, because of its excretion in the urine, although with difficulties and no benefit if compared to urinary cotinine measure to assess a smoking habit. However, the metabolic steps that lead to formation of thiocyanate from hydrogen cyanide produce a chemical compound that is about seven times less toxic than that of the original substance.

It is basic to understand that different signs of cyanide toxicity may occur: from those due to tobacco smoke use, usually of low intensity, to those due to acute poisoning, the final step of which may be death.

Symptoms of cyanide poisoning usually occur from an exposure of 20 to 40 ppm of cyanide vapor phase, a phase that characterizes tobacco smoke as type but with a concentration that is very far to reach in both acute and chronic smoking exposure.

Cyanide poisoning is characterized by different phases with different clinical symptoms.

Headache, drowsiness, vertigo, confusion, and changes in pulse and breathing, that become deeper and more rapid, are the initial symptoms of cyanide intoxication. These symptoms are followed, in case of higher cyanide concentrations or more prolonged exposure, by convulsions, dilated pupils, and clammy skin. A third phase of intoxication is characterized by pulse rate and widely irregular breathing with a fall in body temperature, and then, finally, coma, heart and breath arrest followed by death occur.

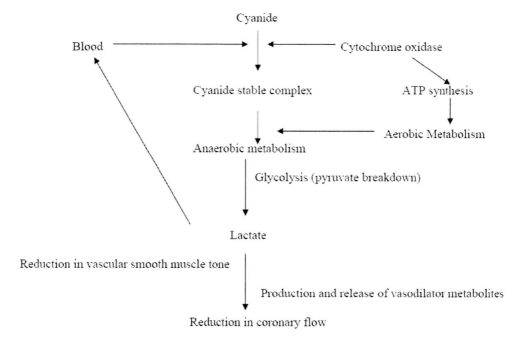

Figure 5.3. The main steps of cyanide metabolism in the body. There is evidence that the original metabolic pathways influence a large series of reactions which stimulate completely all those factors involved in vasomotor coronary regulation. Hydrogen cyanide metabolism occurs mainly in the liver.

Table 5.6. analyzes the symptoms of the different phases that characterize cyanide poisoning to which, however, as previously mentioned, tobacco exposure never gets.

Table 5.6. Symptoms of cyanide intoxication

Phase 1.	General symptoms:	headache, vertigo, drowsiness.
	Cardiorespiratory symptoms:	rapid pulse, rapid and deep breathing,
	Digestive symptoms:	nausea, vomiting.
Phase 2.	Nervous system:	convulsions.
	Eyes:	dilated pupils,
	Skin:	clammy
Phase 3.	Cardiorespiratory symptom	pulse rate and breathing widely irregular,
	Fall in body temperature	
Phase 4.	Coma, cardiorespiratory arrest, death.	

The main characteristic of cyanide compounds, similar to what occurs for nicotine when an individual smokes, is the rapid production of metabolites usually less toxic than those of the original substances and also dosable in the human body. For cyanide, the salts of sodium and/or potassium satisfy particularly such a condition. This property makes different the two chemicals from carbon monoxide which acts directly or indirectly as it is without chemical decomposition.

Smoking Chemicals as Biomarkers

Biomarkers are the molecular indicators of a specific biological process as well as biochemical features or facets that can be used to assess and measure the characteristics of biological phenomena.

Biomarkers may be primarily found in the blood and, generally, in biological fluids or tissues. Significant levels of a biomarker may mean usually that there is a close relationship between the tested biomarker and a specific biological pattern.

Biomarkers may be used also to assess or diagnose and measure a disease and its progress and, therefore, their level is associated with the physiological or pathological state of an individual. There is, therefore, a direct or mediated involvement of a factor (biomarker) – usually a chemical substance to dose – with a response of blood, tissues or organs to its action.

Table 5.7. identifies the main characteristics of a biomarker.

Table 5.7. Characteristics of a biomarker

1	Molecular indicator of specific biological reactions
2	Assessement in biological fluids
3	Close relation with specific biological patterns
4	Diagnostic and prognostic use in specific diseases
5	Metabolic assessment of a physiological or pathological state
6	Chemical substances diluted in biological fluids

Cardiovascular alterations due to smoking as well as smoking exposure can be identified by dosing some biochemical markers which are currently used either for a diagnostic purpose or as markers that permit one to evaluate and/or follow up the course of some specific lesions of the heart and blood vessels including primarily coronary arteries.

Nicotine and its metabolites [35], carbon monoxide and serum thiocyanate [36] are the most widely used biomarkers to assess smoking exposure, both active or passive smoking exposure, although their biochemical measures can undergo unlikely dosage for some of these.

Different methods are used to quantify smoking products, and also there are differences in each method with regard to the type of chemical substance to be dosed. Large-scale epidemiological measures conducted to identify smoking habit in individuals, community, and schools dosed primarily nicotine metabolites, particularly cotinine in urine.

Table 5.8. lists the most frequently used methods for the assessment of tobacco smoke compounds. All these methods measure particularly cotinine [20, 35, 36–44], the main metabolite of nicotine. Its measure may provide data not only about the smoking habit but also to assess the type of exposure to smoke and frequency of exposure. Moreover, the costs to assess the concentrations of cotinine are much less expensive than those of dosing the other smoking compounds, unless carboxyhemoglobin in the blood, and also easier to be estimated in a large majority of cases.

Table 5.8. Methods most frequently used for assessing tobacco smoke compounds and main metabolite dosed

Method		Dosed metabolite
Physico-chemical	Gas Chromatography alone	Cotinine, Nicotine
	Gas Chromatography associated with	
	HPLC (High Pressure Liquid Chromatography)	
	HPLC coupled with mass spectrophotometry	Nicotine, Cotinine, Caffeine
Bio-immunological	RIA (Radioimmunoassay)	Cotinine
	ELISA (Enzyme linked Immunosorbant Assay)	Cotinine
	Fluorescence Polarization Immunoassay	Cotinine

Examining table 5.8, evidence emerges that methods used to assess the markers of smoking exposure can be classified into two main groups: physico-chemical methods and biological- radioimmunoassay methods. All these methods may provide worthy data on both active and passive smoking exposure either in individuals or in epidemiological surveys [45 – 49]. However, methods cannot be used in large-scale epidemiological trials because they need particularly specialized laboratories.

In short, nicotine and cotinine are the biomarkers most widely dosed by the current methods of analysis, although their determination requires specialized laboratories. Moreover, cotinine, a major metabolite of nicotine, is used more widely as a smoking biomarker since its urinary concentration has been considered one of the most specific parameters for tobacco smoke exposure [20, 35, 37–38, 50].

Urinary cotinine values are significantly higher in nonsmokers after their exposure to environmental smoke. Such a fact has been well documented in children [47] exposed to environmental tobacco smoke if they were compared to non-exposed children. Indeed, urinary cotinine concentrations were statistically higher in those children exposed with a statistical significance of a great degree (a P value less than 0.001 was calculated, while a value limit statistically significant is, usually, less than 0.05!).

In a large study that enrolled pregnant women [51], cotinine concentrations were higher in non smoking women who were passively exposed to cigarette smoke than in those who were not exposed, and urinary cotinine levels increased in cases of more prolonged exposure to environmental tobacco smoke. Finally, cotinine levels in those women who smoked were higher after childbirth than during pregnancy.

These results are undoubtedly worthy of two observations: firstly, both active and passive smoking tend to determine higher and prolonged concentrations of smoking metabolites in biologic liquids, and, secondly, dosed metabolites are active metabolites capable of inducing both cardiac muscle and coronary artery alterations.

In conclusion, nicotine and cotinine may affect the cardiovascular system and coronary arteries by a pathologically similar mechanism, although harmful effects of nicotine can be identified primarily after acute exposure to tobacco smoke [50] since they are earlier than those due to cotinine. However, the latter acts longer and it is biochemically easier to be dosed in study samples, particularly large-scale samples.

Carbon Monoxide

Carbon monoxide inhalation from cigarette combustion as well as from passive smoking exposure may be identified by the dosage of carboxyhemoglobin which is easily determined in both arterial and venous blood samples. In contrast, measuring how much higher carboxyhemoglobin levels are due to cigarette smoking alone is often controversial because of the large diffusion of carbon monoxide as an environmental pollutant in different industries, car fuel and other. Thus, one should know the carboxyhemoglobin levels before smoking exposure and then immediately after to determine the effective amount of carboxyhemoglobin due not generically to tobacco smoke but, rather, to a single smoked cigarette. As one can see, it is very hard to identify the amount of damage determined on the cardiovascular system from total tobacco smoke phenomenon by carboxyhemoglobin measures in clinical surveys. In contrast, that is particularly possible under experimental procedures [21] that can provide estimated carboxyhemoglobin measures before and then immediately after acute smoking exposure.

However, as mentioned, carboxyhemoglobin can be satisfactorily dosed in an arterial blood sample or, more easily, in a venous blood sample, which must be collected in a closed container containing an anticoagulant of the type dry sodium heparine or disodium ethylene-diaminotetracetic acid (EDTA). Then, blood samples must be preserved, also for several days, prior to analysis by keeping them cold (4°C) and in the dark. Then, spectrophotometric methods [52–55] are used to assess carboxyhemoglobin.

Another useful approach to estimate the exposure to carbon monoxide [21] may be the analysis of the gas concentration in the expired air after smoking exposure. The percent difference between the amount in gas expired after exposure and that expired before, provides results which can be related to the course of the phenomenon. Should one explain the phenomenon due to a single smoked cigarette to tobacco smoke overall, they would need estimated mathematical calculations.

In conclusion, the importance of carbon monoxide as a biomarker of smoking exposure is worth being estimated only when pre-exposure levels of carboxyhemoglobin are known and other carbon monoxide pollutants excluded. Experimentally, those concentrations of carboxyhemoglobin caused by tobacco smoke which are capable of harming the heart muscle and coronary arteries may be assessed. By that, there is strong evidence that carbon monoxide causes not only functional alterations but, primarily, structural alterations of heart and vessels either when it acts as a product of active smoking or even during passive smoking exposure.

Clinically, it has been well identified that the amount of carboxyhemoglobin in the blood following acute exposure to passive smoking at a concentration of only 30 – 35 ppm of the gas could increase from twice to four times carboxyhemoglobin concentrations [21] measured before exposure.

Thiocyanate

Cigarette smoking commonly releases thiocyanate that has been identified in the smoking vapor phase as hydrogen cyanide.

Both active smokers and nonsmokers exposed to environmental tobacco smoke have a mean blood thiocyanate levels of about 0.4 mcg/ml. These levels are from two to two-times-and-a-half greater than the thiocyanate levels of persons who do not smoke or are not exposed to smoking products. Usually, these people have a normally mean thiocyanate blood concentrations of about 0.15 to 0.20 mcg/ml.

Serum thiocyanate [31–34] has been monitored primarily in the past particularly to assess the effectiveness of cigarette smoking cessation programs and also to estimate its toxicity in experimental animal studies [56]. Its monitoring, however, has been rapidly replaced by the measurement of cotinine or nicotine levels in serum and urine for practical reasons: easier dosage of them and lack of interference with some foods which could and can, otherwise, influence thiocyanate metabolism but not nicotine or cotinine metabolism.

Milk, almonds, garlic, onion, leek, cabbage and cauliflower contribute to a mild elevation in serum thiocyanate concentrations. Such an occurrence could not permit one to separate nonsmokers from smokers or nonsmokers exposed to passive smoke as well as to establish the behaviour of smokers in smoking cessation programs.

Following these observations, the total series of biochemical studies that analyze cigarette smoke chemical concentrations in smokers, past-smokers, and nonsmokers omit to dose serum thiocyanate.

Several other substances have been, time to time, proposed as potential toxics which permitted to assess either smoking exposure or cardiovascular damage [57]: anabasine, anatabine, benzene, hydroxypyrene, aromatic compounds. However, their dosages have been rapidly left since there was evidence of difficulties in their measures and, at the same time, their assessment did not provide clearer results than those obtained by dosing nicotine and, particularly, cotinine. Moreover, coronary artery tree is influenced weakly by the action of these chemicals at the concentrations assessed for cigarette smoking if compared with the harmful action of nicotine or nicotine metabolites and carbon monoxide.

Hematologic Biochemical Markers

Strictly speaking, when a chemical substance determines changes in the routine dosage of hematologic parameters related to a physiological or pathological state, mainly with regard to cardiovascular system, that is the subject treated in this book, one must identify what in these changes is closely associated with harmful effects of the chemical and, consequently, set down a modified parameter as a biomarker of action of the examined substance, specifically cigarette smoking.

Several hematologic parameters, which may be influenced and often changed by a smoking habit, may be estimated as biomarkers of damage [58–62]. These biomarkers may be easily investigated by routine hematologic examinations, although they are not specific markers of smoking alone and, if they are changed from tobacco smoke effects, the exposure, particularly in case of passive exposure, must last for a time long enough to be estimated in many years. However, when the changes in hematologic parameters are caused certainly by smoking exposure, a true clinical problem may arise either to restore baseline measures or remove those biochemical and structural alterations which continue to maintain their characteristics.

The main hematologic parameters, which can be influenced by smoking, are listed in Table 5.9. Some parameters increase their blood concentrations as a direct effect of smoking, whereas some others, always as a consequence of a direct effect of smoking, undergo reduced blood concentrations. Moreover, parameters may change quickly and transiently as a result of acute exposure. Usually, hematologic biomarkers follow a complex series of changes hard to identify since changes may be due also to the close interaction among different coronary risk factors.

Table 5.9. Hematologic parameters mainly related to smoking exposure

Parameters usually increased	Platelet changes (aggregation and adhesiveness)	
	Increased plasma catecholamine levels	
	Increased LDL-Cholesterol	
	Increased fibrinogen level	
	Increased plasma and cell blood components:	Increased Factor VII
		Increased Plasma viscosity
		Increased leukocyte count
	Increased reactive C protein	
Parameters usually reduced	Decreased Plasminogen	
	Decreased serum estrogens	
Immunologic parameters	Increase/decrease	

In conclusion, a smoking habit may be carefully determined by the dosage of cotinine in urine, blood and saliva more than that of other markers. However, also for nicotine and cotinine there are yet limits on their large-scale use.

Blood, urine, and saliva are the samples usually used to dose cotinine and thiocyanate; blood and urine samples are used for measuring nicotine concentrations. Finally, carbon monoxide may be dosed in both blood and expired air.

These biochemical markers due to tobacco smoke exert harmful effects on heart and coronary arteries usually after prolonged chronic exposure to tobacco smoke of individuals, except for some cases in which, experimentally, acute exposure was studied at a standard concentration [7, 21, 63–64].

Chemically, biomarkers of cigarette smoking are, usually, structured with open terminal chains and, therefore, characterized often by a chemical instability as just described particularly for thiocyanate. Such an occurrence can determine more easily chemical reactions with the components of different tissues and organs of the body and production of other chemicals, often less toxic than the original compounds but, sometimes, more harmful, which can potentiate the negative effects of tobacco smoke. However, in the large majority of cases, a hypoxic mechanism with consequent metabolic and structural damage triggers those alterations usually attributed to smoking exposure and that will be described, in detail, in the next chapters.

There is evidence that hypoxia heavily damages different structures of the body, particularly in older individuals and in individuals who suffer from ischemic events. Structural alterations of myocardium and coronary arteries due to direct action of carbon monoxide have also been seen in clinical and animal studies [27, 29–30, 65].

There is a linear relationship between the levels of biochemical markers and level of cardiovascular alterations until a breakdown in the sense that the occurrence of an irreversible lesion usually gets free of the measures of biochemical markers. These parameters could also undergo reduced concentrations, but cardiovascular damage progression could continue independently. Therefore, the evidence of a hypoxic damage in individuals who had been previously exposed to tobacco smoke and later stopped smoking, could be a consequence of a prolonged exposure to smoking even if hematologic or urinary biochemical markers, which were altered, show again normal blood measures.

An example of that is given by the effects of nicotine and carbon monoxide on one of the major risk factors for heart and coronary blood vessels such as blood pressure. Some reports [66] on the relationship between cigarette smoking and blood pressure emphasize tobacco smoke as a factor capable of inducing hypotension, whereas other reports [67–68] identify hypertension as the late result of smoking. There is, therefore, an evident disagreement that could be explained as follows. After a temporary increase in blood pressure due to vasoconstriction for enhanced catecholamine release mediated by nicotine [6, 16-19] as well as autonomic system stimulation, that follows immediately smoking a cigarette, the depressant effects of this metabolite cause vasodilation that determines lower blood pressure levels. At the same time, the heart and blood vessels are damaged because of a direct action of carbon monoxide and, in time, the alterations caused by this gas become irreversible. Therefore, blood pressure tends to reach higher levels again as a consequence of irreversible pathological lesions. Thus, hypertension usually affects elderly people who smoke cigarettes or are exposed to tobacco products for a longer time. At the same time, atherosclerotic coronary lesions as well as systemic artery lesions may develop, maintain and potentiate further vascular changes.

Finally, polycyclic aromatic hydrocarbons [69–73], often involved in studies on cardiovascular and coronary damage from cigarette smoking and, sometimes, identified as biochemical markers of smoking, need a short mention.

Polycyclic aromatic hydrocarbons are a family of hydrocarbons containing two or more closed aromatic ring structures, each based on the structure of benzene, the chemical formula of which is C6H6, and spatial formula as in figure 5.4.

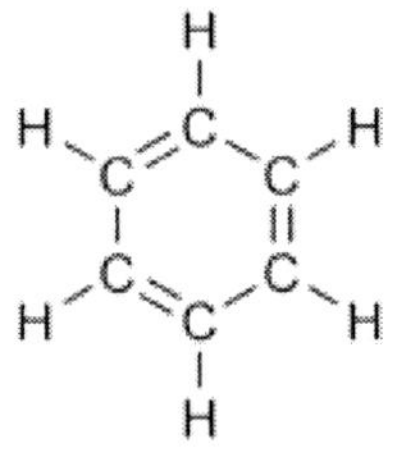

Figure 5.4. Spatial formula of benzene.

These groups of chemicals, the most important of which are benzene, benzopyrene and toluene, potentiate the negative effects on heart and coronary vessels exerted by those smoking chemicals previously analyzed, but they have also been identified as useful susceptibility markers of coronary artery disease, throughout the vitamin D receptor genotype, causing smoking-related DNA damage. It could be involved in the onset of cardiovascular disease. However, these findings are far from being carefully documented and, therefore, the role of these chemical compounds of smoking in causing coronary artery alterations is yet of limited importance.

References

[1]   Kice JL, Marvell EN. *Modern Principles of Organic Chemistry. An Introduction.* 3rd ed, The Macmillan Company, New York, USA, 1967.

[2]   Houseman TH. Studies of cigarette smoke transfer using radioisotopically labelled tobacco constituents. Part II. The transference of radioisotopically labelled nicotine to cigarette smoke. *Beitrage zur Tabakforschung,* 1973; 7: 142 – 7.

[3]   US Department of Health and Human Services. The health consequences of smoking: Nicotine addiction. Washington DC, USA, US Government Printing Office; 1988.

[4]   Armitage AK, Turner DM. Absorption of nicotine in cigarette and cigar smoke through the oral mucosa. *Nature.* 1970; 226: 1231 – 2.

[5]   Armitage AK, Dollery CT, George CF, Houseman TH, Lewis PJ, Turner DM. Absorption and metabolism of nicotine from cigarettes. *BMJ.* 1975; 4: 313 – 6.

[6]   Leone A. Cigarette smoking and health of the heart. *J. Roy. Soc. Health.* 1995; 115: 354 – 5.

[7]   Aronow WS. Effect of passive smoking on angina pectoris. *N. Engl. J. Med.* 1978; 299: 21 – 4.

[8]   Glantz SA, Parmley WW. Passive smoking and heart disease : epidemiology, physiology, and biochemistry. *Circulation.* 1991; 83: 1 – 12.

[9]   Celermejer DS, Sorensen KE, Georgakopoulos D. Cigarette smoking is associated with dose-related and potentially reversible impairment of endothelium-dependent dilation in healthy young adults. *Circulation.* 1993; 88: 2149 – 55.

[10]   Leone A. Relationship between cigarette smoking and other coronary risk factors in atherosclerosis: risk of cardiovascular disease and preventive measures. *Curr. Pharm. Design.* 2003; 9: 2417 – 23.

[11] Glantz SA, Parmley WW. Passive smoking and heart disease. *JAMA.* 1995; 273: 1047 – 53.

[12] Leone A, Giannini D, Bellotto C, Balbarini A. Passive smoking and coronary heart disease. *Current Vascular Pharmacology.* 2004; 2: 175 – 82.

[13] Fielding JE, Phenow KJ. Health effects of involuntary smoking. *N. Engl. J. Med.* 1988; 319: 1452 – 60.

[14] Powell JT. Vascular damage from smoking: disease mechanisms at the arterial wall. *Vasc. Med.* 1998; 3: 21 – 8.

[15] Ball K, Turner R. Smoking and the heart: the basis for action. *Lancet.* 1974; 2: 822 – 6.

[16] Benowitz NL, Jacob P III, Jones RT, Rosemberg J. Interindividual variability in the metabolism and cardiovascular effects of nicotine in man. *J. Pharmacol. Exper. Therapeutics.* 1982; 221: 368 – 72.

[17] Castro de Souza EM, Silva MRE Jr. The release of vasopressin by nicotine: Further studies on its site of action. *J. Physiol.* 1977; 265: 297 – 311.

[18] Cohen AJ, Roe FJC. Monograph on the Pharmacology and Toxicology of Nicotine. Tobacco Advisory Council Occasional Paper 4, 1981; London, UK, 45.

[19] Turner DM, Armitage AK, Briant RH, Dollery CT. Metabolism of nicotine by the isolated perfused dog lung. *Xenobiotica.* 1975; 5: 539 – 51.

[20] Benowitz NL. Cotinine as a biomarker of environmental tobacco smoke exposure. *Epidemiol. Rev.* 1996; 18: 188 – 204.

[21] Leone A, Mori L, Bertanelli F, Fabiano P, Filippelli M. Indoor passive smoking: its effect on cardiac performance. *Int. J. Cardiol.* 1991; 8: 247 – 52.

[22] Adams JD, Erickson HH, Stone HL. Myocardial metabolism during exposure carbon monoxide in the conscious dog. *J. Appl. Physiol.* 1973; 34: 238 – 42

[23] Horwath SM, Raven PB, Dahms TE, Gray DJ. Maximal aerobic capacity at different levels of carboxyhemoglobin. *J. Appl. Physiol.* 1975; 38: 300 – 3.

[24] Lewey FH, Drabkin DD. Experimental chronic carbon monoxide poisoning of dogs. *Am. J. Med. Sci.* 1944; 208: 502 – 11.

[25] Ehrich WE, Bellet S, Lewey FH. Cardiac changes from CO poisoning. *Am. J. Med. Sci.* 1944; 208: 512 – 23.

[26] Musselman NP, Groff WA, Yevich PP, Wilinsky FT, Weeks MH, Oberst FW. Continuous exposure of laboratory animals to low concentration of carbon monoxide. *Aerosp. Med.* 1959; 30: 524 – 9.

[27] Astrup P. Some physiological and pathological effects of moderate carbon monoxide exposure. *BMJ.* 1972; 4: 447 – 52.

[28] Anderson RF, Allensworth DC, DeGroot WJ. Myocardial toxicity from carbon monoxide poisoning. *Ann. Int. Med.* 1967; 11:72 – 82.

[29] Kjeldsen K, Thomsen HK, Astrup P. Effects of carbon monoxide on myocardium. Ultrastructural changes in rabbits after moderate, chronic exposure. *Circ. Res.* 1974; 34: 339 – 48.

[30] Thomsen HK, Kjeldsen K. Threshold limit for carbon monoxide-induced myocardial damage. *Arch. Environ. Health.* 1974; 29: 73 – 8.

[31] Apple FS. Serum thiocyanate concentrations in patients with normal or impaired renal function receiving nitroprusside. *Clin. Chem.* 1996; 42: 1878 – 9.

[32] De la Higuera AJ. Determination of serum thiocyanate in patients with thyroid disease using a modification of the Aldridge method. *J. Anal. Toxicol.* 1994; 18: 58 – 9.

[33] Diagnostic Bulletin. Serum thiocyanate as a marker for exposure to tobacco smoke. *Lab. Report for Physicians*. 1985; 7: 63.

[34] Olea F, Parras P. Determination of serum levels of dietary thiocyanate. *J. Anal. Toxicol.* 1992; 16: 258 – 60.

[35] Benowitz NL, Jacob P. Nicotine and cotinine elimination pharmacokinetics in smokers and nonsmokers. *Clin. Pharmacol. Ter.* 1993; 53: 316 – 23.

[36] Vogt TM, Selvin S, Widdowson G, Hulley SB. Expired air carbon monoxide and serum thiocyanate as objective measures of cigarette exposure. *Am. J. Public Health.* 1977; 67: 545 – 9.

[37] Apselhoff G, Ashton HM, Friedman H, Gerber N. The importance of measuring cotinine levels to identify smokers in clinical trials. *Clin. Pharmacol. Ther.* 1994; 56:460 – 2.

[38] Jarvis MJ, Tunstall-Pedoe H, Feyerabend C, Vesey C, Saloojee Y. Comparison of tests used to distinguish smokers from nonsmokers. *Am. J. Public Health.* 1987; 77: 1435 – 8.

[39] Feyerabend C, Russel MAH. A rapid gas-liquid chromatographic method for the determination of cotinine and nicotine in biological fluids. *J. Pharm. Pharmacol.* 1999; 42: 450 – 2.

[40] James H, Tibazi Y, Taylor R. Rapid method for the simultaneous measurement of nicotine and cotinine in urine and serum by gas-chromatography-mass spectrometry. *J. Chromatogr. B*, 1998; 708: 87 – 93.

[41] Tuomi T, Johnson T, Reijula K. Analysis of nicotine, 3-hydroxycotinine, cotinine and caffeine in urine of passive smokers by HPLC-tandem mass spectrometry. *Clin. Chem.* 1999; 45: 2164 – 72.

[42] Langone JJ, Gjika HB, Van Vunakis H. Nicotine and its metabolites. Radioimmunoassay for nicotine and cotinine. *Biochemistry.* 1973; 12: 5025 – 30.

[43] Langone JJ, Cook G, Bjercke R, Lifshitz MH. Monoclonal antibody ELISA for cotinine in saliva and urine of active and passive smokers. *J. Immunol. Methods.* 1988; 114: 74 – 8.

[44] Ekemin SA, Coxon RE, Colbert DL, Landon J, Smith DS. Urinary cotinine fluoroimmunoassay for smoking status screening adapted to an automated analyser. *Analyst.* 1992; 117: 697 – 9.

[45] Greenberg RA, Haley NJ, Ersel RA, Loda FA. Measuring the exposure of infants to tobacco smoke. *N. Engl. J. Med.* 1984; 310: 1075 – 8.

[46] Strachan DP, Jarvis MJ, Feyerabend C. Passive smoking, salivary cotinine concentrations and middle ear effusion in 7-year-old children. *BMJ.* 1989; 289: 1549 – 52.

[47] Roche D, Callais F, Reungoat P, Momas I. Adaptation of an enzyme immunoassay to assess urinary cotinine in nonsmokers exposed to tobacco smoke. *Clin. Chem.* 2001; 47: 950 –2.

[48] Principles of the Radioimmunoassay - RIA Method - maintained by F Wegner, 2003 University of Wisconsin, USA, System Board of Reagents.

[49] ELISA. Department of Biology, Davidson College, Davidson, NC, USA, 2002.

[50] Leone A. Biochemical markers of cardiovascular damage from tobacco smoke. *Curr. Pharm. Design.* 2005; 11: 2199 – 208.

[51] Spierto FW, Hannon WH, Kendrick JS, Bernert JT, Pirkle J, Gargiullo P. Urinary cotinine levels in women enrolled in a smoking cessation study during and after pregnancy. *J. Smoking-Related Dis.* 1994; 5: 65 – 76.

[52] Drabkin DL, Austin JH. Spectrophotometric studies. II. Preparation from washed blood cells; nitric oxide hemoglobin and sulfhemoglobin. *J. Biol. Chem.* 1935; 112: 51 – 65.

[53] Malenfant AL, Gambino SR, Waraska AJ, Roe EL. Spectrophotometric determination of hemoglobin concentration and percent oxyhemoglobin and carboxyhemoglobin saturation. *Clin. Chem.* 1968; 14: 789.

[54] Small KA, Radford EP, Frazier JM, Rodkey FL, Collison HA. A rapid method for simultaneous measurement of carboxy and methemoglobin in blood. *J. Appl. Physiol.* 1971; 31: 154 – 60

[55] Lily REC, Cole PV, Hawkins LH. Spectrophotometric measurements of carboxyhemoglobin. *Br. J. Ind. Med.* 1972; 29: 454 – 7.

[56] Rogers WR, Bass III RL, Johnson DE, Kruski AW, McMahan CA, Montiel MM, Mott GE, Wilbur RL, McGill HC Jr. Atherosclerosis-related responses to cigarette smoking in the baboon. *Circulation.* 1980; 61: 1188 – 93.

[57] Hatsukami DK, Hecht SS, Hennrikus DJ, Joseph AM, Pentel PR. Biomarkers of tobacco exposure or harm: Application to clinical and epidemiological studies. *Nicotine and Tobacco Research.* 2003;5: 387 – 96.

[58] Muscat JE, Harris RE, Haley NY, Wynder EL. Cigarette smoking and plasma cholesterol. *Am. Heart J.* 1991; 121: 141 – 7.

[59] Imaizumi T, Satoh K, Yoshida H, Kawamura Y, Hiramoto M, Takamatsu S. Effect of cigarette smoking on the levels of platelet-activating factor-like lipid(s) in plasma lipoproteins. *Atherosclerosis.* 1991; 87: 47 – 55.

[60] Becker C, Dubin T. Activation of Factor XII by tobacco glycoprotein. *J. Exp. Med.* 1977; 146: 457 – 67.

[61] Saba S, Mason R. Some effects of nicotine on platelet. *Thromb. Res.* 1975; 7: 819 – 24.

[62] Ou X, Ramos K. Benzo(a)pyrene inhibits protein kinase C activity in subcultured rat aortic smooth muscle cells. *Chem. Biol. Interact.* 1994; 91: 29 – 40.

[63] McMurray RG, Hicks LL, Thompson DL. The effects of passive inhalation of cigarette smoke on exercise performance. *Eur. J. Appl. Physiol.* 1985; 54: 196 – 200.

[64] Pimm PE, Silverman F, Shepard RJ. Physiolgical effects of acute passive exposure to cigarette smoke. *Arch. Environ. Healt.* 1978; 33: 201 – 13.

[65] Lough J. Cardiomyopathy produced by cigarette smoke. Ultrastructural observations in guinea pigs. *Arch. Pathol. Lab. Med.* 1978: 102: 377 – 80.

[66] Smoking and Health. Report of the Surgeon General. US Department of Health, Education, and Welfare. 1979.

[67] Leone A. The heart: a target organ for cigarette smoking. *J. Smoking-Related Dis.* 1992; 3: 197 – 201.

[68] Leone A, Lopez M, Picerno G. Il ruolo del fumo nel determinismo della cardiopatia coronarica. *Min. Cardiang.* 1984; 32: 435 – 9.

[69] Hajimiragha H, Ewers U, Brockhaus A, Boettger A. Levels of benzene and other volatile aromatoic compounds in the blood of non-smokers and smokers. *Int. Arch. Occup. Environ. Health.* 1990; 61: 513 – 8.

[70] Colmsjo AL, Zebuhr YU, Ostman CE. Polycyclic aromatic compounds in curing smoke. *Zeitschrift fur Lebensmitteluntersuching und forschung A*, 1984; 179: 308 – 10.

[71] Harwey RG. *Polycyclic aromatic hydrocarbons.* VCH Publication 1997.

[72] Dor F, Dab W, Empereur-Bissonnet P, Zmirou D. Validity of biomarkers in environmental health studies: the case of PHAs and benzene. *Crit. Rev. Toxicol.* 1999; 29: 129 – 68.

[73] Van schooten FJ, Hirvonen A, Maas LM, De mol BA, Kleinjans JCS, Bell DA, Durrer JD. Putative susceptibility markers of coronary artery disease: association between VDR genotype, smoking, and aromatic DNA adduct levels in human right atrial tissue. *FASEB J.* 1998; 12: 1409 – 17.

[74] Hummel T, Hummel C, Pauli E, Kobal G. Olfactory discrimination of nicotine-enantiomers by smokers and non-smokers. *Chemical Senses.* 1992; 17: 13 – 21.

[75] Man S, Potàcek M, Necas M, Zak Z, Dostàl J. Molecular and crystal structures of three berberine derivates. *Molecules.* 2001; 6: 433 – 41.

Chapter VI

Types of Coronary Vessel and Heart Damage

Abstract

Four types of coronary artery damage have been described: functional damage, closely related to cigarette smoking; clinical damage, characterized by the appearance of clinical symptoms of coronary artery disease as a consequence of a pre-existing coronary artery alteration; anatomical damage where coronary artery changes of different type, degree and extension may occur; and, finally, a combined damage which is the result of the simultaneous action of the three previous types of damage.

Main determinants of these types of damage are primarily atherosclerotic plaque formation as well as a series of artery wall changes closely related to arterial aging or coronary involvement due to diseases not linked to an atherosclerotic plaque. There is evidence that both phenomena interact among them to induce coronary artery disease although a markedly stronger effect is exerted by atherosclerotic plaque and its complications.

The major coronary risk factors act to potentiate particularly the development of atherosclerotic plaque and, therefore, increasing the rate of appearance of coronary artery disease.

Among the major coronary risk factors, tobacco smoke in all its types, smoking actively a cigarette or following passive exposure, plays a strong role in stimulating both functional and structural changes of the coronary artery wall because of the multiple effects of its compounds.

Keywords: Anatomical damage, functional damage, clinical damage, combined damage, atherosclerotic plaque, arteriosclerosis, coronary artery wall, arterial lumen dilation, intima-media thickening, arterial stiffness, endothelium, arterial compliance, coronary vasospasm, coronary stenosis, coronary ostia, arteritis, periarteritis nodosa, coronary aneurysm, aortic aneurysm, aortic medionecrosis, thoracic compression, trauma, neoplasm, radiotherapy, hematologic alteration, substance abuse, cocaine, heart metabolism.

Coronary artery damage in smokers and nonsmokers is usually of the atherosclerotic type and that contributes primarily to the appearance of ischemic changes of cardiac muscle [1–2].

In both humans and animals, function and anatomical structure of coronary arteries experience changes throughout their lifetime [3]. These changes develop those characteristics of the arteries defined as sclerotic type that differs deeply by vessel atherosclerosis due to pathological injuries as an effect primarily of a response to major coronary risk factors.

As a consequence of both phenomena, coronary involvement closely related to age and pathological arterial damage due to different types of stimuli, particularly risk factors, complex mechanisms may trigger, maintain, and, moreover, develop coronary alterations which will be different for each individual since the level of change of artery wall structure will be of a different degree.

Epidemiologically, dilation of arterial lumen, arterial coat changes, increased arterial stiffness, reduced artery compliance, and metabolic and structural changes of endothelium (table 6.1.) characterize senile involution of vessel structures. These changes increase arterial susceptibility to harmful stimuli although they do not cause, independently or together, pathological events. In contrast, superimposed damage due to coronary risk factors (figure 6.1.) stimulates atherosclerotic plaque formation.

**Table 6.1. Main factors which influence, physiologically,
senile involution of coronary arteries**

1	Arterial lumen dilation
2	Intimal thickening (focal or irregularly diffuse)
3	Medial thickening (usually diffuse, fibrosis, reduced elastic and muscular fibers)
4	Adventitia changes (fibrosclerosis and vasa vasorum twisting)
5	Increased arterial stiffness
6	Endothelial functional or structural changes (endothelial dysfunction)
7	Reduced arterial compliance (vascular tone deregulation)

Thus, it is worthy to note that the phenomena that these factors determine on the arterial wall need to be analyzed since they often are associated with coronary artery damage. And, the latter is the primary factor capable of inducing cardiovascular disease.

Finally, some differences characterize coronary damage in smokers if compared to past or never smokers with arterial changes which can be, sometimes, of an important significance.

Arterial Lumen Dilation

Arterial lumen changes may characterize artery aging, primarily of those arteries which have a prevailing elastic structure, with an increase in lumen size [4].

Different mechanisms contribute to produce arterial lumen dilation, the end result of which is, physiologically, the consequence of a balanced activity of many factors without any

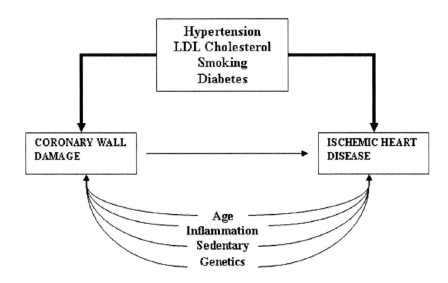

Figure 6.1. Schematic description of those factors capable of inducing both functional and structural changes in the coronary artery wall.

appearance of pathological events. In contrast, changes in arterial lumen dilation with possibly superimposed alterations may occur when pathological events may act. The latter alternative determines, often, reduction or occlusion of a dilated arterial lumen since narrowing phenomena due to the pathologic stimulus exert their effects on the arterial wall causing harmful results to its structure.

Coronary lumen dilation usually associated with diffuse tortuosity of the coronary arteries is primarily a consequence of aging since those proliferative alterations which characterize inflammatory and hyperplastic phenomena are, usually, lacking. Moreover, pathological occurrences like heart atrophy may induce coronary lumen dilation.

Coronary lumen dilation is also associated with increased thickness of the artery wall, and a constant enlargement involves the total diameter of the coronary artery along its circumference as well as the internal diameter of its lumens [5].

Twisting coronary tree and major distance between coronary vessels and myocardial fibers are the pathogenetic bases capable of inducing artery lumen dilation. Indeed, heart atrophy, which may be defined as a decrease in size of the cardiac muscle with reduced thickening and complete disappearance of myocardial fibers due to autolytic phenomena [6], determines a major distance between intramyocardial coronary arteries and limiting membrane of cardiocytes allowing an expansion of coronary vessels with consequent lengthening and lumen dilation.

Increased distance in intramyocardial vessel and cardiocyte space influences negatively oxygen transport and diffusion with a further impairment in heart size and function. A reduced amount of subepicardial fat, which undergoes degenerative changes as a consequence of atrophy often associated with edema, may cause involvement of epicardial coronary arteries.

These changes in arterial lumen diameter associated with vessel twisting are weakly associated with coronary artery disease [7] but they are mainly a consequence of vessel aging and, therefore, present in both old smokers and nonsmokers.

In conclusion increased intra-arterial lumen diameter is a vascular parameter which plays a weak role in inducing coronary damage, although it may be associated with other possible mechanisms of coronary pathology, and, then, potentiate coronary alterations in this way.

Artery Wall Thickening

As one can see from table 6.1, all artery coats may undergo coronary changes which are primarily correlated with a senile involution of coronary arteries [7]. Therefore, intimal-medial thickening would be an age-related phenomenon away from atherosclerosis, as experimental findings on animal models seem to indicate [8–11].

Coronary atherosclerosis has been also associated with pre-existing artery wall thickening, namely arteriosclerosis, which, however, is capable of potentiating those changes in coronary blood flow usually attributable to atherosclerotic lesions [12–17].

Structurally, changes in coronary wall coats consist of diffuse but irregular thickening due to the action of some physical factors related to pressure and cardiac wall tension which influence the coronary tree. Because of these reasons, the coronary intima is the coat more heavily thickened and the thickening is exceeding that observed in muscular arteries of systemic vascular districts. In some conditions, the intima of the coronary arteries is as thick as the medial coat.

Thickening processes are the result of active mechanisms which determine splitting of some vascular structures like internal elastic lamina and development of collagenous connective tissue into the arterial wall [18] particularly at the sites of main coronary arteries as well as where the major coronary branches arise.

Histologically, the coronary artery wall meets a progressive deterioration of the elastic tissue associated with no characteristic microscopic change [19] unless when inflammatory and degenerative processes, which belong to atherosclerosis, are involved.

In human arteries, there is evidence [20] that, with age, the elastic tissue of arterial media undergoes degeneration and calcification even if pathologic events do not affect artery vessels. When atherosclerotic stimuli occur, the breakdown of medial elastic tissue may accelerate and potentiate those hyperplatic-degenerative phenomena which characterize the plaque formation.

In conclusion, when a superimposed pathology is absent, the structural features, which may be observed on the coats of the coronary arteries and lead to arterial dilation and twisting, do not cause, usually, ischemic events and, therefore, they also could be identified as patterns of vessel senile involution.

Arterial Stiffness

The increase in arterial wall thickening is one of the most important mechanisms capable of inducing changes in arterial stiffness.

Arterial stiffness [21–23] changes are the result of two main factors: age and atherosclerotic processes. Therefore, changes in arterial stiffness cannot be only considered as a marker of vascular aging, like the previously analyzed factors, but they should also be included among those markers of developing atherosclerotic disease and, consequently, of increased cardiovascular risk.

Coronary arteries are involved in changes of their stiffness either throughout mechanical events or by functional stimuli. However, one of the major determinants of increased risk for coronary artery disease is the evidence of increased aortic stiffness.

Coronary artery stiffness is influenced also by some major cardiovascular risk factors like diabetes mellitus and oxidative stress [24]. Results [25–28] also demonstrated that large coronary vessels not only responded passively to changes in distending pressure but underwent active changes in cross-sectional area following a different series of pharmacological stimuli. Indeed, nitroglycerin, and, generally, nitrates induced and maintained prolonged coronary dilation, whereas alpha-adrenergic stimulation reduced, experimentally, cross-sectional area of large coronary arteries even when distending pressure was markedly increased.

Large epicardial coronary arteries are, usually, primarily involved in stiffness changes although changes have been well identified also in small coronary arteries. Totally, isolated changes in coronary artery stiffness need the action of factors, including, among other things, cigarette smoking, which trigger an atherosclerotic mechanism. In this way, changes in coronary artery stiffness may be identified as a risk factor for ischemic heart disease.

Endothelial Dysfunction

This parameter of coronary damage has been widely discussed in chapter 4 of this book where endothelial function has been analyzed on its physiologic and pathologic characteristics.

Here, it is worthy noting only that endothelial activation should be considered the sliding door to atherosclerosis [29] since it triggers those inflammatory and proliferative processes that lead to this disease.

Reduced Arterial Compliance

Compliance is the property of the artery vessels, primarily large elastic arteries but also large musculo-elastic arteries, to undergo dilation under, usually, increasing pressure stimuli and, then, restore baseline parameters when the applied stimulus has stopped.

As just described, increased stiffening of the large arteries, including coronary arteries, is associated with increased risk or presence of coronary heart disease [30–33]. Coronary artery compliance is, however, depending on systolic compression and atherosclerotic plaque. The latter modifies coronary arteriosclerosis in a type of athero-arteriosclerosis lesion and, in this way, coronary alterations may induce ischemic heart pathology.

It is known that reduction of plaque area in systole probably recognizes mechanisms related to physical properties of conduit arteries, although epicardial coronary arteries are stretched weakly during systole. Also a reduction in tissue blood volume could play a role in regulating coronary artery compliance [34–35].

In conclusion coronary artery compliance is dependent on both arterial senile involution associated often with the presence of atheroma which contributes actively to promote coronary artery disease.

In summary, factors listed in table 6.1. do not determine, usually, cardiac ischemic alterations mediated by the coronary tree. In contrast, such an occurrence could be met when a significant increase in cardiac work or events due to systemic diseases which affect negatively heart function, are superimposed on those coronary vessels which display namely arteriosclerotic alterations.

At most, the examined factors able to induce arteriosclerosis can potentiate the negative effects on the heart caused by coronary atherosclerosis.

Type of Cardiovascular Damage

Four types of heart damage (table 6.2.) may be determined by coronary alterations through a combined action of the major coronary risk factors, including cigarette smoking: a functional damage usually transient but also repeated; a clinical damage in individuals acutely but, primarily, chronically exposed to coronary risk factors; an anatomical damage typical of an acute or pre-existing ischemic heart disease; and a different combination of all types of damage.

Table 6.2. Type of cardiovascular damage and its characteristic

Type of damage	Risk factor	Characteristic	Changes
1.Functional damage	Smoking	Transient, repeated	Functional disorders; no anatomical altration.
2.Clinical damage	All	Acute, chronic	Functional disorders and symptoms of heart disease.
3.Anatomical damage	All	Acute, previous ischemic heart disease	Structural alterations.
4.Combined damage (1+2+3)	All	1 + 2 + 3	1 + 2 + 3.

Functional damage of the coronary tree and heart is usually related to the action of toxic chemicals which exert their effects acutely. Thus, acute exposure to cigarette smoking, like actively smoking a cigarette or following an exposure to environmental tobacco smoke, may induce, even in the first phases of exposure, a transient alteration to the cardiovascular system. Functional alterations usually recognize sympathetic nerve stimulation and endothelial dysfunction as main pathogenetic factors [36–39] which may be repeated and, therefore, cause structural changes of the coronary artery wall in the long run.

Some parameters rather than others are influenced negatively by a functional damage: heart rate and systolic blood pressure usually increase, exercise tolerance usually worsens, and cardiac rhythm disorders may appear. All these disorders are functional changes which are also maintained by the increased catecholamine levels usually associated with acute smoking exposure. Functional damage is specifically harmful for those subjects who suffer from ischemic heart disease as well as for those who are chronically exposed to passive smoking, being autonomic system and catecholamine release factors, in themselves, capable of causing spontaneously detrimental effects on both heart and blood vessels.

Coronary vessels may be influenced negatively, and also heavily, by functional damage since it is capable of causing coronary vasospasm which could cause angina pectoris, acute myocardial infarction or sudden death.

Clinical damage affects primarily those individuals who are displaying, customary, major coronary risk factors. Among these, primarily high LDL-cholesterol concentrations and hypertension play a significant role, but also cigarette smoking and diabetes mellitus exert negative effects not to be underestimated. Symptoms of angina pectoris, myocardial infarction, arrhythmias and respiratory disease [40–41] may be seen or worsened when this type of damage exists. When an anatomical damage is associated, the latter may act as an underlying disease and, then, there will be signs correlated with both events.

Clinical damage may be also associated with a transiently functional damage, that may appear particularly after acute exposure to tobacco smoke. Exposed individuals worsen clinical damage with symptoms related, mainly, to coronary and cerebrovascular disease.

Anatomical damage is the final and, in one way, unavoidable result of chronic and prolonged action of an atherosclerotic coronary lesion. It develops, usually, slowly but progressively until it attains the characteristics of irreversibility. Stable alterations that are associated with an anatomical damage may involve not only coronary arteries and, then, myocardium but often systemic arteries causing stable systolic and diastolic hypertension and cerebrovascular disease [1-2; 42].

In several cases, anatomical alterations support or aggravate pre-existing clinical symptoms. Impairment of clinical symptoms in individuals affected by major coronary risk factors and with a previous heart disease could be a useful, even if indirect, marker to follow-up further worsening and progression of underlying anatomical damage.

As mentioned, the main determinant to support anatomical damage is the progression of an atherosclerosis lesion that can be triggered by all types of coronary artery changes, particularly repeated functional events. Then, a functional damage causing endothelial dysfunction, platelet function changes and altered fibrinogen levels potentiates and determines a progression in atherosclerotic plaque formation or, when atherosclerotic plaque exists, its complications. Therefore, as one can see, all those factors capable of determining coronary artery and cardiac alterations are involved in the causative mechanism of the anatomical damage.

Anatomical damage may be, then, followed by those complications that induce severe and, sometimes fatal, cardiovascular events.

A cause-effect relationship would regulate anatomical damage and cigarette smoking as it will be described in detail in the next chapters, leading to the identification of tobacco smoke as an etiolgic more than a risk factor of coronary disease.

Coronary Artery Vasospasm

Coronary vasospasm has been firstly described as a clinical syndrome characterized by chest pain at rest associated with ST-segment elevation at the electrocardiogram by Prinzmetal and co-workers [43]. Authors interpreted the disease as a consequence of an increased coronary vasomotor tone which acted transiently on a pre-existing coronary narrowing capable of inducing an acute reduction in coronary blood flow.

The typical syndrome is characterized by symptoms attributable to angina pectoris, but it may be also associated with acute myocardial infarction, life threatening arrhythmias and sudden death. Exercise stress testing in these individuals evokes, usually, normal responses, since, even if some patients may have underlying coronary artery disease, there are others who have normal coronary arteries. However, patients who display different degrees of atherosclerosis of coronary arteries are widely present, and about 18 percent of them die or develop an acute myocardial infarction within three months after symptoms have begun according to the observations of Waters et al.[44].

However, the excellent findings of Maseri and his co-workers [45–51] have identified systematically either the clinical or bio-humoral and instrumental characteristics which belong to this ischemic syndrome.

Variant angina is a pathological event caused by a coronary spasm which, usually, involves a segment of an epicardial coronary artery, a vascular district where functional disorders may be induced by different factors, as it has been described in the previous chapter.

Coronary vasospasm recognizes primarily two mechanisms. Firstly, a segmental change in sensitivity [48] of an epicardial coronary artery without, probably, any initial alterations in receptorial responses, and, secondly, the action of different vasoconstrictor stimuli that exert their action on the altered coronary segment.

These two mechanisms would contribute to clarify the appearance of a coronary spasm, although other factors may act. Hypothetically, since the pathogenesis of this disorder is yet unknown [52], other factors, evoked time by time, could explain how vascular altered sensibility may affect a coronary segment. Table 6.3. summarizes the main factors which could be capable of modifying local sensitivity of an epicardial coronary segment.

Necropsy findings [53–61], even if conducted on relatively few observations, would seem to identify more extensive coronary artery alterations than those seen by angiographic studies in vivo which showed frequently normal arteriographic patterns of the coronary tree.

Observed alterations would consist of markedly sclerotic narrowings of epicardial coronary arteries with lumen reduction due to atherosclerotic plaque particularly at the site where vasospasm had been demonstrated by angiographic examination during life in some cases. Also intimal ridges have been demonstrated at the autopsy in a patient deceased from acute myocardial infaction following coronary vasospasm [62]. Histologically, intimal ridges showed a typical atherosclerotic plaque [63] and changes in smooth muscle cells capable of determining altered coronary wall thickness.

Table 6.3. Main factors evoked to explain altered vascular sensitivity of a coronary segment

Endothelial damage
Eccentric pre-existing atherosclerotic narrowing
Fixed coronary lumen narrowing
Luminal concentric plaque with predominance of smooth muscle cells
Intimal coronary ridges
Increased growth factor production
Platelet function changes
Focal arterial wall fibrosclerosis

Interesting observations have been provided by the examination of those vasospams superimposed to an eccentric atherosclerotic plaque [64]. Eccentric atherosclerotic plaque is a vessel lesion characterized by incomplete circled lumen narrowing and, therefore, the artery segment affected will have a wall site where atherosclerotic plaque exists with a different degree of thickness and extension and the opposite site without plaque, but, however, weakened by the presence of the opposite atherosclerotic plaque itself. Thus, this site could be more vulnerable to vasospasm.

Studies have demonstrated [65] that coronary vasospasm is a consequence of an endothelial damage. As previously documented, there is a close relationship between endothelial function and major coronary risk factors, including cigarette smoking which is capable of inducing endothelial changes either functionally – and these types of changes are earliest although transient – or structurally. Normal endothelium, in response to increases in shear stress or platelet stimulation, releases vasodilator endothelium-derived factors. In contrast, when endothelium is damaged, the reduced production of vasodilator substances leads to platelet aggregation with release, primarily, of serotonin and thromboxane A2. These substances cause contraction of smooth mucle cells and such an event may trigger an endothelial activation with consequent endothelial damage of the arterial wall.

Finally, changes in platelet function, bio-humoral factor production, and multiple foci of arterial wall fibrosis could predispose the arterial wall to those stimuli which may trigger coronary vasospasm.

Among triggering factors, there are stimuli of different types [66–74] capable of inducing coronary vasospasm by their action on an altered coronary segment. The main ones are summarized in table 6.4.

It must be mentioned, however, that major coronary risk factors play a crucial role either in inducing stable coronary alteration or coronary vasospastic phenomena. Moreover, all main compounds of cigarette smoking are capable of evoking those stimuli that trigger coronary vasospasm.

Table 6.4. Main stimuli capable of inducing coronary vasospasm

1	Adreno-sympathetic stimulation
2	Alpha-agonistic drugs
3	Physical exercise
4	Cold pressure test
5	Increased or decreased vagal activity
6	General anesthesia
7	Bromocryptine (in pregnancy-induced hypertension)
8	Interventional coronary procedures
9	Histamine (allergic angina)

Coronary Damage Due to Structural Changes

Structural changes that may be observed on coronary arteries are primarily those capable of causing ischemic heart disease in the presence, but even in the absence, of coronary risk factors.

The basic features of coronary structural damage are those which characterize the atherosclerotic lesion which occurs almost exclusively in the large conduits of the coronary tree. Atherosclerotic changes identify typically the anatomical damage. Small coronary artery disease has been also documented but due to different pathogenetic mechanisms which involve mainly a pathology of microvascular type as seen, among other things, in diabetes mellitus.

Atherosclerotic lesions will be discussed widely in Chapter 7. Here, it is worthy to note that coronary atherosclerosis is the most frequent factor causing coronary heart disease particularly in association with the major coronary risk factors. However, several other occurrences different from atherosclerosis may lead to heart ischemic pathology. Some of these are closely related to cigarette smoking.

Observations have emerged [40] that structural changes which involved the coronary wall and were following or pre-existing to ischemic heart pathology were similar for the coronary tree of smokers, past smokers or never smokers, although the degree and extension of the alterations would seem to be of a major gravity in active smokers and in past smokers or never smokers exposed passively to tobacco smoke, if compared to the alterations observed in non-exposed never smokers.

A superimposed functional damage which may be also transiently associated with anatomical damage does not change structurally the characteristics of the coronary lesions even if clinical course of ischemic heart disease may be, sometimes, worsened for the appearance of new non-fatal [75] or, in any cases, also fatal events. The reasons why a cardiac event following a superimposed damage on a pre-existing coronary damage is non-fatal or fatal are far from being identified or interpreted. Probably, that could depend on the type of event that triggers the heart attack since there are some, like life- threatening ventricular arrhythmias, which accompany a fatal occurrence with a significantly major incidence than others like chest pain without associated rhythm disorders.

Among those coronary lesions associated with ischemic heart pathology but differing from atherosclerotic plaque, there are some worthy to be analyzed since they have been documented in both clinical and experimental findings conducted on humans or animals exposed, in some cases, to tobacco smoke [76–82].

Stenosis of coronary ostia associated or not with incomplete or complete occlusion of one or both coronary arteries has been also documented in patients with ischemic heart disease. Nowadays, the most frequent cause of this alteration has been identified to be atherosclerotic disease, particularly in the elderly, or a complication following surgical replacement of aortic valve [83]. However, in the past syphilitic arteritis associated with other manifestations of cardiovascular syphilis determined stenosis of coronary ostia [84–87]. These reports, even if timely dated, provide a good correlation between ischemic cardiac pathology and structural coronary damage documented autoptically.

Epicardial coronary arteritis [88], etiologically depending on viral, bacterial, parasitic or allergic causes, is a rare event which can result in coronary heart pathology with or without occlusive alterations of the coronary tree, but with well documented coronary lesions consisting of focal artery wall necrosis associated or not with calcification, possible rupture of the vessel wall not due to trauma or interventional procedures, coronary artery wall thickening with secondary luminal narrowing and possible associated thrombosis, and aneurysm formation. Arteritis (vasculitic) syndromes rarely recognize harmful effects due to cigarette smoking. In contrast, they may recognize a pathogenetic immunologic mechanism due to circulating immuno-complexes in some cases [89–92]. The earliest vasculitis syndrome named periarteritis nodosa [93–94] develops nodules along the course of small arteries as a possible consequence of necrotizing and hyperplastic vascular alterations.

External compression of the epicardial coronary arteries as a consequence of traumatic events, chronic aortic dissection due to aortic medionecrosis or coronary aneurysms, primitive or metastatic thoracic neoplasms [95–97] have been identified as causes of ischemic heart pathology throughout a mechanism of coronary vessel damage, although of a different type with regard to coronary atherosclerotic plaque. Also all these diseases are completely not influenced by cigarette smoking, unless neoplastic thoracic pathology, and such an occurrence further underlines the significant role of the main compounds of tobacco smoke in inducing primarily atherosclerotic plaque formation and, then, ischemic heart disease.

Finally, non-atherosclerotic causes of coronary tree alterations with consequently possible ischemic heart disease [98–101] have been documented in several hematologic diseases, thoracic radiation therapy, and cocaine abuse. Several observations of artery thrombosis and spasm have been reported in these events.

Table 6.5. summarizes structural damages of the coronary tree mainly observed in the absence of an atherosclerotic pathology.

Currently, there is a general agreement that structural changes in coronary arteries, particularly epicardial coronary arteries, capable of inducing ischemic heart pathology are due to two types of alterations which may closely interact among themselves: atherosclerotic phenomena which play a basic role potentiated possibly by major coronary risk factors, and arteriosclerotic alteration. The latter, sometimes, may cause cardiac coronary events directly, although with a lower incidence in view of the type of structural damage of the coronary artery wall that it, usually, causes.

Table 6.5. Non-atherosclerotic structural damages of the coronary tree

Stenosis of coronary ostia
Arteritis
Periarteritis nodosa
Aortic and coronary aneurysms
Aortic medionecrosis
Thoracic compression (trauma, neoplastic pathology)
Hematologic diseases (thrombocytopenic purpura, leukemia, primary thrombocytosis, polycitemia)
Radiotherapy
Substance abuse (cocaine)

Those alterations which are related to arteriosclerosis are mainly linked to arterial aging rather than to a mechanism triggered by coronary risk factors, including smoking. Therefore, when one estimates the damage caused by coronary risk factors on the coronary tree, one has yet to estimate those events, some of these physiological occurrences, which can contribute to modify arterial wall structure independently from smoking.

Finally, since heart metabolism is almost totally of the aerobic type with a great amount of oxygen extracted at resting, limited increases in oxygen extraction may occur during exercise [102]. Consequently, increased oxygen demand particularly under stress conditions must be obtained throughout proportional increases in coronary blood flow, and an altered coronary tree could fail this function.

References

[1] Glantz SA, Parmley WW. Passive smoking and heart disease : epidemiology, physiology, and biochemistry. *Circulation.* 1991; 83: 1 – 12.

[2] Leone A. Relationship between cigarette smoking and other coronary risk factors in atherosclerosis: risk of cardiovascular disease and preventive measures. *Curr. Pharm. Design.* 2003; 9: 2417 – 23.

[3] Naijar SS, Scuteri A, Lakatta EG. Arterial aging: is it an immutable cardiovascuar risk factor? *Hypertension.* 2005; 46: 454 – 62.

[4] Gerstenblith G, Frederiksen J, Yin FC, . Echocardiographic assessment of a normal adult aging population. *Circulation.* 1977; 56: 273 – 8.

[5] Ehrich W, De La Chapelle C, Cohn AE. Anatomical ontogeny. B. Man: I. A study of the coronary arteries. *Am. J. Anat.* 1931; 49: 241 – 82.

[6] Karsner HT, Saphir O, Todd TW. The state of the cardiac muscle in hypertrophy and atrophy. *Am. J. Path. Bact.* 1925; 1: 351 – 71.

[7] Adams MR, Nakagomi A, Keech A, Robinson J, McCredie R, Bailey BP, Freedman SB, Celermajer DS. Carotid intima-media thickness is only weakly correlated with the extent and severity of coronary artery disease. *Circulation.* 1995; 92: 2127 – 34.

[8] Li Z, Froehlich J, Galis ZS, Lakatta EG. Increased expression of matrix metalloproteinase-2 in the thickened intima of aged rats. *Hypertension.* 1999; 33: 116 – 23.

[9] Wang M, Lakatta EG. Altered regulation of matrix metalloproteinase-2 in aortic remodeling during aging. *Hypertension.* 2002; 39: 865 – 73.

[10] Wang M, Takagi G, Asai K, Resuello RG, Natividad FF, Vatner DE, Vatner SF, Lakatta EG. Aging increases aortic MMP-2 activity and angiotensin II in nonhuman primates. *Hypertension.* 2003; 41: 1308 – 16.

[11] Lakatta EG. Central arterial aging and the epidemic of systolic hypertension and atherosclerosis. *JASH.* 2007; 1: 302 – 40.

[12] Regan IT, Hellems HK, Bing RJ. Effect of cigarette smoking on coronary circulation and cardiac work in patients with arteriosclerotic coronary disease. *Ann. N.Y. Acad. Sci.* 1960; 90: 186 – 9.

[13] Bellet S, West JW, Muller OF, Manzoli UC. Effect of nicotine on the coronary blood flow and related circulatory parameters: Correlative study in normal dogs and dogs with coronary insufficiency. *Circ. Res.* 1962; 10: 27 – 34.

[14] Zeiher AM, Drexler H, Wollschlager H, Just H. Endothelial dysfunction on the coronary microvasculature is associated with coronary blood flow regulation in patients with early atherosclerosis. *Circulation.* 1991; 84: 1984 – 92.

[15] Gorlin R. Regulation of coronary blood flow. *Br. Heart J.* 1971; 33: S9 – 14.

[16] Anderson TJ, Uehata A, Gerhard MD, Meredith IT, Knab S, Delagrange D, Lieberman EH, Ganz P, Creager MA, Yeung AC. Close relation of endothelial function in the human coronary and peripheral circulation. *J. Am. Coll. Cardiol.* 1995; 26: 1235 – 41.

[17] Nabel EG, Selwyn AP, Ganz P. Large coronary arteries in humans are responsive to changing blood flow: an endothelium-dependent mechanism that fails in patients with atherosclerosis. *J. Am. Coll. Cardiol.* 1990; 16: 349 – 56.

[18] Wolkoff K. Uber die atherosklerose der coronararterien des herzens. *Beitr. Path. Anat.* 1929; 82: 555 – 96.

[19] Movat HZ, Haust MD, More R. The morphologic elements in the early lesions of arteriosclerosis. *Am. J. Path.* 1959; 35: 93 – 102.

[20] Leary T. Atherosclerosis: the important form of arteriosclerosis, a metabolic disease. *JAMA.* 1935; 105: 475 – 81.

[21] Cohn JN. Arteries, myocardium, blood pressure and cardiovascular risk: towards a revised definition of hypertension. *J. Hypertension.* 1998; 16: 2117 – 24.

[22] Glasser SP, Arnett DK, Mc Veigh GE, Finkelstein SM, Bank AJ, Morgan DJ, Cohn JN. Vascular compliance and cardiovascular disease: a risk factor or a marker? *Am. J. Hypertension.* 1997; 10: 1175 – 89.

[23] Duprez DA, De Buyzere MM, De Bruyne L, Clement DL, Cohn JN. Small and large artery elasticity indices in peripheral arterial occlusive disease (PAOD). *Vasc. Med.* 2001; 6: 211 – 4.

[24] Katz PS, Rocic P, Souza FM, Matrougui K, Lord KC, Lucchesi PA. Increased oxidative stress modulates coronary artery remodeling and passive stiffness in db/db diabetic mice. *FASEBJ.* 2007; 21: 959 – 63.

[25] Vatner SF, Pagani M, Manders TW, Pasipoularides AD. Alpha adrenergic vasoconstriction and nitroglycerin vasodilation of large coronary arteries in the conscious dog. *J. Clin. Invest.* 1980; 65: 5 – 14.

[26] Winbury MM, Howe BB, Hefner MA. Effect of nitrates and other coronary dilators on large and small coronary vessels: an hypothesis for the mechanism of action of nitrates. *J. Pharmacol. Exp. Ther.* 1969; 168: 70 – 95.

[27] Douglas JE, Greenfield JC Jr. Epicardial coronary compliance in the dog. *Circ. Res.* 1970; 27: 921 – 9.

[28] Patel DJ, Janicki JS. Static elastic properties of the left coronary circumflex artery and the common carotid artery in dogs. *Circ. Res.* 1970; 27: 149 – 58.

[29] Desideri G, Ferri C. Endothelial activation. Sliding door to atherosclerosis. *Curr. Pharm. Design.* 2005; 11: 2163 – 75.

[30] Dart AM, Lacombe F, Yeoh JK, Cameron JD, Jennings GL, Laufer E, Esmore DS. Aortic distensibility in patients with isolated hypercholesterolaemia, coronary artery disease, or cardiac transplant. *Lancet.* 1991; 338: 270 – 3.

[31] Gatzka CD, Cameron JD, Kingwell BA, Dart AM. Relation between coronary artery disease, aortic stiffness, and left ventricular structure in a population sample. *Hypertension.* 1998; 32: 575 – 8.

[32] Cameron JD, Jennings GL, Dart AM. Systemic arterial compliance is decreased in newly diagnosed patients with coronary heart disease: implications for prediction of risk. *J. Cardiovasc. Risk.* 1996; 3: 495 – 500.

[33] Shaw JA, Kingwell BA, Walton AS, Cameron JD, Pillay P, Gatzka CD, Dart AM. Determinants of coronary artery compliance in subjects with and without angiographic coronary artery disease. *J. Am. Coll. Cardiol.* 2002; 39: 1637 – 43.

[34] Carew TE, Vaishnav RN, Patel DJ. Compressibility of the arterial wall. *Circ. Res.* 1968; 23: 61 – 8.

[35] Depre C, Havaux X, Wijns W. Neovascularization in human coronary atherosclerotic lesions. *Cathet. Cardiovasc. Diagn.* 1996; 39: 215 – 20.

[36] Westfall T, Cipolloni P, Edmundowicz A. Influence of propranolol on hemodynamic changes and plasma catecholamine levels following cigarette smoking and nicotine. *Proc. Soc. Biol. Med.* 1966; 123: 174 – 9.

[37] White S, McRitchie R. Nasopharyngeal reflexes: integrative analysis of evoked respiratory and cardiovascular effects. *Aust. J. Exp. Biol. Med. Sci.* 1973; 51: 17 – 31.

[38] McMurray RG, Hicks LL, Thompson DL. The effects of passive inhalation of cigarette smoke on exercise performance. *Eur. J. Appl. Physiol.* 1985; 54: 196 – 200.

[39] Leone A. The heart : a target organ for cigarette smoking. *J. Smoking-Related Dis.* 1992; 3: 197 – 201.

[40] Leone A, Bertanelli F, Mori L, Fabiano P, Battaglia A. Features of ischaemic cardiac pathology resulting from cigarette smoking. *J. Smoking-Related Dis.* 1994; 5: 109 – 14.

[41] Hole DJ, Gillis CR, Chopra C, Hawthorne VM. Passive smoking and cardiorespiratory health in a general population in the West of Scotland. *BMJ.* 1989; 299: 423 – 7.

[42] Barnoya J, Glantz SA. Cardiovascular effects of secondhand smoke. Nearly as large as smoking. *Circulation.* 2005; 111: 2684 – 98.

[43] Prinzmetal M, Kennamer R, Merliss R, Wada T, Bor N. A variant form of angina pectoris. *Am. J. Med.* 1959; 27: 375 – 88.

[44] Waters DD, Szlachcic J, Miller DD, Theroux P. Clinical characteristics of patients with variant angina complicated by myocardial infarction or death within one month. *Am. J. Cardiol.* 1982; 49: 658 – 64.

[45] Maseri A, Mimmo R, Chierchia S, Marchesi C, Pesola A, L'Abbate A. Coronary spasm as a cause of acute myocardial ischemia in man. *Chest.* 1975; 68: 625 – 33.

[46] Maseri A, Severi S, Nes MD, L'Abbate A, Chierchia S, Marzilli M, Ballestra AM, Parodi O, Biagini A, Distante A. "Variant" angina: one aspect of a continuous spectrum of vasospastic myocardial ischemia. *Am. J. Cardiol.* 1978; 42: 1019 – 35.

[47] Maseri A, L'Abbate A, Baroldi G, Chierchia S, Marzilli M, Ballestra AM, Severi S, Parodi O, Biagini A, Distante A, Pesola A. Coronary vasospasm as a possible cause of myocardial infarction. A conclusion derived from the study of "preinfarction" angina. *N. Engl. J. Med.* 1978; 299: 1271 – 7.

[48] Kaski JC, Crea F, Meran D, Rodriguez L, Araujo L, Chierchia S, Davies G, Maseri A. Local coronary supersensitivity to diverse vasoconstrictive stimuli in patients with variant angina. *Circulation.* 1986; 74: 1255 – 65.

[49] Chierchia S, Davies G, Berkenboom G, Crea F, Crean P, Maseri A. Alpha-adrenergic receptors and coronary spasm: an elusive link. *Circulation.* 1984; 69: 8 – 14.

[50] Chierchia S, Patrono C, Crea F, Ciabattoni G, De Caterina R, Cinotti GA, Distante A, Maseri A. Effects of intravenous prostacyclin in variant angina. *Circulation.* 1982; 65: 470 – 7.

[51] Maseri A, Parodi O, Fox KM. Rational approach to the medical therapy of angina pectoris: the role of calcium antagonists. *Prog. Cardiovasc. Dis.* 1983; 15: 269 – 78.

[52] Roberts WC, Curry RC, Isner JM, Waller BF, McManue MB, Mariani- Constantini R, Ross AM. Sudden death in Prinzmetal's angina with coronary spasm documented by angiography: Analysis of 3 necropsy patients. *Am. J. Cardiol.* 1982; 50: 203 – 10.

[53] Silverman ME, Flamm MD. Variant angina pectoris: Anatomic findings and prognostic implications. *Ann. Intern. Med.* 1971; 75: 339 – 43.

[54] Dhurandhar RW, Watt DL, Silver MD, Trimble AS, Adelman AS. Prinzmetal's variant form of angina with arteriographic evidence of coronary arterial spasm. *Am. J. Cardiol.* 1972; 30: 902 – 5.

[55] Kaski JC, Tousoulis D, Gavrielides S, McFadden E, Galassi AR, Crea F, Maseri A. Comparison of epicardial tone and reactivity in Prinzmetal's variant angina and chronic stable angina pectoris. *J. Am. Coll. Cardiol.* 1991; 17: 1058 - 62.

[56] Cheng TO, Bashour T, Kelser GA, Weiss L, Baos J. Variant angina of Prinzmetal with normal coronary arteriograms: A variant of the variant. *Circulation.* 1973; 47: 476 – 85.

[57] Brown BF. Coronary vasospasm: Observations linking the clinical spectrum of ischemic heart disease to the dynamic pathology of coronary atherosclerosis. *Arch. Intern. Med.* 1981; 141: 716 – 22.

[58] Donsky MF, Harris MD, Curry GC, Blomquest CG, Willerson JT, Mullins CB. Variant angina pectoris: A clinical and coronary arteriographic spectrum. *Am. Heart J.* 1975; 89: 571 – 8.

[59] Bromberg-Marin G, Mahmud E, Tsimikas S. Spontaneous multivessel coronary vasospasm leading to cardiogenic shock. *J. Invasive Cardiol.* 2007; 19: E85 – 8.

[60] Isner JM, Donaldson RF, Katsas GC. Spasm at autopsy: A prospective study. *Circulation.* 1983; 68: III – 1028.

[61] Halper J, Factor SM. Coronary lesions in neurofibromatosis associated with vasospasm and myocardial infarction. *Am. Heart J.* 1984; 108: 420 2.

[62] El-Maraghi NRH, Sealey BJ. Recurrent myocardial infarction in a young man with coronary arterial spasm, demonstrated at the autopsy. *Circulation.* 1980; 61: 199 – 207.

[63] Isner JM, Fortin AH, Fortin RV. Depletion of smooth muscle from the media of atherosclerotic coronary arteries: A potential factor in the pathogenesis of myocardial ischemia and the variable response to anti-anginal therapy. *Clin. Res.* 1983; 31: 193A.

[64] Waller BF. The eccentric coronary atherosclerotic plaque : morphologic observation and clinical relevance. *Clin. Cardiol.* 1988; 12: 14 – 20.

[65] Shepherd JT, Katusik ZS, Vedernikov Y, Vanhoutte PM. Mechanisms of coronary vasospasm: role of endothelium. *J. Mol. Cell Cardiol.* 1991; 23: 125 – 31.

[66] Yasue H, Touyama M, Kato H, Tanaka S, Akiyama F. Prinzmetal's variant form of angina as a manifestation of alpha-adrenergic receptor mediated coronary artery spasm: documentation by coronary arteriography. *Am. Heart J.* 1976; 91: 148 – 55.

[67] Yasue H, Horio Y, Nakamura N, Fujii H, Imoto N, Sonoda R, Kugiyama K, Obata K, Morikami Y, Kimura T. Induction of coronary artery spasm by acetylcholine in patients with variant angina: possible role of the parasympathetic nervous system in the pathogenesis of coronary artery spasm. *Circulation.* 1986; 74: 955 – 63.

[68] Specchia G, De Servi S, Falcone C, Bramucci E, Angoli L, Mussini A, Marinoni GP, Montemartini C, Bobba P. Coronary arterial spasm as a cause of exercise-induced ST-segment elevation in patients with variant angina. *Circulation.* 1979; 59: 948 – 54.

[69] Raizner AE, Chahine RA, Ishimori T, Verani MS, Zacca N, Jamal N, Miller RR, Luchi RJ. Provocation of coronary artery spasm by the cold pressure test. Hemodynamic, arteriographic and quantitative angiographic observations. *Circulation.* 1980; 62: 925 – 32.

[70] Lanza GA, Pedrotti P, Pasceri V, Lucente M, Crea F, Maseri A. Autonomic changes associated with spontaneous coronary spasm in patients with variant angina. *J. Am. Coll. Cardiol.* 1996; 28: 1249 – 56.

[71] Zainea M, Duvernoy VF, Chauhan A, David S, Soto E, Small D. Acute myocardial infarction in angiographically normal coronary arteries following induction of general anesthesia. *Arch. Intern. Med.* 1994; 154; 2495 – 8.

[72] Ruch A, Duhring JL. Postpartum myocardial infarction in a patient receiving bromocryptine. *Obstet. Gynecol.* 1989; 74: 448 – 51.

[73] Fischell TA. Coronary artery spasm after percutaneous transluminal coronary angioplasty: Pathophysiology and clinical consequences. *Cathet. Cardiovasc. Diagn.* 1990; 19: 1 – 3.

[74] Kounis NG, Zavras GM. Histamin induced coronary artery spasm: The concept of allergic angina. *Br. J. Clin. Prac.* 1991; 45: 121 –8.

[75] Leone A, Bertanelli F, Mori L, Fabiano P, Bertoncini G. Ventricular arrhythmias by passive smoke in patients with pre-existing myocardial infarction. *J. Am. Coll. Cardiol.* 1992; 19: 256A.

[76] Eliot RS, Baroldi G, Leone A. Necropsy studies in myocardial infarction with minimal or no coronary luminal reduction due to atherosclerosis. *Circulation.* 1974; 49: 1127 – 31.

[77] Auerbach O, Carter HW, Garfinkel L, Hammond EC. Cigarette smoking and coronary artery disease: a macroscopic and microscopic study. *Chest.* 1976; 70: 697 – 706.

[78] Doyle JT, Dawber TR, Kannell WB. The relationship of cigarette smoking to coronary heart disease. *JAMA.* 1964; 190:886 – 90.

[79] Sandler DP, Comstock JW, Helsing KJ, Shore DL. Death from all causes in non-smokers who lived with smokers. *Am. J. Public Health.* 1989; 79: 163 – 7.

[80] Leone A. Cardiovascular damage from smoking: a fact or belief? *Int. J. Cardiol.* 1993; 38: 113 – 7.

[81] Zhu BQ, Sun HP, Sievers RE, Isenberg WM, Glantz SA, Parmley WW. Passive smoking increases experimental atherosclerosis in cholesterol-fed rabbits. *J. Am. Coll. Cardiol.* 1993; 21: 225 – 32.

[82] Gvozdjakova A, Bada V, Sany L, Kucharska J, Kruty F, Bozek P, Trstansky L, Gvozdjak J. Smoke cardiomyopathy: disturbance of oxidative processes in myocardial mitochondria. *Cardiovasc. Res.* 1984; 18: 229 – 32.

[83] Yates JD, Kirsh MM, Sodeman TM, Walton JA, Brymer JF. Coronary ostial stenosis: A complication of aortic valve replacement. *Circulation.* 1974; 49: 530 – 4.

[84] Bruenn HG. Syphilitic disease of the coronary arteries. *Am. Heart J.* 1934; 9: 421 – 36.

[85] Moritz AR. Syphilitic coronary arteritis. *Arch. Path.* 1931; 11: 44 – 59.

[86] Wearn JT. The relationship of the thebesian circulation to coronary occlusion. *Am. Heart J.* 1931; 7: 119 – 20.

[87] Bruenn HG, Turner KB, Levy RL. Notes on cardiac pain and coronary disease. Correlation of observations made during life with structural changes found at autopsy in 476 cases. *Am. Heart J.* 1936; 11: 34 – 40.

[88] Lie JT. Coronary vasculitis:A review in the current scheme of classification of vasculitis. *Arch. Pathol. Lab. Med.* 1987; 111: 224 – 33.

[89] Cristian CL, Sergent JS. Vasculitis syndromes: Clinical and experimental models. *Am. J. Med.* 1976; 61: 385 – 92.

[90] Fauci AS, Hayne BF, Katz P. The spectrum of vasculitis: clinical, pathogenic, immunologic, and therapeutic considerations. *Ann. Intern. Med.* 1978; 89: 660 – 76.

[91] Soter NA, Austen KF. Pathogenetic mechanisms in necrotizing vasculitides. *Clin. Rheum. Dis.* 1980; 6: 233 – 53.

[92] McCluskey RT, Fienberg R. Vasculitis in primary vasculitides, granulomatoses, and connective tissue diseases. *Hum. Pathol.* 1983; 14: 305 – 15.

[93] Dickson WE. Polyarteritis acuta nodosa and periarteritis nodosa. *J. Pathol. Bacteriol.* 1908; 12: 31 – 57.

[94] Zeek PM. Periarteritis and other forms of necrotizing angiitis. *N. Engl. J. Med.* 1953; 248: 764 – 72.

[95] Giritsky AS, Ricci MT, Reitz BA, Shumway NE. Extrinsic coronary artery obstruction by chronic aortic dissection. *Ann. Thorac. Surg.* 1981; 32: 289 – 93.

[96] Gardia-Rinaldi R, Von Koch L, Howell JP. Aneurysm of the sinus of Valsalva producing obstruction of the left main coronary artery. *J. Thorac. Cardiovasc. Surg.* 1976; 72: 123 – 6.

[97] Kopelson G, Herwig KJ. The etiologies of coronary artery disease in cancer patients. *Int. J. Radiat. Oncol. Biol. Phys.* 1978; 4: 895 – 906.

[98] Om A, Ellahham S, Vetrovec GW. Radiation induced coronary artery disease. *Am. Heart J.* 1992; 124: 1598 – 1602.

[99] Spach MS, Howell DA, Harris JS. Myocardial infarction and multiple thrombosis in a child with primary thrombocytosis. *Pediatrics.* 1963; 31: 268 – 76.

[100] Virmani R, Robinowitz M, Smialek JE, Smyth DF. Cardiovascular effects of cocaine: An autopsy study of 40 patients. *Am. Heart J.* 1988; 115: 1068 – 76.

[101] Goldman BI, Wurzel J. Hematopoiesis/erythropoiesis in myocardial infarcts. *Mod. Pathol.* 2001; 14: 589 – 94.

[102] Hastings AB, White FC, Sanders TM, Bloor CM. Comparative physiological responses to exercise stress. *J. Appl. Physiol.* 1982; 52: 1077 – 83.

Chapter VII

Coronary Atherosclerosis

Abstract

Estimating the significance of atherosclerotic plaque formation as well as its effects on heart pathology is not yet a well-defined pattern, although morpho-functional features of the atherosclerotic process have been widely studied and identified.

Coronary atherosclerosis is a degenerative-hyperplastic disease of large and medium-sized epicardial coronary arteries characterized by the presence of two main pathological alterations: the fatty streaks and an atheromatous or fibrofatty plaque. Fatty streaks are characterized by lipid deposition in the intima, whereas fibrous plaque is localized to the intima and consists of lipid-laden smooth muscle cells and macrophages associated with hard connective tissue including collagen, intracellular and extracellular lipid deposits.

Fibrous plaque is not a stable lesion but may undergo remodeling with appearance of complications like ulceration, thrombosis, calcification, and hemorrhage which can lead to non-fatal or fatal cardiovascular events.

Endothelial cell injuries, that determine endothelial activation and related inflammatory responses, are associated particularly with lipid material infiltration as pathogenetic mechanisms explaining the type of observed alterations. However, multifactorial etiology is believed to be responsible for the disease.

Various factors, namely coronary risk factors like, particularly, hypertension, lipid disorders, diabetes mellitus and cigarette smoking, usually contribute to raise both incidence and severity of coronary atherosclerosis with consequent imparment in coronary blood flow supply and appearance of ischemic heart pathology.

Keywords: Coronary atherosclerosis, ischemic heart disease, coronary occlusion, coronary narrowing(s), risk factor(s), remodeling, lipid, fibrous cap, fatty streak(s), vulnerable plaque, intimal cushion, gelatinous lesion, vessel enlargement, ulceration, calcification, hemorrhage, hypertension, HDL-Cholesterol, LDL-Cholesterol, oxidative stress, homocysteine, smoking, platelet, coagulation-fibrinolysis system, fibrinogen, metabolic syndrome.

The purpose of this chapter goes beyond a detailed description of the atherosclerotic coronary disease since this subject has been widely described, and in an excellent way by several textbooks of cardiovascular medicine [1–5]. It sets the goal of characterizing all those metabolic mechanisms and physiopathologic features which may be identified as a consequence of the complex relationship between coronary risk factors and coronary artery changes that influence the appearance of clinical syndromes of ischemic heart disease.

The previous chapters had shown the different types of responses of coronary circulation to provide arterial blood supply to the heart according to its metabolic and functional request. Indeed, structural characteristics of the coronary arteries influence closely this function.

A crucial problem in assessing the type of ischemic pathology of the heart seems to depend on two main factors: the degree of developing coronary collateral circulation and the type of occlusion of a coronary artery, which evokes different responses whether it occurs slowly or suddenly as well as can determine a complete or incomplete artery lumen stenosis. Generally, gradual but progressive narrowing of a coronary artery leads to chronic degenerative alterations in cardial muscle, whereas sudden occlusion of coronary circulation as a consequence, primarily, of thrombotic phenomena may cause, usually, a myocardial infarction, that is, pathologically, an area in which the whole tissue of cardiac muscle has been killed by the sudden ischemia, or sudden death in some individuals.

As one can see, the structural characteristics of coronary arteries and, primarily, the degree of patency of their lumen play a strong role in regulating coronary blood flow and, then, type of cardiac responses. Unfortunately, the coronary circulation is frequently affected by atherosclerotic lesions. These lesions narrow the lumen of the vessels and predispose affected individuals to thrombosis and occlusion.

Narrowings may be, usually, seen with a major incidence in older age and with a major severity in men rather than in women. They recognize also a multifactorial etiology since various risk factors may exert a predisposing role of different amounts.

Coronary artery remodeling [6] usually follows atherosclerotic changes and coronary procedures conducted as diagnostic and/or therapeutic approaches.

The term atherosclerosis, firstly used by Marchand [7], means, literally, " mushy and hard arteries". It was deriving from the Greek language, where "athero" means gruel or porridge and sclerosis means hardening. It was identified, at that time, as the synthesis of two separate pathologic manifestations named atherosis and sclerosis.

Atherosclerotic Lesion

Atherosclerosis is a chronic immunoinflammatory, fibroproliferative disease which involves primarily lipid metabolism [8]. The pathognomonic feature of athrosclerotic disease is the formation of a lesion called atherosclerotic plaque, which should be interpreted as the final development of a large series of phenomena that weaken artery wall structure, but also the initial step of appearance of complications, which influence negatively and heavily those body organs where altered arteries provide blood flow. Indeed, coronary flow feels, particularly, the negative effects of reduced blood supply determined, particularly, by two factors: degree of narrowing and vulnerable plaque.

Atherosclerotic plaque is an artery wall lesion which consists primarily of both lipids and "hard" substances like calcium and fibrous tissue. Veins do not undergo atherosclerotic alterations, unless they are involved in surgical procedures like aorto-coronary bypass and, therefore, would function as artery conduits.

Histologic composition and structure of a coronary atherosclerotic plaque [9–20] permit one to identify more easily the clinical course that lesion may determine and, so, they can lead to a possible estimate of a future type of cardiac pathology. A great amount of components deriving from vessel wall, blood cells, metabolites, and immunologic substances contribute to atherosclerotic plaque composition.

Atherosclerosis is a timely dated disease but, in time, has changed some characteristics. Therefore, it is worthy defining briefly the main changes met as time went.

First observations in atherosclerotic pathology date back to Egyptian mummies and B.C. population, as reported by several authors [21–30]. Lipids were demonstrated in the artery wall by histologic and immunochemical methods and consisted of adipose deposits irregularly distributed into the arterial wall of different body districts, including the heart and brain. Deposits differed widely from a typical atherosclerotic plaque and were attributed to lifestyle, nutrition, social conditions and working of examined corpses.

In the following centuries, further investigations conducted by several authors confirmed two features which involved both systemic and coronary arteries: fatty deposits in the arterial layers intima and media associated with an evident hardening of the vessel. These changes, even if not yet interpreted as having the structural characteristics of the "actual" atherosclerotic plaque, permitted, however, the identification of that disease called arteriosclerosis.

From these observations, in the past three main pathogenetic mechanisms of atherosclerosis development had been hypothesized: incrustation or blood dyscrasia theory formulated by von Rokitansky in 1852 [27], inflammatory theory formulated by Virchow in the mid 1850s [25], and imbibition theory formulated by Ignatowsky [28] in the first years of 1900 and improved by Anitschow and Chalatov [29-31] a few years later.

Incrustation theory recognized atherosclerotic plaque as a result of excessive deposits of blood material, particularly fibrin, following dyscrasic phenomena into the arterial wall. Observed patterns were a consequence of fibrin-induced alterations. This theory could partially explain the thrombus formation which may be often superimposed an atherosclerotic plaque.

Inflammatory theory supported its hypothesis on the observation that proliferative and degenerative phenomena involved arterial wall coats. These phenomena consisted of connective tissue formation associated with arterial wall calcification and fatty degeneration. This theory better than incrustation theory explained the first as well as final manifestations that characterize, pathologically, atherosclerotic plaque, although both crucial mechanisms and specific types of lipids involved were not completely clarified.

Finally, imbibition theory meets closely some basic mechanisms recognized nowadays in atherosclerotic plaque development. The theory hypothesized that atheroma formation was the result of cholesterol imbibition and filtration through the intimal coat and, consequently, lipid infiltration as a pathogenetic mechanism was formulated. Several observations derived from the findings conducted on the subject [29–31]:

1. In the earliest lesions - the fatty streaks- most of the lipid was found inside cells containing large numbers of lipid-containing vacuoles (foam cells). These elements were Sudan positive and contained birefringent droplets (the liquid crystals of cholesterol esters). Initially, there was evidence that the endothelium over the lesion appeared to be intact.

2. Lesions could be seen at the root of the aorta and in the aortic arch and then proceeded caudally.

3. Lesions were distributed mainly within those sites which underwent hemodynamic stress.

4. Animals, who had undergone cholesterol feeding over a long period, finally displayed deposits of connective tissue and development of a fibrous cap.

5. Only early lesions were reversible but only some of the lipids could be mobilized from advanced lesions, leaving behind the fibrous cap and some cholesterol crystals. Such a statement is well consistent with the phenomenon called reverse cholesterol transport that will be described below.

6. The extent and amount of lesions were proportional to blood cholesterol concentrations which entered arterial wall from the blood.

7. The cholesterol-loaded cells were probably white blood cells that had infiltrated the artery wall.

As one can see, from the studies of Anitschkow and coworkers, several features that explain fully the structure and formation of an atherosclerotic lesion, emerge although some of the hypotheses formulated by inflammatory and incrustation theories help to complete atherosclerotic patterns. Therefore, a synthesis of the three hypotheses better support today our knowledge on the subject.

Macroscopic Changes

Findings of Wolkoff [32] describe systematically atherosclerotic changes of coronary arteries macroscopically.

Grossly, five types of alterations, which are equivalent of histologic features, may be, usually, identified (table 7.1.): fatty streaks with or without yellow deposits of lipids bulging vascular lumen; elevated fibrous plaques which may cause eccentric or concentric narrowings of the coronary artery wall with possible reduction in vascular lumen diameter; plaques complicated by hemorrhagic phenomena or ulcerations which characterize the internal surface of intima of an irregularly pigmented ploughing; and, then, calcified plaques usually more stable and, usually, far from causing embolization.

Complicated plaques are most frequently identified in populations who have a high incidence of fatal coronary artery disease [33], whereas superficial deposits of lipids may be found early in arteries of children aged six months and are a constant pattern after three years of age [34–35]. The significance of these phenomena is still under investigation since there are not unanimous opinions on their relation with the development of a future atherosclerotic plaque.

Table 7.1. Macroscopic changes in coronary atherosclerotic arteries

Type	Possible feature
Fatty streaks	No deposits
	Yellow lipid deposits bulging lumen
Elevated fibrous plaque	Narrowing arterial lumen
	Reduction in arterial lumen
Hemorrhagic phenomena	Embolization
Ulcerations	Embolization
Artery wall hardening	Calcification

The first macroscopic alterations may be seen as yellow streaks on the inner surface of the arterial walls which run irregularly along the course of epicardial coronary arteries. These streaks, usually, reduce minimally arterial lumen. They may be seen firstly on the left anterior descending artery [36] which is usually that coronary vessel most often involved in plaque formation.

Macroscopically (figure 7.1.), fibrous plaque is usually identified as a rounded or irregular formation of white color, easily visible in the context of artery wall, which gets up the intimal coat. Not infrequently fibrous plaques may exhibit red purple foci due to hemorrhagic phenomena developing towards arterial lumen, ulcerations, visible as splits of the inner surface of intima coat, and calcifications often felt as hardened conduits.

The first third of the left anterior descending artery as well as the main left coronary artery along all its course are the most frequent localizations of a coronary atherosclerotic plaque which is, also, characterized by a strong degree of severity since it undergoes occlusion or complications more easily than what occurs for other coronary districts. Such a fact is worth noting to understand and clearly estimate ischemic pathology of the heart in the presence of coronary atherosclerosis.

Microscopic Changes

A complex series of features may be seen when coronary atherosclerosis is examined histologically. Various steps of developing the atherosclerotic plaque with specific features for each step have been described. They initiate from simple alterations equivalent to isolated fatty streaks documented macroscopically to the final specific changes which characterize a stable or, conversely, vulnerable plaque. Other types of histologic alterations have been also described and defined as intimal cushion and gelatinous lesions, although they have a weak role in estimating correctly atherosclerosis.

Atherosclerotic plaque has been identified as the basic alteration. The American Heart Association Committee [20] on Vascular Lesions of the Council on Arteriosclerosis classified the basic histologic characteristics of the advanced atherosclerotic plaque in 1995, deferring to its first report [37] the features of initial steps of atherosclerotic plaque.

As previous mentioned, there is evidence that atherosclerosis is a dynamic process and atherosclerotic plaque often is followed by complications (vulnerable plaque) as a result of a final pathway. Therefore, its development requires much time to reach the final feature and, moreover, different steps of lesions have been identified on the wall of the same artery at the same time. Such a feature makes it very difficult to hypothesize the final result of those pathologic changes which may be observed in a body organ supplied by an atherosclerotic vessel, particularly for what is determined by coronary atherosclerosis.

It is worth noting that similar coronary atherosclerotic changes may give different patterns of ischemic heart disease, except in those circumstances where there is an atherosclerotic plaque completely and acutely occluding coronary vessels not associated with a proportional development of collateral circulation and, moreover, undergone complications.

The main characteristics which may be seen in the development of an atherosclerotic plaque are reported in table 7.2.

Table 7.2. Main features observed in the development of an atherosclerotic plaque

Atherosclerotic plaque	Type of Lesion
1. Type I	Accumulation of monocytes from the blood into the arterial intima across an intact endothelium.
2. Type II	Fatty streak: multifocal accumulation of lipid-foam cells beneath an intact endothelium.
3. Type III	Different size, but small, pools of extracellular lipid.
4. Type IV	Appearance of smooth muscle cells within the lesion beneath endothelium and formation of "lipid core" for coalescence of lipid pools.
5. Type V	Formation of a fibrous capsule containing the "lipid core" due to deposition of connective tissue (type Va), hard calcification (type Vb), and collagen, lipids and smooth muscle cells (type Vc).
6. Type VI	Complicated plaque with hemorrhage, thrombosis, rupture or embolization.

(Reproduced, with permission, from: *Passive Smoking and Cardiovascular Pathology: Mechanisms and Physiopathological Bases of Damage*. A. Leone ed, Nova Science Publishers; Inc., New York, 2007).

The dynamics of the atherosclerotic process directed to plaque formation is characterized by initial phases of cell migration [38-39] beneath an intact endothelium. Monocytes reach the intima where they undergo an activation and consequently conversion to macrophages. They catch lipids leading to formation of lipid-foam cells. These first steps are followed by multiple phases of accumulation and proliferation which are phenomena capable of determining several alterations consisting of fibrous capsule formation, lipid coalescence, calcification and smoth muscle cell disruption. These alterations are associated with endothelial activation, consequences of inflammatory processes, and, then, loss in function. Fibrous capsule formation is a basic step of atherosclerotic plaque since it determines the following features which may be plaque stabilization or progression towards the appearance of complications.

Therefore, atherosclerotic plaque has three main components (table 7.3.): 1. a cellular component with macrophages, smooth muscle cells, leukocytes and lipid-foam cells; 2. a fibrous matrix with connective tissue, collagen and elastic fibers; 3. a deposit of lipids coming from the intracellular and extracellular matrix, the amount of which varies widely and determines the structural characteristic of the plaque.

Table 7.3. Main components of a coronary plaque

1. Cellular component	macrophages, smooth muscle cells, leukocytes, lipid-foam cells.
2. Lipid deposit	cholesteryl esters
3. Fibrous component	connective tissue, collagen, disrupted elastic fibers.
4. Complication component	hemorrhagic material, calcium, cholesterol emboli, thrombi.

Observing the dynamic events of the atherosclerotic lesion, observations worthy to be analyzed emerge. There is evidence that initial alterations occur with an intact endothelium. Normal endothelial function, as mentioned in Chapter 4, impedes initially the progression of atherosclerotic injury since vasodilator metabolites, particularly NO, are capable of preventing the harmful effects. On the contrary, whether endothelial dysfunction occurs frequently, even in case of transiently acute events, atherosclerotic plaque tends to form more quickly since coronary endothelial dysfunction may be followed by endothelial activation. There is evidence that functional disorders, particularly those caused by cigarette smoking, are triggering factors of atherosclerosis.

At a microscopy light, atherosclerotic plaque appears to have different characteristics according to its prevailing composition. Usually, a fibrous cup with central lipid core rich in cholesterol and cholesteryl ester is localized to the intima and protrudes into arterial lumen giving different degrees as well as types of vessel narrowings. Lipid deposits characterize particularly atherosclerotic plaque which, however, in some cases displays a great amount of connective material and smooth muscle cells. Fibrin deposits may also be identified as endothelial covering. In the presence of an advanced lesion, coronary artery lumen is often almost totally occluded and internal elastic lamina disappears beneath atherosclerotic plaque. Dystrofic and atrophic phenomena of the media coat begin to be documented. Sometimes, internal elastic lamina shows its normal structure, but media coat atrophy will be seen. Such a feature could explain some different mechanisms evoked in developing atherosclerosis.

Complicated atherosclerotic plaques [40–45] may be also documented microscopically. Almost always, advanced plaques display calcifications which, in some cases, may involve massively arterial wall. Ulceration of lumen surface with debris of hemorrhagic material as well as superimposed thrombi may characterize light microscopy observations.

Figures 7.2 to 7.4 show a widely different spectrum that may characterize the atherosclerotic plaque.

In conclusion, microscopic observation of an atherosclerotic plaque, primarily an advanced coronary plaque, permits one to identify a different degree of thickening of endothelial cells protruding and reducing vascular lumen immediately upon a subintimal fibrous cup containing proliferated smooth muscle cells, various amounts of collagen and intracellular lipids including foam-cells. A necrotic center into the plaque displays cell debris, cholesterol crystal and esters, and, most often, calcium deposits with different distribution.

Fatty streaks are pathologic alterations which need some explanations either for their histologic profile or pathogenetic significance. Usually, they do not cause hemodynamic disorders, but are believed to be the main precursors of an atherosclerotic plaque, particularly for the coronary circulation, although not unanimous opinions exist on the subject.

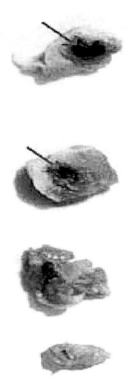

Figure 7.1.

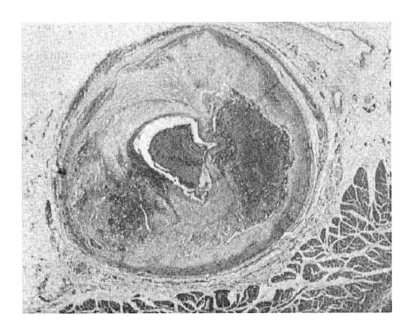

Figure 7.2.

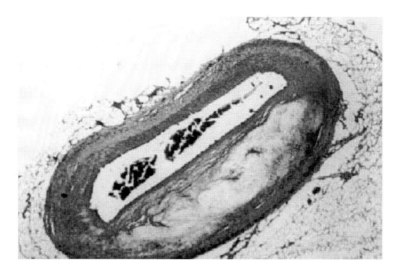

Figure 7.3.

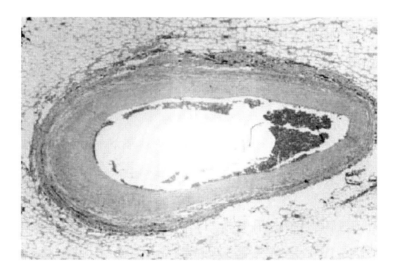

Figure 7.4.

Figure 7.1 to 7.4. Different alterations of coronary arteries due to atherosclerotic lesions of different degree and type. Figure 7.1 shows, macroscopically, the vessel lumen totally occluded by an old thrombus (red arrow); the thrombus narrows almost totally (95 percent of narrowing) vessel lumen on the coronary segment immediately below (red arrow). It is also showing the arterial wall with calcification. Histologically, the lumen of the vessel is occluded for about 95 percent by an old thrombus and arterial wall shows calcific deposits (figure 7.2.). Figure 7.3. shows an eccentric narrowing with incomplete occlusion of the vessel lumen by an atherosclerotic plaque that is filled by lipid material and irregular calcium deposits. Figure 7.4. shows minimal atherosclerosis changes. One can see that the vessel lumen is almost totally patent and irregular breaking of intima may be observed. Observing these different figures, there is evidence of the "mosaic" of alterations that can characterize atherosclerotic disease. (Reproduced, with permission, from: *Passive Smoking and Cardiovascular Pathology: Mechanisms and Physiopathological Bases of Damage*, A. Leone ed., Nova Science Publishers, Inc. New York, 2007).

Microscopically, the fatty streaks appear to be formed by small fusiform or stellate cells of probable myo-intimal matrix containing poor amounts of lipid drops as well as by a series of bigger poligonal cells containing lipophagic vacuoles and a dense nucleus in contrast with the cytoplasmic paleness due to vacuoles themselves. Such a composition makes very probable the hypothesis that fatty streaks can be one of the first manifestations of the metabolic lipid alteration which characterizes plaque development.

Now, an important question arises: are the fatty streaks really the first precursors of an atherosclerotic plaque?

Different opinions exist since the abdominal aorta, that is the structure where fatty streaks are not particularly encountered, is the main localization of the atherosclerotic plaque. Conversely, fatty streaks are mainly localized along the course of thoracic aorta and their regression may be identified in humans [46–48]. In contrast, for the coronary circulation an atherosclerotic plaque develops almost always where fatty streaks had appeared [49].

The question is still widely debated. However, there is evidence that fatty streaks are widely diffused on the arterial wall and may undergo reduction in size or disappearance particularly on aorta as it has been well documented. In the coronary artery, particularly in individuals with major coronary risk factors, they usually are active precursors of an atherosclerotic plaque.

Finally, minor atherosclerotic coronary lesions inconstantly described have been identified as alterations that may influence plaque growing [50], although their role is far from being completely assessed.

Histologically, these minor lesions like an intimal cushion with prevailing muscoloelastic structure without lipids and gelatinous lesions, which contain a large amount of lipids, particularly cholesterol, do not occlude vessel lumen, and, yet, when they may be identified, are, usually, localized at the artery braching.

There is also evidence that atherosclerotic arteries tend to undergo compensatory vessel enlargement to respond to the progressive atherosclerotic plaque growth that characterizes plaque formation [51–53]. The extension and size of this enlargement varies according to different factors, and failure in this compensatory mechanism of coronary artery could determine the development of significant coronary lesions [54] with, consequently, crucial changes in coronary blood flow which are similar to what occurs in several vascular districts of the body. Indeed, atherosclerosis affects elastic and larger muscular arteries with a stronger prevalence for those vessels which supply blood to heart, brain, kidney and legs.

Atherosclerotic change leads, absolutely, to final coronary artery remodeling. It influences significantly physiological responses of these vessels with reduced blood flow supply to myocardium under stress or, sometines, even at rest.

Pathogenesis of Atherosclerosis

As just mentioned, three major components belong to atherosclerotic lesions. Firstly, a cellular component consisting particularly of smooth muscle cells and macrophages; secondly, a matrix of connective tissue in different amounts and extracellular lipids; thirdly, intracellular lipids distributed diffusely but primarily accumulating into macrophages which are converted into foam-cells. Pathogenetic mechanisms of a multifactorial disease like atherosclerosis are directed towards lesion components.

Two theories have been hypothesized to explain the basic mechanisms of atherosclerosis: 1. A primary marked lipid role capable of initiating the disease, and 2. A repeated acute or chronic endothelial injury, largely based on the Virchow's insudation theory, which suggested that the lesions that led to atherosclerosis were a consequence of an initial abnormal response to repeated endothelial stressing stimuli [25, 55]. These two theories may, probably, explain together the multifactorial etiology of the disease.

The lipid hypothesis involves primarily a disorder of lipid metabolism as a basic mechanism of fatty accumulation which will conduct to atherosclerosis.

Elevated plasma LDL-Cholesterol concentrations cause penetration of the substance into the arterial wall as well as its accumulation in smooth muscle cells and macrophages with a consequent lipid-foam cell formation.

This phase is followed by all those dynamic processes which lead to fibrous cap formation as a final result. Lipid role in atherosclerosis will be discussed more widely in the section of this chapter on coronary risk factors related to atherosclerosis.

The lipid theory, once identified as the main initiating mechanism of atherosclerotic plaque formation has been, nowadays, replaced by the endothelial injury theory that formulates a primary endothelial change to develop the atherosclerotic process. However, accumulation of lipids is a basic factor for the development of those alterations that lead to a definite plaque as well as embolic complications. Embolization due to cholesterol or, generally, lipid debris may be a consequence of complications which may affect a vulnerable plaque resulting in ulceration. Usually, lipid debris may produce microemboli which, however, tend to occlude distally coronary branches.

Moreover, data that suggest a strong role of lipid metabolism in inducing coronary lesions are derived from both experimental and clinical observations. Experimentally, diets rich in lipid components are able to increase both plasma cholesterol concentrations and formation or progression of an atherosclerotic alteration. Similarly, in human pathology, there is evidence that increased blood cholesterol, particularly LDL-Cholesterol, is usually associated with markedly more severe atherosclerosis and, also, heart ischemic pathology.

Endothelial injury theory is well related to the Virchow hypothesis. It postulates that different factors may induce endothelial dysfunction, and, consequently, adhesion of platelets to subendothelium, increased platelet aggregation, monocyte chemotaxis with release of a monocyte-derived growth factors that move smooth muscle cells from the media into the intima. Then, smooth muscle cells replicate and synthesize the fibrous material, like connective tissue, collagen and proteoglycans, which stimulates fibrous plaque formation. Figure 7.5. displays the factors of Virchow's theory to explain endothelial activation following an abnormal stimulus.

Independently of the two hypotheses, there is no doubt that triggering factors, primarily major coronary risk factors, including smoking exposure [56] can activate those atherosclerotic mechanisms of damage proposed by the two theories.

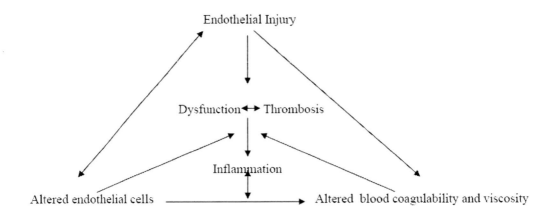

Figure 7.5. Virchow' theory for atherosclerotic plaque formation.. Endothelial integrity is the basic factor to avoid a triggering mechanism for atherosclerosis. Injured endothelial cells can activate all those mechanisms which lead to atherosclerotic plaque formation.

In addition to endothelial damage, smoking accelerates the development of atherosclerosis because its negative effects on lipid metabolism [57]. Moreover, early studies suggest that there are specific agents derived from cigarette smoking able to damage the arterial wall [58] as well as free radicals or different mutagens that activate smooth muscle cell proliferation [59].

Pathogenetic mechanisms which could explain both atherosclerosis and its complications [60–65] are, therefore, the result of an interaction among those structural components which are involved in the process.

A short mention is necessary of the role of inflammatory phenomena which influence atherosclerotic plaque formation. They, most often, are involved in explaining some atherosclerotic features although they seem to be factors which play their role once the atherosclerotic process has begun and are related primarily to endothelial activation, that would follow endothelial dysfunction. However, some reports would identify inflammation as a factor mediating all stages of atherosclerosis from the initiation through a progression and, ultimately, thrombotic complications [66].

Inflammatory marker elevation [67–73], primarily C-reactive protein, serum amyloid A, fibrinogen, and pro-inflammatory cytokines like interleukin-6 and interleukin-1 produced by lymphocyte-T-cells, has been identified, and would predict outcomes of acute coronary syndromes, independently of type and extension of myocardial damage. It is worth noting that lymphocyte-T-cells mediate actively the particular type of immunity called cell mediated immunity that, sometimes, is depressed in current smokers, particularly when they are heavy smokers.

Both intralesional or extralesional inflammation [66] could hasten atheroma evolution and precipitate acutely ischemic events.

In conclusion, the different pathogenetic hypotheses described as capable of explaining structural changes of atherosclerosis suggest a multifactorial etiology for this disease. Once begun, the atherosclerotic process develops in various steps through disruption and repair phenomena involving simultaneously the same or a different segment of the coronary artery wall. Therefore, lesions with a different degree of development may be seen to characterize the structure of the same plaque and, also, of the same coronary artery.

Risk Factors for Coronary Atherosclerosis

Epidemiologic findings have identified some risk factors which are capable of increasing the likelihood and incidence of atherosclerotic lesions as well as risk of non-fatal or fatal coronary pathology [74–79]. Therefore, idntifying and treating coronary risk factors are essential procedures to reduce coronary atherosclerosis and, then, prevent an atherothrombotic coronary event. The latter, however, can continue to appear without any known reason as to why its occurrence may be non-fatal or fatal.

The proven risk factors for atherosclerosis are listed in table 7.4. Among them, hypertension, lipoprotein changes, diabetes mellitus associated with obesity (metabolic syndrome), and cigarette smoking have been identified as major coronary risk factors and, therefore, will be described for their main characteristics in this chapter. These factors are closely linked to large-scale epidemiologic studies which would prove undoubtedly their role in atherosclerosis beginning and its progression. Moreover, individuals who display major coronary risk factors have also a greater incidence of ischemic cardiovascular events independent from the extension of atherosclerotic lesions.

Indeed, some limits exist when we analyze singularly the specific influence of a risk factor alone since, often, there is a variable association among them and that makes it hard to estimate its crucial role. However, the association of the major risk factors with atherosclerotic plaque is a markedly strong occurrence although with a variable degree for each individual.

The role of minor coronary risk factors has to be yet completely defined not for what is their role as risk factor for atherosclerosis, as, primarily, for their potential effect in inducing the disease.

Finally, there is a group, always increasing numerically, which includes all those risk factors not yet fully interpreted in their specific role. Among them, mental and/or physical stress, homocysteine and oxidative stress seem to play a significant role. However, primarily, observations on homocysteine would seem to identify a significant association of this substance with ischemic heart disease.

Hypertension

Hypertension has been proven undoubtedly to be a strong cardiovascular risk factor [80] also capable of promoting atherosclerosis. Indeed, individuals with elevated blood pressure show acceleration of both systemic and coronary atherosclerotic processes with a significantly major incidence of cardiac and cerebrovascular events.

Table 7.4. Proven risk factors for atherosclerosis

Major coronary risk factors	Hypertension
	Lipid metabolism disorders
	Smoking
	Diabetes mellitus
	Metabolic syndrome
Minor coronary risk factors	Male sex
	Pre- menopausal female + contraceptive drugs
	Age
	Family history
	Sedentary life
Risk factors to be fully interpreted	Mental or physical stress (chronic, acute?)
	Homocysteine
	Oxidative stress

Nowadays, emerging opinion is that hypertension is not the causative factor of the atherosclerosis but, on the contrary, a factor capable of stimulating and aggravating an atherosclerotic lesion when blood pressure is not satisfactorily controlled. Clinical trials have shown that lowering blood pressure below 140 mmHg for systolic and 90 mmHg for the diastolic measures determines both clinical and prognostic benefits [81]. Moreover, just recently, blood pressure measures from 120/80 mmHg to 139/89 mmHg have identified a pattern called prehypertension that is considered a precursor of stage 1 hypertension and predictor of excessive cardiovascular risk [82].

Mechanisms capable of accelerating and potentiating atherosclerosis through hypertension are of a different type: physical, metabolic, and biohumoral factors. There is evidence, however, that endothelial alterations play a crucial role [83–84].

Among physical factors, the shear stress on the arterial wall exerted by increased blood pressure particularly where vessels branch, associated with eddy currents of the blood, has been identified as a mechanism capable of aggravating atherosclerosis [85]. In coronary circulation, hypertension induces changes that accelerate atherosclerotic lesion progression associated also with plaque complications.

There is also evidence that various biochemical and humoral factors like renin, angiotensin, adrenergic substances, and others may induce either an increase in blood pressure or a direct damage of endothelial cells that predisposes to atherosclerosis, as described in Chapter 4.

Finally, hypertension coupled with an atherosclerotic diet [86] has been shown to increase the extent of aortic and coronary lesions in proportion to the elevation in arterial blood pressure and, furthermore, modified and impaired structural characteristics of the lesions.

A factor that plays a crucial role in linking coronary atherosclerosis and hypertension is the increase in the heart working determined by elevated blood pressure. Such an occurrence requires a major amount in oxygen availability for cardiac function and atherosclerotic coronary arteries may supply poorly when evident limits exist to adjust coronary blood flow because of coronary lesions. This mechanism, although it is an indirect mechanism of further damage, potentiates, however, the effects described in the relationship between coronary atherosclerosis and hypertension.

Finally, it is worth noting that all these mechanisms, by which hypertension may influence negatively atherosclerotic disease, are the same exerted by cigarette smoking in both current smokers or individuals exposed passively to burned tobacco.

Lipid Disorders

Metabolic disorders of lipoproteins are probably the strongest risk factor which influences type, extension and complications of atherosclerotic disease.

Metabolically, lipoproteins [87] are the result of an interaction between body adipose tissue and diet. These two factors form fatty acids which are esterified into triglycerides in the liver. Moreover, the liver may synthesize directly a variable amount of fatty acids using acetate as a substrate. Triglycerides produce esterified cholesterol and, then, cholesterol-lipoprotein through a series of enzymatic reactions involving mainly a metabolic process of esterification.

Five types of lipoproteins differing primarily in fatty compound, size and density are those components of lipid metabolism involved in the atherosclerotic process, although with a different degree and role. Also differences linked to the association with other risk factors have been identified. Smoking, including also passive exposure [88–92], would seem to lower HDL-Cholesterol levels. Indeed, HDL-Cholesterol higher blood concentrations play evident antiatherogenic effects.

The types of lipoproteins classified according to their increase in size and decrease in density are as follows: 1. Chylomicrons, where triglycerides are the major lipid component; 2. Very low-density lipoproteins (VLDL), where triglycerides are, again, the major lipid component; 3. Intermediate-density lipoproteins (IDL) with cholesteryl ester as a major component; 4. Low-density lipoproteins (LDL) containing mainly cholesteryl ester; 5. High-density lipoproteins (HDL), where a mixture of cholesteryl ester and phospholipids may be found.

Among those lipoproteins which exert an atherogenic effect, LDL-Cholesterol plays a strong role.

Oxidized LDL-Cholesterol is the major precursor of atherogenesis entering various stages of those processes which lead to plaque formation as well as complications. Oxidation of LDL-Cholesterol leads monocytes to bind endothelial cells and, therefore, a successive migration of them into the intima of the arterial wall occurs. This process contributes to form foam cells within the fatty streaks.

Then, the foam cells begin to secrete proinflammatory cytokines that maintain a chemotactic stimulus for adherent leukocytes, augment expression of scavenger receptors, and promote macrophage replication [8]. Circulating lymphocytes are also involved in forming atherosclerotic plaque through the interaction with endothelial adhesion molecules [93]. Then, these phenomena lead to the formation of the "lipid core" that induces a progression of the atherosclerotic lesion as one can see from table 7.2. Lipid core size is a basic feature that can influence the composition of an atherosclerotic plaque.

In contrast, HDL-Cholesterol develops its preventive effects on atherosclerotic plaque through an inhibition of foam cell formation and LDL-Cholesterol oxidation. Also the appearance of endothelial dysfunction is hindered by HDL-Cholesterol. These effects of HDL-Cholesterol may be explained by two main mechanisms [91, 94].

Firstly, HDL-Cholesterol removes cholesterol excess from blood vessels, moves cholesterol excess into the liver where it may be excreted by bile. This property of HDL-Cholesterol transport has been defined as reverse cholesterol transport.

Secondly, HDL-Cholesterol impedes induced-LDL-Cholesterol oxidation following an oxidative stress and, therefore, exerts antioxidant properties.

Oxidative stress is a term used to describe the level of structural damage caused by free oxygen radicals in a cell, tissue or organ. Free oxygen radicals are a group of substances produced by chemical reactions that involve oxygen metabolism, and exist in all aerobic organisms. Usually, endogenous sources originate these compounds. There are, however, free oxygen radicals derived from exogenous sources like cigarette smoking [95], that plays a crucial role, although not the strongest, in inducing free oxygen radical formation. Formation of free radicals is the metabolic result of oxidative reactions that characterize intracellular respiratory phenomena [96-97].

Generally, free oxygen radicals determine an excessive LDL-Cholesterol oxidation with possible triggering of atherosclerotic process. Moreover, there is evidence [97] that children exposed to passive smoking are damaged as a consequence of oxidative stress at different levels, including atherosclerosis. Therefore, one can conclude that the large majority of lipoproteins has pro-atherogenic effects unless HDL-Cholesterol. Thus, establishing those HDL-Cholesterol and LDL- Cholesterol concentrations respectively below or above which there is a close relationship respectively with atherosclerotic regression or progression, would be a benefit to prevent effectively atherosclerosis development as suggested by reports [98].

When HDL-Cholesterol, defined generically as "good cholesterol", reaches a blood concentration below 40 mg/dL, it seems to increase the risk of coronary heart disease and worsens atherosclerotic lesions since excess cholesterol from atherosclerotic coronary plaque is not removed.

Similarly, but with much more negative results, LDL-Cholesterol in high blood concentrations build up in the inner walls of coronary arteries determining lesion growth and raising the incidence of heart attacks. Table 7.5. analyzes blood LDL-Cholesterol levels estimated as effective or not to control atherosclerosis progression.

Table 7.5. LDL-Cholesterol levels and their role in inducing atherosclerosis

LDL-Cholesterol Concentrations (mg/dL)	Risk of atherosclerosis
Less than 100	Weak
100 to 129	Borderline/mild
130 to 159	Moderate/high
160 to 189	High
190 and up	Highest

Diabetes Mellitus and Insulin Resistance Syndrome

Diabetes mellitus is an independent modifiable risk factor of atherosclerosis as well as insulin resistance [99–100], that is strongly related to glucose metabolism alterations, although some other metabolic and humoral patterns are, usually, involved negatively for the pathogenesis of this syndrome.

Large-scale studies on populations showed an association of hyperglycemia with coronary atherosclerosis, although the levels of increase in blood glucose did not relate grossly to the degree of development of atherosclerotic lesion [101].

Not only are individuals affected by diabetes mellitus at an increased risk of developing coronary atherosclerosis, but the atherosclerotic process also tends to be, usually, accelerated, more severe and more widespread.

Since atherosclerosis damages primarily large and medium blood vessels, the term macroangiopathy, that is considered as a pathology of large and medium caliber arteries and a consequence of the damage caused by diabetes on atherosclerotic arteries, is often used to identify the association of atherosclerosis and diabetes. Also microangiopathy that affects, conversely, small vessels and capillaries in diabetic patients may contribute to aggravate coronary atherosclerosis of large-medium vessels since it determines a further impairment of coronary blood flow because of the reduction in patency of the vascular bed.

A complex series of factors would regulate the interaction which exists among the two diseases.

Moreover, one most keep in mind that almost all major coronary risk factors are often associated in diabetic patients, and such an occurrence makes it hard to establish which type and degree of coronary altarations are due to diabetes alone rather than association with other factors.

The relationship between atherosclerosis and diabetes, however, does not provide unanimous results. In an autopsy study [102] that examined both coronary vessel and myocardial lesions in diabetic patients, there was evidence that men with mild atherosclerosis had smaller and larger myocardial lesions not associated with a proportional increase in atherosclerosis. Therefore, myocardial alterations of diabetic patients would develop independently from atherosclerosis progression.

Thus, hyperglycemia and atherosclerosis are usually associated, since there is a significant prevalence of large vessel disease in studied populations who display diabetes mellitus and, on the other hand, an increased incidence of hyperglycemia is associated with atherosclerosis.

It is also worth noting that increased release of catecholamines may be seen in diabetics, and the role of catecholamines in inducing atherosclerotic lesions has been well established and described previously in this book.

Increased insulin resistance is also recognized as an independent risk factor for coronary heart disease [103].

Such an assessment leads to establishing either a definition of insulin resistance syndrome or its potential role as risk factor for coronary heart disease [95, 104–113].

Insulin resistance syndrome, also called metabolic syndrome or syndrome X, has been widely described by Reaven. The syndrome is characterized by various clinical and metabolic disorders (table 7.6.) consisting of obesity, increased blood pressure, changes in lipid profile with elevated LDL-Cholesterol and low HDL-Cholesterol, increased triglyceride blood concentrations, and elevated blood insulin levels which are recognized as the main pathogenetic mechanism.

Metabolic syndrome is highly prevalent in some countries worldwide, among these the United States and North East Asia as if there was a racial predisposition.

Metabolic syndrome has been identified as a disease capable of increasing the risk for developing type 2 diabetes and cardiovascular disease, and it is also associated with an all-cause mortality.

Also a relationship with cigarette smoking has been hypothesized.

Cigarette smoking can stimulate and impair those metabolic alterations that characterize the syndrome in view of the multiple mechanisms capable of negatively influencing, by its chemical compounds, the different structures deputed to the control of the main steps of the biochemical and hormonal metabolism, the changes of which are the pathogenetic substrate of the disease.

Table 7.6. Main clinical and metabolic signs of metabolic syndrome

Metabolic changes	Clinical signs	Involved parameter
Glucose metabolism	Type 2 diabetes mellitus	Hyperglycemia
	Abdominal obesity	Hyperinsulinemia
	Sub-clinical inflammation	Insulin resistance
Lipid metabolism	Coronary atherosclerosis	LDL-C increase
		HDL-C decrease
		Triglyceride increase
	Endothelial dysfunction	All
Coagulation-fibrinolysis	Thrombo-embolic events	Fibrinogen
		Other hematologic factors

Pathogenesis of this syndrome recognizes a various, but elevated, degree of insulin resistance in two levels: adipose tissue and muscle. Syndrome may be also associated with endothelial dysfunction and thrombo-embolic phenomena.

Physical inactivity, excess weight gain, high alcohol intake, and certain dietary components have been identified as modifiable risk factors for metabolic syndrome and its complications.

Evidence indicates, however, that metabolic syndrome is a clinical pattern capable of accelerating and aggravating coronary atherosclerosis at any step of development. Its basic type of action would involve metabolic mechanisms that can determine either functional or structural changes in coronary arteries.

Cigarette Smoking

There are consistent data that permit one to recognize cigarette smoking as one of the major risk factors for atherosclerotic plaque formation and appearance of ischemic heart disease.

Both types of smoking, active smoking and passive smoking, damage heart and coronary [114–136] arteries by a double mechanism: a direct action of tobacco smoking toxics, particularly nicotine and carbon monoxide, on the structural constituents of the arterial wall, and an indirect mechanism mediated by systemic structures like sympathetic system, adrenergic system, and endothelium which are all together primarily involved in triggering the atherosclerotic process. Therefore, the cardiovascular system must be considered a target organ for smoking, and the type of damage produced on the coronary arteries recognizes multiple pathogenetic mechanisms.

Mechanisms of damage are known to be a repeated occurrence of endothelial dysfunction, changes in blood coagulation cascade and platelet function [127, 130-133–136], lipid metabolism disorders [137], and, however, all those functional and biochemical factors which can favor the development of thrombosis [136]. Also current association of passive smoking exposure with other major cardiovascular risk factors accelerates the progression of atherosclerosis.

However, atherosclerotic plaque formation related to passive smoking exposure usually tends to appear late and pathologic events, particularly of the ischemic type, are due to complications of an atherosclerotic lesion that more often has become an irreversible structural alteration [136].

A strong interaction exists between smoking and other coronary risk factors. Among these, a closer relationship links cigarette smoking with lipid disorders and some hemostatic parameters.

Smoking is often associated with lower HDL-Cholesterol and increased LDL-Cholesterol and triglycerides. At the same time, smoking raises plasma fibrinogen levels. Both these parameters influence strongly either atherosclerotic plaque formation and growth or appearance of plaque complications. Moreover, changes in platelet function [127] may initiate, accelerate and also aggravate atherosclerosis, and there is evidence that cigarette smoking can raise either acutely or chronically platelet adhesiveness and aggregation.

Finally, smoking causes specific lesions on the coronary circulation that will be analyzed in Chapter 9.

About the appearance of clinical symptoms related to smoking alone or smoking associated with other coronary risk factors, three pathogenetic mechanisms have been postulated: firstly, occlusive thrombosis superimposed at a level of an atherosclerotic plaque; secondly, plaque growing without occlusive thrombi and, consequently, production of a significant narrowing of the arterial lumen; thirdly, blood flow reduction due to external factors that precipitate an unstable coronary vascular response.

All these mechanisms can cause impairment in arterial blood flow but, however, they may act, to do it, only when the atherosclerotic plaque is formed. Therefore, it is usual that clinical events will appear several years later from the origin of the lesions as well as influence of risk factors, unless functional disorders due to experimentally acute exposure to smoking [114].

Atherosclerotic Plaque Evolution and Instability

During plaque evolution, changes in fibrous cap thickness have been documented [8, 38, 66]. They are mediated particularly by inflammatory phenomena at the site of atheroma where inflammatory cells release a number of proinflammatory agents like cytokines and some others. Degradation in arterial extracellular matrix formed particularly by connective tissue is associated with "plaque inflammation" and these events together weaken the structure of fibrous cap determining also its instability and, consequently, a greater incidence of complications.

Plaque instability is, therefore, one of the major determinants of ischemic acute events appearing. Continuous phenomena of plaque damage and repair associated often with cardiovascular risk factors exert a detrimental impact on coronary artery wall, and, then, further impair those adjustments of coronary blood flow that the heart could demand.

A reduction in fat intake, avoidance of obesity, smoking cessation, physical activity, and drugs in some cases [138–139], are recommended to control both coronary atherosclerosis development and plaque instability.

Also thrombus formation follows plaque instability. Vulnerable plaque [140] easily undergoes rupture which occurs more frequently as its volume is bigger and macrophage content elevated.

The events that follow plaque disruption lead to the appearance of hemorrhagic or thrombotic phenomena that may determine a stronger degree of coronary narrowings, thrombo-embolic complications or, in some cases, newer plaque healing. Plaque cap final structure, therefore, may change continuously as a result of intercurrent destructive-degenerative or repair processes, that are usually grown by hard collagen deposition.

A balance between pro-atherosclerotic and antiatherosclerotic factors regulate, probably, plaque formation, although the causes of triggering and progressing mechanisms are yet far from being fully clarified.

References

[1]   Ross R. Factors influencing atherogenesis. In: *Hurst's The Heart* 9th Edition, Alexander WR, Schlant RC, Fuster V, eds., McGraw-Hill, New York, NY,USA 1998; 1139 – 59.

[2]   Gould SE, Ioannides G. Diseases of the Coronary Vessels. In: *Pathology of the Heart and Blood Vessels* 3rd Edition, Gould SE ed, Charles C Thomas, Springfield, Ill, USA 1968; 545- 600.

[3]   Libby P. The vascular biology of atherosclerosis. In: *Braunwald's Heart Disease- A textbook of cardiovascular medicine* 7th Edition, Zipes DP, Libby P, Bonow RO, Braunwald E eds., Elsevier Saunders, Philadelphia, Penn, USA 2005; 921 – 37.

[4]   Falk E, Shah PK, Fuster V. Atherothrombosis and thrombosis-prone plaques. In: *Hurst's The Heart* 11th Edition, Fuster V, Alexander WR, O'Rourke RA eds, McGraw-Hill, New York, NY, USA 2004; 1123 – 39.

[5] Fuster V, IP JHJ , Kiung Jang IK, Chesebro JH. Antithrombotic therapy in cardiac disease. In: *Cardiology* 7th Edition, Parmley WW and Chatterjee K eds, Lippincott-Raven, Philadelphia-New York, USA 1994; Vol 1(25): 1 – 40.

[6] Varnava A. Coronary artery remodelling. *Heart.* 1998; 79: 109 – 10.

[7] Marchand F (1904). In:Aschoff L, Introduction. *Arteriosclerosis: A survey of the problem.* Cowdry EV ed, McMillan, New York, NY, USA 1933; 1 – 18.

[8] Libby P. Inflammation in atherosclerosis. *Nature.* 2002; 420: 868 – 74.

[9] Stary HC, Chandler AB, Glagov S, Guyton JR, Insull W Jr, Rosenfeld ME, Schaffer A, Schwartz CJ, Wagner WD, Wissler RW. A definition of initial, fatty streak, and intermediate lesions of atherosclerosis: a report from the Committee on Vascular Lesions of the Council on Arteriosclerosis, American Heart Association. Special report. *Arterioscler. Thromb.* 1994; 14: 840 – 56.

[10] Dartsch PC, Bauriedel G, Schinko I, Weiss HD, Hofling B, Betz E. Cell constitution and characteristics of human atherosclerotic plaques selectively removed by percutaneous atherectomy. *Atherosclerosis.* 1989; 80: 149 – 57.

[11] Simons M, Leclerc G, Safian RD, Isner JM, Weir L, Baim DS. Relation between activated smooth-muscle cells in coronary-artery lesions and restenosis after atherectomy. *N. Engl. J. Med.* 1993; 328: 608 – 13.

[12] Hofling B, Welsch U, Heimerl J, Gonschior P, Bauriedel G. Analysis of atherectomy specimens. *Am. J. Cardiol.* 1993; 72: E96 – 107.

[13] Rosenschein U, Ellis SG, Haudenschild CC, Yakubov SJ, Muller DW, Dick RJ, Topol EJ. Comparison of histopathologic coronary lesions obtained from directional atherectomy in stable angina versus acute coronary syndromes. *Am. J. Cardiol.* 1994; 73: 508 – 10.

[14] Stary HC. Evolution and progression of atherosclerotic lesions in coronary arteries of children and young adults. *Arteriosclerosis.* 1898; 9 (Suppl 1): I-19 – 32.

[15] Glagov S, Weisenberg E, Zarins CK, Stankunavicius R, Kolettis GJ. Compensatory enlargement of human atherosclerotic coronary arteries. *N. Engl. J. Med.* 1987; 316: 1371 – 5.

[16] Ross R, Wight TN, Strandness E, Thiele B. Human atherosclerosis, I: cell constitution and characteristics of advanced lesions of the superficial femoral artery. *Am. J. Pathol.* 1984; 114:79 – 93.

[17] Pouchlev A, Youroukova Z, Kiprov D. A study of changes in the number of mast cells in the human arterial wall during the stages of development of atherosclerosis. *J. Atheroscler. Res.* 1966; 6: 342 – 51.

[18] Pomerance A. Peri-arterial mast cells in coronary atheroma and thrombosis. *J. Pathol. Bact.* 1958; 76: 55 – 70.

[19] Glagov S, Zarins C, Giddens DP, Ku DN. Hemodynamics and atherosclerosis: insights and perspectives gained from studies of human arteries. *Arch. Pathol. Lab. Med.* 1988; 112: 1018 – 31.

[20] Stary HC, Chandler AB, Dinsmore RE, Fuster V, Glagov S, Insull W Jr, Rosenfeld ME, Schwartz CJ, Wagner WD, Wissler RW. A definition of advanced types of atherosclerotic lesions and a histological classification of atherosclerosis: a report from

the Committee on Vascular Lesions of the Council on Arteriosclerosis, American Heart Association. *Circulation.* 1995; 92: 1355 – 74.

[21]   Sandison AT. Persistence of sudanophilic lipid in sections of mummified tissue. *Nature.* 1959; 183: 196 – 7.

[22]   Ruffer MA. Histological studies on Egyptian Mummies. *Mem à l'Institut Egyptien.* 1911; 6: Fasc. 3.

[23]   Ruffer MA. On arterial lesions found in Egyptian mummies (1580 B.C. – 525 A.D.). *J. Path. Bact.* 1911; 15: 453 – 462.

[24]   Shattock SG. A report upon the pathological condition of the aorta of King Memeptah. *Proc. Roy Soc. Med.* (Pathological Section) 1909; 2: 122 – 7.

[25]   Virchow R. Phlogose und thrombose im Gefassystem. In: *Gesammelte Abhanndlugen zur wissensehaftlichen medizin.* F Meidinger Sohn and Company, Frankfurt-am- Main, German, 1856; 458 – 521.

[26]   Tapp E, Wildsmith K. The autopsy and endoscopy in the Leeds mummy. In: *The Mummy Tale.* David AR and Tapp E eds., Michael O'Mara Books, London, UK 1992; 132 – 53.

[27]   Fejfar Z, Hlavackova L. Profiles in cardiology. Karl Rokitansky. *Clin. Cardiol.* 1997; 20: 816 – 8.

[28]   Ignatowski AC. Influence of animal food on the organism of rabbits. *Izv. Imp. voyenno- Med. Akad. Peter.* 1908; 16: 154 – 73.

[29]   Anitschkow NN, Chalatov S. Ueber experimentelle Choleserinsteatose und ihre bedeutung fur die entstehung einiger pathologischer prozesse. *Zentralbl. Allg. Pathol.* 1913; 24: 1 – 9.

[30]   Anitschkow N. Ueber die veranderungen der kaninchenaorta bei experimenteller cholesterinsteatose. *Beitr. Pathol. Anat.* 1913; 56: 379 – 404.

[31]   Anitschkow N. Experimental atherosclerosis in animals. In: *Arteriosclerosis*, Cowdry EV ed, McMillan, New York, NY, USA, 1933; 271 – 322.

[32]   Wolkoff K. Uber die atherosklerose der coronararterien des herzens. *Beitr. Path. Anat.* 1929; 82: 555 – 96.

[33]   Gore I, Robertson WB, Hirst AE, Hadley GG, Koseki Y. Geographic differences in the severity of aortic and coronary atherosclerosis: the U.S., Jamaica, W.L., South India, and Japan. *Amer. J. Path.* 1960; 36: 559 – 74.

[34]   Zinserling WD. Untersuchungen uber atherosclerose. I. Uber die aortenverfettung bei kindern. *Virchow Arch. Path. Anat.* 1925; 225: 677 – 705.

[35]   Holman RL, McGill HC Jr, Strong JP, Geer JC. The natural history of atherosclerosis. The early aortic lesions as seen in New Orleans in the middle of the 20th century. *Am. J. Path.* 1958; 34: 209 – 35.

[36]   Monckenberg JG. Mediaverkalkung und atherosklerose. *Vircows Arch. Path. Anat.* 1914; 216: 408 – 16

[37]   .Stary HC, Blankenhorn DH, Chandler AB, Glagov S, Insull W Jr, Richardson M, Rosenfeld ME, Schaffer SA, Schwartz CJ, Wagner WD, Wissler RW. A definition of the intima of human arteries and of its atherosclerosis-prone regions: a report from the Committee on Vascular Lesions of the Council on Arteriosclerosis. American Heart Association. Special Report. *Circulation.* 1992; 85: 391 – 405.

[38] Ross R. The pathogenesis of atherosclerosis: A perspective for the 1990s. *Nature.* 1993; 362: 801 – 9.

[39] Faggiotto A, Ross R, Harker L. Studies of hypercholesterolemia in the non-human primate: I. Changes that lead to fatty streak formation. *Arteriosclerosis.* 1984; 4: 323 – 40.

[40] Tracy RE, Devaney K, Kissling G. Characteristics of the plaque under a coronary thrombus. *Virchows Arch. A Pathol. Anat. Histopathol.* 1985; 405: 411 – 27.

[41] Davies MJ, Thomas AC. Plaque fissuring: the cause of acute myocardial infarction, sudden ischemic death, and crescendo angina. *Br. Heart J.* 1985; 53: 363 – 73.

[42] Falk E. Morphologic features of unstable atherothrombotic plaques underlying acute coronary syndromes. *Am. J. Cardiol.* 1989; 63: E114 – 120.

[43] Falk E. Why do plaques rupture? *Circulation.* 1992; 86: SIII 30 – 42.

[44] Richardson PD, Davies MJ, Born GV. Influence of plaque configuration and stress distribution on fissuring of coronary atherosclerotic plaques. *Lancet.* 1989; 2: 941 – 4.

[45] Van der Wal AC, Becker AE, Van der Loos CM, Das PK. Site of intimal rupture or erosion of thrombosed coronary atherosclerotic plaques is characterized by an inflammatory process irrespective of the dominant plaque morphology. *Circulation.* 1994; 89: 36 – 44.

[46] Wissler RW, Vesselinovitch D. Regression of atherosclerosis in experimental animals and man. *Mod. Conc. Cardiovasc. Dis.* 1977; 46: 27 – 32.

[47] Nissen SE, Tuzcu EM, Schoenahangen P, Brown BG, Ganz P, Vogel RA, Crowe T, Howard G, Cooper CJ, Brodie B, Grines CL, De Maria AN, for the REVERSAL Investigators. Effect of intensive compared with moderate lipid-lowering therapy on progression of coronary atherosclerosis: a randomized controlled trial. *JAMA.* 2004; 291: 1071 – 80.

[48] Ballantyne CM, Herd JA, Dunn JK, Jones PH, Farmer JA, Gotto AM Jr. Effects of lipid-lowering therapy on progression of coronary and carotid artery disease. *Curr. Opin. Lipidol.* 1997; 8: 354 – 61.

[49] Moore S, Friedman RJ, Gent M. Evolution of fatty streak to fibrous plaque in injury-induced atherosclerosis. *Fed. Proc.* 1975; 34: 875A.

[50] Smith EB. Molecular interactions in human atherosclerotic plaques. *Am. J. Pathol.* 1977; 86: 665 -

[51] von Birgelen C, Mintz GS, de Vrey EA, Kimura T, Popma JJ, Airiian SG, Leon MB, Nobuyoshy M, Serruys PW, de Feyter PJ. Atherosclerotic coronary lesions with inadequate compensatory enlargement have smaller plaque and vessel volumes: observations with three dimensional intravascular ultrasound in vivo. *Heart.* 1998; 79:137 – 42.

[52] Bond MG, Adams MR, Bullock BC. Complicating factors in evaluating coronary arterial atherosclerosis. *Artery.* 1981; 51: 434 – 9.

[53] Armstrong ML, Heistad DD, Marcus ML, Megan MB, Piegors DJ. Structural and hemodynamic response of peripheral arteries of macaque monkeys to atherogenic diet. *Arteriosclerosis.* 1985; 5: 336 – 46.

[54] Clarkson TB, Prichard RW, Morgan TM, Petrick GS, Klein KP. Remodeling of coronary arteries in human and nonhuman primates. *JAMA.* 1994; 271: 289 – 94.

[55] Ross R, Glomset JA. The pathogenesis of atherosclerosis, an update. *N. Engl. J. Med.* 1976; 295: 369 – 77.

[56] Leone A. Cigarette smoking and cardiovascular damage: analytic review of the subject. *Singapore Med. J.* 1994; 35: 492 – 4.

[57] Barnoya J, Glantz SA. Cardiovascular effects of secondhand smoke: nearly as large as smoking. *Circulation.* 2005; 111:2684 – 98.

[58] Becker CG, Dubin T, Wiedemann HP. Hypersensitivity to tobacco antigen. *Proc. Natl. Acad. Sci. USA.* 1976; 73: 1712 – 6.

[59] Stafford RS, Becker CG. Cigarette smoking and atherosclerosis. In: Fuster V, Ross R, Topol EJ eds. *Atherosclerosis and Coronary Artery Disease*; Lippincott-Raven, Philadelphia, USA, 1996: 303 – 25.

[60] Abrams J. Role of endothelial dysfunction in coronary artery disease. *Am. J. Cardiol.* 1997; 79: 2 – 9.

[61] Davies MJ, Woolf N, Rowles PM, Pepper J. Morphology of the endothelium over atherosclerotic plaques in human coronary arteries. *Br. Heart J.* 1988; 60: 459 – 64.

[62] Davies MJ. A macro and micro view of coronary vascular insult in ischemic heart disease. *Circulation.* 1990; 82 (Suppl 3): II38 – 46.

[63] Danenberg HD, Szalai AJ, Swaminathan RV, Peng L, Chen Z, Seifert P, Fay WP, Simon DI, Edelman ER. Increased thrombosis after arterial injury in human C-reactive protein-transgenic mice. *Circulation.* 2003; 108: 512 – 5.

[64] Kolodgie FD, Gold HK, Burke AP, Fowler DR, Kruth HS, Weber DK, Farb A, Guerrero LJ, Hayase M, Kutys R, Narula J, Finn AV, Virmani R. Intraplaque hemorrhage and progression of coronary atheroma. *N. Engl. J. Med.* 2003; 349: 2316 – 25.

[65] Kockx MM, Cromheeke KM, Knaapen MWM, Bosmans JM, De Meyer GRY, Herman AG, Bult H. Phagocytosis and macrophage activation associated with hemorrhagic microvessels in human atherosclerosis. *Arterioscler. Thromb. Vasc. Biol.* 2003; 23: 440 – 6.

[66] Libby P, Ridker P, Maseri A. Inflammation and atherosclerosis. *Circulation.* 2002;105: 1135 – 43.

[67] Berk BC, Weintraub WS, Alexander RW. Elevation of C-reactive protein in "active" coronary artery disease. *Am. J. Cardiol.* 1990; 65: 168 – 72.

[68] Liuzzo G, Biasucci LM, Gallimore JR, Grillo RL, Rebuzzi AG, Pepys MB, Maseri A. The prognostic value of C-reactive protein and serum amyloid A protein in severe unstable angina. *N. Engl. J. Med.* 1994; 331: 417 – 24.

[69] Rebuzzi AG, Quaranta G, Liuzzo G, Caligiuri G, Lanza GA, Gallimore JR, Grillo RL, Cianflone D, Biasucci LM, Maseri A. Incremental prognostic value of serum levels of troponin T and C-reactive protein on admission in patients with unstable angina pectoris. *Am. J. Cardiol.* 1998; 82: 715 – 9.

[70] de Vinter RJ, Heyde GS, Koch KT, Fischer J, van Straalen JP, Bax M, Schotborgh CE, Mulder KJ, Sanders GT, Piek JJ, Tijssen JGP. The prognostic value of pre-procedural plasma C-reactive protein in patients undergoing elective coronary angioplasty. *Eur. Heart J.* 2002; 23: 960 – 6.

[71] Morrow DA, Rifai N, Antman EM, Weiner DL, McCabe CH, Cannon CP,Braunwald E. Serum amyloid A predicts early mortality in acute coronary syndromes: A TIMI IIA substudy. *J. Am. Coll. Cardiol.* 2000; 35: 358 – 62.

[72] Toss H, Lindahl B, Siegbahn A, Wallentin L, for the FRISC Study Group. Prognostic influence of increased fibrinogen and C-reactive protein levels in unstable coronary artery disease. *Circulation.* 1997; 96: 4204 – 10.

[73] Heeschen C, Hamm CW, Bruemmer J, Simoons ML. Predictive value of C-reactive protein and troponin T in patients with unstable angina: a comparative analysis. CAPTURE investigators. Chimeric C7e3 Antiplatelet Therapy in Unstable Angina Refractory to Standard Treatment Trial. *J. Am. Coll. Cardiol.* 2000; 35: 1535 – 42.

[74] McGill HC Jr. Risk factors for atherosclerosis. *Adv Exp Med Biol* 1978; 104: 273 – 80.

[75] Martin MJ, Hulley SB, Browner WS, Kuller LH, Wentworth D. Serum cholesterol, blood pressure, and mortality: implications from a cohort of 361,662 men. *Lancet.* 1986; 25: 933 – 6.

[76] Stamler J, Wentworth D, Neaton JD. Is relationship between serum cholesterol and risk of premature death from coronary heart disease continuous and graded? Findings in 356,222 primary screenes of the Multiple Risk Factor Intervention Trial (MRFIT). *JAMA.* 1986; 256: 2823 – 8.

[77] Solberg LA, Strong JP. Risk factors and atherosclerotic lesions: a review of autopsy studies. *Arteriosclerosis.* 1983; 3: 187 – 98.

[78] Kuller LH, Tracy RP, Shaten J, Meilahn EN. Relation of C-reactive protein and coronary heart disease in the MRFIT nested case-control study. Multiple Risk Factor Intervention Trial. *Am. J. Epidemiol.* 1996; 144: 537 – 47.

[79] Schaefer EJ, Levy RI. Pathogenesis and management of lipoprotein disorders. *N. Engl. J. Med.* 1985; 312: 1300 – 10.

[80] Lewington S, Clarke R, Qizilbash N, Peto R, Collins R. Age-specific relevance of usual blood pressure to vascular mortality: a meta-analysis of individual data for one million adults in 61 prospective studies. *Lancet.* 2002; 360: 1903 – 13.

[81] Collins R, Peto R, MacMahon S, Hebert P, Fiebach NH, Eberlein KA, Godwin J, Qizilbash N, Taylor JO, Hennekens CM. Blood pressure, stroke, and coronary heart disease.Part 2, Short-term reductions in blood pressure: overview of randomised drug trials in their epidemiological context. *Lancet.* 1990; 335: 827 – 38.

[82] Julius S, Nesbitt SD, Egan BM, Weber MA, Michelson EL, Kaciroti N, Black HR, Grimm RH Jr, Messerli FH, Oparil S, Schork AM, for the Trial of Preventing Hypertension (TROPHY) Study Investigators. Feasibility of treating prehypertension with an angiotensin-receptor blocker. *N. Engl. J. Med.* 2006; 354: 1685 – 97.

[83] John S, Schmieder RE. Impaired endothelial function in arterial hypertension and hypercholesterolemia: potential mechanisms and differences. *J. Hypertens.* 2000; 18: 363 – 74.

[84] Ghiadoni L, Taddei S, Virdis A, Sudano I, Di Legge V, Meola M, Di Venanzio L, Salvetti A. Endothelial function and common carotid artery wall thickening in patients with essential hypertension. *Hypertension.* 1998; 32: 25 – 32.

[85] Fry DL. Hemodynamic forces in atherogenesis. In: *Cerebrovascular Disease,* Scheinberg, P. ed., Raven Press, New York, NY, USA, 1976; 77 – 95.

[86]   Pick R, Johnson PJ, Glick G. Deleterious effects of hypertension on the development of aortic and coronary atherosclerosis in stumptail macaques (macaca speciosa) on an atherogenic diet. *Circ. Res.* 1974; 35: 472 – 82.

[87]   Havel RJ, Kane JP. Structure and metabolism of plasma lipoproteins. In: *The Metabolic and Molecular Bases of Inherited Disease II*, Scriver CR, Beaudet AL, Sly WS, Valle D eds, 7th Ed, Mc-Graw-Hill, New York, NY, USA, 1995; 1841 – 51.

[88]   Mizoue T, Ueda R, Hino Y, Yoshimura T. Workplace exposure to environmental tobacco smoke and high density lipoprotein cholesterol among nonsmokers. *Am. J. Epidemiol.* 1999; 150: 1068 – 72.

[89]   Moffat RJ, Stamford BA, Biggerstaff KD. Influence of worksite environmental tobacco smoke on serum lipoprotein profiles of female non-smokers. *Metabolism.* 1995; 44: 1536 – 9.

[90]   Moffat RJ, Chelland SA, Pecott DL, Stamford BA. Acute exposure to environmental tobacco smoke reduces HDL1-C and HDL2-C. *Prev. Med.* 2004; 38: 637 – 41.

[91]   Kwiterovich PO Jr. The antiatherogenic role of high-density lipoprotein cholesterol. *Am. J. Cardiol.* 1998; 82: Q13 – 21.

[92]   Azizi F, Raiszadeh F, Salehi P, Rahmani M, Emami H, Ganbarian A, Hajipour R. Determinants of serum HDL-C level in a Tehran urban population: the Tehran Lipid and Glucose Study. *Nutr. Metab. Cardiovasc. Dis.* 2002; 12: 80 – 9.

[93]   Hansson GK, Libby P, Schonbeck U, Yan ZQ. Innate and adaptive immunity in the pathogenesis of atherosclerosis. *Circ. Res.* 2002; 91: 281 – 91.

[94]   Tall AR. An overview of reverse cholesterol transport. *Eur. Heart J.* 1998; 19: A31 – 5.

[95]   Block G, Dietrich M, Norkus EP, Morrow JD, Hudes M, Caan B, Packer L. Factors associated with oxidative stress in human population. *Am. J. Epidemiol.* 2002; 156: 274 – 85.

[96]   Harrison D, Griendling KK, Landmesser U, Hornig B, Drexler H. Role of oxidative stress in atherosclerosis. *Am. J. Cardiol.* 2003; 91: 7A – 11A.

[97]   Kosecik M, Erel O, Sevinc E, Selek S. Increased oxidative stress in children exposed to passive smoking. *Int. J. Cardiol.* 2005; 100: 61 – 4.

[98]   Barter P, Gotto AM, LaRosa JC, Maroni J, Szarek M, Grundy SM, Kastelein JJP, Bittner V, Fruchart JC, for the treating to New Targets Investigators. HDL cholesterol, very low levels of LDL cholesterol, and cardiovascular events. *N. Engl. J. Med.* 2007; 357: 1301 – 10.

[99]   Kendall DM, Sobel BE, Coulston AM, Peters-Harmel AL, McLean BK, Peregallo-Dittko V, Buse JB, Fonseca VA, Hill JO, Nesto RW, Sunyer FX. The insulin resistance syndrome and coronary artery disease. *Coron. Artery Dis.* 2003; 14: 335 – 48.

[100] Reaven GM. The insulin resistance syndrome: Definition and dietary approaches to treatment. *Annu. Rev. Nutr.* 2005; 25: 391 – 406.

[101] Gordon T, Castelli WP, Hjortland MC, Kannel WB, Dawber TR. Diabetes, blood lipids, and the role of obesity in coronary heart disease risk for women. The Framingham Study. *Ann. Intern. Med.* 1977; 87: 393 – 7.

[102] Burchfield CM, Reed DM, Marcus EB, Strong JP, Hayashi T. Association of diabetes mellitus with coronary atherosclerosis and myocardial lesions. An autopsy study from the Honolulu Heart Program. *Am. J. Epidemiol.* 1993; 137: 1328 – 40.

[103] Feskens EJ, Kromhout D. Cardiovascular risk factors and the 25-year incidence of diabetes mellitus in middle-aged men: the Zutphen Study. *Am. J. Epidemiol.* 1989; 130: 1101 – 8.

[104] Ronnemaa T, Ronnemaa EM, Pukka P, Pyorala K, Laakso M. Smoking independently associated with high plasma insulin levels in nondiabetic men. *Diabetes Care.* 1996; 19: 1229 – 32.

[105] Henkin L, Zaccaro D, Haffner S, Karter A, Rewers M, Sholinsky P, Wagenknecht L. Cigarette smoking, environmental tobacco smoke exposure and insulin sensitivity : The Insulin Resistance Atherosclerosis Study. *Ann. Epidemiol.* 1999; 9: 290 – 6.

[106] Hanson RL, Imperatore G, Bennett PH, Knowler WC. Components of the "metabolic syndrome" and the incidence of type 2 diabetes. *Diabetes.* 2002; 51: 3120 – 7.

[107] Isomaa B, Almgren P, Tuomi T, Forsen B, Lahti K, Nissen M, Taskinen MR, Groop L. Cardiovascular morbidity and mortality associated with the metabolic syndrome. *Diabetes Care.* 2001; 24: 683 – 9.

[108] Reaven GM, Tsao PS. Insulin Resistance and compensatory hyperinsulinemia: the key player between cigarette smoking and cardiovascular disease? *J. Am. Coll. Cardiol.* 2003; 41: 1044 – 7.

[109] Lakka H-M, Laaksonen DE, Lakka TA, Niskanen LK, Kumpusalo E, Tuomilehto J, Salonen JT. The metabolic syndrome and total and cardiovascular disease mortality in middle-aged men. *JAMA.* 2002; 288: 2909 – 16.

[110] Carnethon MR, Loria CM, Hill JO, Sidney S, Savage PJ, Liu K. Risk factors for the metabolic syndrome: the Coronary Artery Risk Development in Young Adults (CARDIA) Study, 1985 – 2001. *Diabetes Care.* 2004; 27: 2707 – 15.

[111] Yoo S, Niklas T, Baranowski T, Zakeri IF, Yang SJ, Srinivasan SR, Berenson GS. Comparison of dietary intakes associated with metabolic syndrome risk factors in young adults: the Bogalusa Heart Study. *Am. J. Clin. Nutr.* 2004; 80: 841 – 8.

[112] Ford ES, Giles WH, Dietz WH. Prevalence of the metabolic syndrome among US adults: findings from the third National Health and Nutrition Examination Survey. *JAMA.* 2002; 287: 356 – 9.

[113] Yoon YS, Oh SW, Baik HW, Park HS, Kim WY. Alcohol consumption and the metabolic syndrome in Korean adults: the 1998 Korean National Health and Nutrition Examination Survey. *Am. J. Clin. Nutr.* 2004; 80: 217 – 24.

[114] Leone A. Cardiovascular damage from smoking: a fact or belief? *Int. J. Cardiol.* 1993; 38: 113 –7.

[115] Sherman CB. Health effects of cigarette smoking. *Clin. Chest. Med.* 1991 Dec;12(4):643-58.

[116] Leone A. The heart: a target organ for cigarette smoking. *J. Smoking-Related Dis.* 1992; 3: 197 – 201.

[117] US Department of Health, Education, and Welfare: The health consequences of smoking: a report of the Surgeon General. Cardiovascular disease. Rockville, MD: US

Department of Health and Human Services, Public Health Service Office of Smoking and Health. DHHS Publication NO (PHS) 84-50204,1983.

[118] Leone A. Cigarette smoking and health of the heart. *J. Roy Soc. Health.* 1995; 115: 354 – 5.

[119] Hammond EC, Garfinkel L. Coronary heart disease, stroke and aortic aneurysm. *Arch. Environ. Health.* 1969; 19: 167 – 82.

[120] McBride PE. The health consequences of smoking. Cardiovascular diseases. *Medical Clinics of North America.* 1992; 76: 333 – 53.

[121] Aronow WS: Effect of passive smoking on angina pectoris. *N. Engl. J. Med.* 1978; 299: 21 – 4.

[122] Sparrow D, Dawber TR, Colton T. The influence of cigarette smoking on prognosis after a first myocardial infarction. *J. Chronic Dis.* 1978; 31: 425 – 32.

[123] Leone A, Bertanelli F, Mori L, Fabiano P, Bertoncini G. Ventricular arrhythmias by passive smoke in patients with pre-existing myocardial infarction. *J. Am. Coll. Cardiol.* 1992; 3: 256 (A).

[124] Wilhelmsson C, Vedin JA, Elmfeldt D, Tibblin G, Wilhelmsen L. Smoking and myocardial infarction. *Lancet.* 1975; 1: 415 – 20.

[125] Auerbach O, Carter HW, Garfinkel L, Hammond EC. Cigarette smoking and coronary heart disease, a macroscopic and microscopic study. *Chest.* 1976; 70: 697 – 705.

[126] Reid DD, Hamilton PJS, McCartney P, Rose G. Smoking and other risk factors in coronary heart disease in British civil servants. *Lancet.* 1976; 11: 979 – 84.

[127] Glantz SA, Parmley WW. Passive smoking and heart disease. *JAMA.* 1995; 273: 1047 – 53.

[128] Wells AJ. Passive smoking as a cause of heart disease. *J. Am. Coll. Cardiol.* 1994; 24: 546 – 54.

[129] Meinert CL, Forman S, Jacobs DR, Stamler J. Cigarette smoking as a risk factor in men with a prior history of myocardial infarction. *J .Chronic Dis.* 1979; 32: 415 – 25.

[130] Glantz SA, Parmley WW. Passive smoking and heart disease : epidemiology, physiology, and biochemistry. *Circulation.* 1991; 83: 1 – 12.

[131] Baer L, Radichevich I. Cigarette smoking in hypertensive patients. Blood pressure and endocrine responses. *Am. J. Med.* 1985; 78: 564 – 8.

[132] Celermajer DS, Adams MR, Clarkson P, Robinson J, McRedie R, Donald A, Deanfield JE. Passive smoking and impaired endothelium-dependent arterial dilatation in healthy young adults. *N. Engl. J. Med.* 1996; 334: 150 – 4.

[133] Leone A, Lopez M. Oral contraception, ovarian disorders and tobacco in myocardial infarction of woman. *Pathologica.* 1986; 78: 237 – 42.

[134] Pojola S, Siltanen P, Romo M. Five-year survival of 728 patients after myocardial infarction. *Br. Heart J.* 1980; 43: 176 – 83.

[135] Leone A. Relationship between cigarette smoking and other coronary risk factors in atherosclerosis: risk of cardiovascular disease and preventive measures. *Curr. Pharm. Design.* 2003; 2417 – 23.

[136] Leone A. Biochemical markers of cardiovascular damage from tobacco smoke. *Curr. Pharm. Design.* 2005; 11: 2199 – 2208.

[137] Tsiara S, Mikhailidis DP, Elisaf M. Influence of smoking on vascular risk factors. *Angiology.* 2003; 54: 507 – 30.

[138] Canner PL, Berge KG, Wenger NK, Stamler J, Friedman L, Prineas RJ, Friedwald W. Fifteen year mortality in Coronary Drug Project patients: long-term benefit with niacin. *J. Am. Coll. Cardiol.* 1986; 8: 1245 – 55.

[139] Glueck CJ, Mattson F, Bierman EL. Diet and coronary heart disease: Another view. *N. Engl. J. Med.*1978; 298: 1471 – 3.

[140] Mann JM, Davies MJ. Vulnerable plaque: Relation of characteristics to degree of stenosis in human coronary arteries. *Circulation.* 1996; 94: 928 – 31.

Chapter VIII

Coronary Circulation in Nonsmokers

Abstract

Nonsmoker individuals may be divided into four groups: never smokers who have been never exposed to smoking (environmental smoking); never smokers who have been partially or totally exposed to environmental tobacco smoke; past smokers who have been never exposed to environmental tobacco smoke after their smoking cessation; past smokers partially or totally exposed to environmental tobacco smoke after their smoking cessation. Moreover, in their turn, past smokers may be divided in recent past-smokers or old-past smokers.

Coronary circulation in nonsmoker individuals show some features closely related to environmental tobacco exposure like smoking cessation in past-smokers, physiologic parameters related to age, health status and lifestyle of the nonsmoking population.

Usually, the types of coronary alterations observed are similar to those of smokers although with lesser severity, extension and some pathologic characteristics: similar fatty streaks and atherosclerotic plaque. The latter, however, which narrows partially arterial lumen, is less frequently vulnerable and, more frequently, may undergo reversibility. Moreover, phenomena of calcification and segmental extension may be seen, histologically, in a limited number of observations.

Keywords: Nonsmokers, Past-smokers, coronary circulation, passive smoking, smoking cessation, fatty streak, atherosclerotic plaque, environment, mainstream smoke, sidestream smoke, age, health status, lifestyle, children, elderly, diet.

Nonsmoking individuals may be divided into four groups (table 8.1.): never smokers who have never been exposed to smoking (environmental smoking); never smokers who have been partially or totally exposed to environmental tobacco smoke; past smokers who have been never exposed to environmental tobacco smoke after their smoking cessation; past smokers partially or totally exposed to environmental tobacco smoke after their smoking cessation. Moreover, in their turn, past smokers may be divided into recent past-smokers or old-past smokers.

Table 8.1. Classification of nonsmokers according to their smoking habit

Nonsmokers		Smoking exposure
1. Never smokers		Never-exposed
2. Never smokers		Exposed
3. Past smokers	Recent past-smokers	Never-exposed
	Old past-smokers	Never -exposed
4. Past smokers	Recent past-smokers	Exposed
	Old past-smokers	Exposed

All these groups of individuals need to be carefully studied in an attempt to establish the type and extension of alterations that can involve coronary circulation.

Firstly, the distribution of never smokers in groups as indicated in table 8.1. plays a basic role since some main observations have to be analyzed: existence or not of coronary circulation improvement in past smokers following their smoking cessation and benefit of smoking cessation; coronary circulation in never smokers with or without ischemic heart pathology; characteristics of coronary circulation in past or never smokers never exposed to environmental tobacco smoke compared with similar characteristics of the same group of individuals who have been partially or totally exposed passively; main features of passive smoking; physiological status that could influence the characteristics of coronary circulation; and, finally, the type and extension of structural coronary alterations.

Some data on these findings derive from autopsy studies since they provide an effective control of the changes that may involve coronary circulation. In the large majority of cases of ischemic heart disease, atherosclerotic changes are present in the coronary tree.

Assessing better the features of coronary circulation in nonsmokers requires, in my opinion, the need to analyze firstly the effects produced by smoking cessation and characteristics of environmental tobacco smoke.

Smoking Cessation

Since there is evidence [1–5] of harmful effects that smoking is able to exert on several tissues and organs of our body, an always greater amount of current smokers become past-smokers particularly when they suffered from an ischemic heart attack. Therefore, the number of past-smokers is increasing continuously.

Benefits of smoking cessation and better techniques to reach this goal have been estimated differently in various findings [6–15]. However, the results of smoking cessation depend on the balance between two opposing forces: motivation to stop smoking and degree of nicotine dependence.

Strong motivation to stop smoking may derive from the knowledge of harmful effects of smoking particularly for those individuals who become frightened following health problems and are persuaded that positive outcomes may occur by avoiding smoking.

Nicotine dependence, on the contrary, may require, sometimes, a specific treatment.

After an ischemic event, particularly acute myocardial infarction, risk associated with smoking, in presence of smoking cessation, declines rapidly [16], although some concepts must be kept in mind. The decline is maximum within the first three years following smoking cessation, and coronary risk due to cigarette smoking halves its harmful effects on the cardiovascular system. Conversely, a further decline in cardiovascular risk occurs slowly after this time period so that the total cessation of the risk needs from five to fifteen years depending on the number of smoked cigarettes and previous duration of smoking habit. These factors could influence negatively coronary circulation as well as regression of an atherosclerotic coronary lesion.

In the Parisian Prospective Study [17], among a cohort of 7,746 men with ages from 45 years to 54 years at the beginning of the enrollment into the study protocol, there was evidence, after a twenty year follow-up, that a daily consumption of 11 cigarettes increased the incidence of ischemic heart disease by 40 percent, and stopping smoking could reduce this observed incidence of more than a quarter. However, large-scale studies on smoking cessation are yet a limited number and, therefore, do not permit certain conclusions.

Differences of time in disappearing coronary risk after smoking cessation could be related also to the presence or not of associated coronary risk factors, and, often, the role of the other risk factors continue to maintain in the time those coronary changes that stopping smoking would have, probably, reduced in severity and extension.

Globally, cigarette smoking consumption has undergone a reduction although through cyclic phases of increase/decrease/ and again increase [18]. Particularly in women, decline in cardiovascular risk after smoking cessation does not provide positive results and it is worthy noting that women are unlikely stop smoking as reports seem to demonstrate [19–20]. Moreover, there are some categories of women at very high risk of developing severe coronary alteration particularly when cigarette smoking is associated with contraceptive drug use [21–22]. Two reports identified a fatal myocardial infarction in a young female smoker who used contraceptive drugs and a non-fatal myocardial infarction complicated by postinfarction aneurysm in a middle-aged female smoker with ovarian disorders. Cardiac surgery improved the health status in the latter woman who stopped smoking.

From these data, it emerges that the results obtained after smoking cessation may vary widely according to different factors.

In conclusion, coronary arteries in past smokers may present a large spectrum of alterations, which will be described with a major detail. They may consist of irreversible lesions due to previous smoking habit when smoking had produced an irreversible atherosclerotic plaque, reversible lesions when decrease particularly in LDL-cholesterol concentrations may be seen after smoking cessation and an atherosclerotic plaque did not have features of irreversibility, and, finally, increasing lesions of different severity and extension in a decreased atherosclerotic alteration in "situ" or on adjacent segments of the coronary arteries when past smokers undergo environmental tobacco smoke exposure. This wide spectrum of alterations may cause variable responses in coronary circulation as findings seem to demonstrate [23–25]. However, there is opinion that, totally, intensive multifactor risk reduction, including smoking cessation, conducted over 4 years reduced the rate of luminal narrowing in coronary arteries of men and women affected by coronary artery disease and decreased hospitalizations for clinical cardiac events [26]. Moreover, other major coronary risk factors, particularly lipid disorders, respond favorably to smoking cessation also [27-28]. Therefore, all recommendations [29–30] on the prevention of coronary artery disease suggest needing smoking cessation for the reduction of the risk of both non-fatal and fatal coronary events, since smoking cessation would influence positively the level and extension of lesion in coronary circulation.

Passive Smoking

Passive smoking is probably the most important determinant of the vessel alterations in coronary circulation for nonsmokers [14, 31–36].

About passive smoking, two main questions arise: what really is environmental tobacco smoke (a term that is also defined as involuntary smoking, passive smoking, or secondhand smoking), and what is its role in influencing coronary circulation?

Empirically, one could hypothesize that passive smoking may exert different but, however, harmful effects in never smokers or in past smokers exposed. Conversely, strongly statistical observations move this hypothesis from an empiric level to a level of documented scientific certainty since definitive data about the different but harmful effects caused by passive smoking exposure on the two groups of individuals, nonsmokers and past smokers, exist.

Environmental tobacco smoke is a mixture of particles derived from the burning end of cigarettes, but also cigars and pipes, and smoke exhaled by smokers. Therefore, almost all those toxic compounds, which number more than 4,000 [37] and are a volatile phase of smoking, play a harmful role in exposed individuals. Toxics reach body structures where they exert their negative effects particularly through inhalation and then diffuse into the body through blood. Inhalation occurs, usually, involuntarily in exposed nonsmokers and voluntarily in active smokers who inhale the smoke of their cigarette as they are smoking.

The process of cigarette smoking produces three types of tobacco smoke, the main characteristics of which are reported in table 8.2.

Table 8.2. Types and main composition of environmental tobacco smoke

Smoking Type	Composition
1. Mainstream smoke	Chemical carcinogens and other toxics.
2. Exhaled mainstream smoke	Carcinogens and other toxics partly altered.
3. Sidestream smoke	Same toxics in smaller particles.

The first type of passive smoking is the mainstream smoke, which is the smoke inhaled directly through the burning cigarette by the smokers. The second type, called exhaled mainstream smoke, is the smoke breathed out by the smokers from their lungs. The composition of these two types of passive smoking is likely to differ since some of the compounds in smoke are, usually, retained by the smoker or, otherwise, altered by the mechanisms involved by the process. The third type is called sidestream smoke which is the smoke drifting from the end of the lit cigarette.

Indeed, environmental tobacco smoke is defined as an exposure to sidestream smoke from the burned cigarettes which lie in an environment as well as mainstream smoke exhaled by smokers. Both types of smoking contain a large number of toxic compounds including carbon monoxide and formaldehyde. Passive smoking compounds have carcinogenic and negative cardiovascular effects. The particles of sidestream smoke are smaller that those of mainstream smoke, meaning that they can be inhaled more deeply into the lungs [38].

It has been estimated that 85 percent of the smoke which pollutes an environment is, on the average, composed of sidestream smoke. Therefore, passive smokers have a lower exposure to the harmful components of tobacco smoke than active smokers, who draw smoke directly into their lungs.

Quantification of exposure by the nonsmokers depends on a number of factors including the filtration, tar level and cigarettes smoked, environment size and architecture, ventilation rate, and duration of exposure as well as characteristics and healthy or pathologic status of exposed individuals [2, 39–40].

Exposure to passive smoking may cause two types of effects: acute effects, which involve primarily respiratory system as well as cardiac performance [41] and also coronary blood flow [42], and long-term effects, which are responsible for an increased risk of heart disease and lung cancer [43]. Long-term exposure influences the changes that have been documented in coronary circulation since prolonged and repeated exposure to passive smoking triggers those mechanisms of cardiovascular damage that lead to atherosclerotic plaque formation. Notwithstanding a large number of findings that demonstrate the harmful effects of passive smoking on heart and coronary circulation, there are some reports, which are, however, not related to specific findings but to an "artfully chosen" meta-analysis on a limited number of epidemiologic studies that would document a lack of association between environmental tobacco smoke and coronary heart syndromes [44]. It is worth noting that a discussion without bias on cardiovascular damage due to passive smoking exposure identifies environmental tobacco smoke as a risk factor for cardiovascular disease, as also the American Heart Association suggests [33, 36, 45].

About the mechanism of damage that exposure to passive smoking can cause on coronary circulation, there is evidence that undoubtedly endothelial dysfunction may play a triggering mechanism. However, disorders in lipid metabolism as well as those risk factors up to now examined play their role in determining atherosclerotic plaque formation of different type and extension. Indeed, this is the main alteration which one can observe in coronary circulation of exposed never or past smokers.

Coronary Circulation in Past Smokers

Past smokers may be divided into two groups: past smokers who stopped smoking many years ago (more than 5 years), and past smokers whose stopped smoking less than 5 years ago. The statement of this division is correlated with findings on smoking cessation that estimated these times responsible, respectively, for the almost complete or not the end of cardiovascular risk due to smoking.

Once established in what type of group past smokers belong, a further subdivision may be applied to identify those individuals who are not exposed from those who have a continuous or partial exposure to environmental tobacco smoke, since the type of exposure is a strong determinant of harmful effects [46–47] as shown in table 8.3. Similarly, never smokers may be also influenced by factors listed in the same table.

Table 8.3. Major determinants of harmful effects due to passive smoking exposure

1. Passive smoking features	Duration of exposure (partial or total)
	Type of exposure (acute or chronic)
	Environmental concentration of pollutants
2. Indoor architecture	Cubic metres
	Ventilation
	Workplace or Home
3. Exposed individual	Age, sex
	Health status
	Coronary risk factors associated
4. Others	Factors able to influence those in 1,2,3.

The "mosaic" of physiopathologic mechanisms through which cigarette smoking may cause ischemic heart pathology, including coronary alterations observed in past smokers, is related strictly to the factors listed in table 8.3. Among these, there are some prevailing ones for what concerns the damage to coronary vessels. Duration and type of exposure as well as smoking pollutant concentrations into the environment play a stronger action than that of the other factors.

Both carbon monoxide and nicotine polluting the environment cause coronary vessel damage in exposed past smokers particularly through the endothelial dysfunction.

A wide spectrum of changes may be seen in the coronary circulation of past smokers. Alterations may consist [2, 45] of no or minimal coronary lumen reduction identified in individuals with or without coronary events up to the appearance of an atherosclerotic plaque occluding totally or, more often, partially arterial lumen. Moreover, plaque complications have been also documented although they occurred occasionally and, generically, with lesser calcium deposits.

Atherosclerotic plaque reversibility may be identified in past smokers never exposed, but also in past smokers partially exposed although with a lower incidence.

In a scientific field, the concept of a reverse alteration is established by the capacity of going through a well-defined series of changes either backward or else forward in the progression of a studied phenomenon. Usually, positive results are obtained when any specific alteration meets a backward.

Atherosclerotic plaque reversibility has been postulated in the past and furtherly suggested nowadays in both experimental and clinical findings [48–50]. Several factors, primarily related to dietary intake but also to spatial features of the plaque [51], play a role in determining plaque regression.

Experimental studies [48] identified that cholesterol lowering alone did not cause reversibility of an atherosclerotic plaque but only when reduction in cholesterol was added to a dietary supplementation of vitamin C.

Also therapeutic reduction in total and LDL-cholesterol may reach similar results [49–50].

Two studies, the Cholesterol Lowering Atherosclerosis Study (CLAS) and the Monitored Atherosclerosis Regression Study (MARS), explored by imaging techniques the reversibility of atherosclerosis with lipid lowering therapy in coronary and systemic vascular bed as well as in coronary artery bypass grafts. Results indicated that both very early lesions confined to the arterial wall and established lesions late in the atherosclerotic process could be reversed by lipid-lowering therapy. Moreover, beneficial effects on atherosclerotic plaque regression were obtained when individuals, particularly those with lipid metabolism disorders, received statin therapy.

Reversibility could be also favored by the spatial orientation of the atherosclerotic plaque which develops more frequently on the myocardial side of the vessel wall, where, usually, shear-stress is lower, although plaque size is similar on the epicardial and myocardial side. These observations would further underline the role of hemodynamic factors in regulating atherosclerotic plaque development, regulation that is more effective in nonsmokers, even if partially exposed to environmental tobacco smoke, than that in current smokers.

All these structural changes that the coronary tree may meet in past smokers can determine a newer coronary circulation remodeling that, however, is usually a positive occurrence since the degree and extension of coronary alterations diminish with beneficial effects on coronary blood flow.

The assessment of tobacco smoke exposure and, thus, the objective cardiovascular risk in individuals, who were smokers in the past, is a basic factor to be known in an attempt to follow up the degree and extension of coronary circulation changes. Follow up is possible using laboratory quantitative measurements of those biomarkers related to tobacco smoke exposure [37], and among these, particularly nicotine and urinary cotinine [52–55].

In conclusion, the spectrum of coronary circulation changes related to smoking in past smokers identifies minimal or no coronary artery lesions associated or not with functional disorders, the main of which is coronary vasospasm, structural lesions that may be conducted to fatty streak development as well as coronary atherosclerotic plaque with narrowings of different degree and extension, pre-existing stable or vulnerable plaque, and, finally, similar lesions not due to smoking exposure but to other coronary events determined by the action of other major risk factors. Moreover, coronary vessel pathology due to non-atherogenic mechanisms (congenital alteration, inflammation and so on), and also not linked to smoke, may affect coronary circulation of past smokers and determine complex pathologic manifestations of cardiovascular damage.

Coronary Circulation in Never Smokers

This group of individuals recognizes anatomical features of coronary circulation depending on the fact that examined subjects are or are not exposed to passive smoking.

Never smokers, who have never been exposed to environmental tobacco, obviously may display coronary circulation changes not related to smoking.

Several reports have been published on the relationship between passive smoking and non-fatal and fatal episodes of coronary heart disease [3, 8, 40, 56–57] in exposed subjects. A large majority of findings concerned fatal coronary events in never smoker women who were, usually, exposed at home to smoke from their husbands' cigarettes. In addition, epidemiologic data may be deduced through the analysis of two cross-sectional studies of prevalent disease [58].

Other findings [59–62] documented a relationship between passive smoking and coronary heart disease that was statistically significant at a P value less than 0.05 in three reports [59–61] whereas a fourth study was significant statistically at a level of P less than 0.01, but only for women married to men smoking at least 20 cigarettes/day. The analysis of these reports would seem to demonstrate the relationship between coronary events and passive smoking, since there would be evidence that when increasing the number of cigarettes smoked, there was, at the same time, an evident increase in coronary disease with a significantly major statistical value. Also, the study of Kawachi and al.[63] documented a 71 percent increase in risk of coronary heart disease with a P value less than 0.05 among women exposed passively to cigarette smoke at home or work.

Case-control studies [35, 64–66] better identified the relationship between coronary heart disease and environmental tobacco smoke exposure. However, both cross-sectional and case-control studies resulted in inconsistent findings in the association between passive smoking and coronary events, although a very interesting finding [66], which investigated the number of coronary stenoses in women following chronic exposure to passive smoking and occurrence of coronary heart disease, concluded that the number of stenotic coronary arteries increased with the amount of exposure to passive smoking from the husband and, moreover, passive smoking could be causally associated with ischemic heart disease.

On the contrary, there are many cohort-studies, some of which conducted by meta-analysis, that found exposure to passive smoking strongly related to coronary heart disease [67–68].

Additional evidence of the coronary damage from passive smoking comes experimentally through animal findings. Passive smoking accelerated atherosclerosis in rabbits and cockerels [25, 32, 69]. Exposed cockerels in an environment polluted by passive smoking components at a concentration usually found in living places showed an increase in size of atherosclerotic plaque particularly in the aorta. Passive smoking also worsened endothelial function in lipid-fed rabbits leading to inappropriate vasoconstriction which could be avoided by dietary supplementation of L- arginine.

These experimental observations support the role of endothelial changes caused by passive smoking exposure as well as progression in atherosclerotic lesions.

Thus, there is evidence that long-term effects of passive smoking exposure in never smokers include damage to coronary endothelium, increased plaque formation and reduced HDL-cholesterol, which, in turn, leads to a progression of atherosclerosis [45, 70]. Both heightened platelet aggregation and the presence of carcinogenic agents can increase plaque formation as observed in avian and animal models. Moreover, other findings [71] supported an acceleration in atherosclerotic plaque formation following exposure to passive smoking.

Also acute exposure to passive smoking induces endothelial changes consisting of impaired artery wall dilation [72–74] that, however, is transient but reproducible under similar experimental type of exposure even in healthy young individuals. Impaired endothelium-dependent dilation has been documented particularly by brachial ultrasonography, but there is evidence that endothelial alterations in the systemic arterial bed may be transferred to similar changes in the coronary tree [42].

Exposure to passive smoking raises carboxyhemoglobin blood concentration. According to Glantz and Parmley [45] elevated carboxyhemoglobin levels reduce exercise performance in coronary patients as well as in normal individuals, adversely affect platelet function, and damage the coronary endothelium. Thus, environmental tobacco smoke may exert both short-term effects by inducing coronary vasoconstriction and platelet aggregation, and long-term effects sustained by structural damage of the endothelium and atherosclerotic plaque formation. Patients with established coronary heart disease have been shown to develop angina and electrocardiographic changes sooner when they exercised in environments where carbon monoxide was added at a low concentration (from 1 to 40 ppm) rather than in environments not polluted by the carbon monoxide [41, 75–83]. The precise mechanisms by which exposure causes impairment in coronary circulation remain yet unclear, although they seem to be a direct consequence of environmental carbon monoxide concentrations since more negative coronary responses are, usually, seen when the level of gas in the environment is higher.

Structural coronary changes observed from autopsy studies [84–85] show an increase in atherosclerotic lesions in individuals exposed to smoking either active smoking or passive smoking, when they are compared to non exposed never smokers. At autopsy, atherosclerotic coronary lesions, estimated macroscopically by radiographs and histologically by coded specimens, were severe in heavy smokers and the least in serious nonsmokers, either nonsmokers with cardiac pathology or those without cardiovascular involvement.

Structurally, fatty streaks associated with a different degree of fibrosis in the arterial wall in epicardial and myocardial coronary arteries are prevailing alterations almost always documented in nonsmokers. About atherosclerotic plaque and degree of arterial lumen narrowing, there was evidence that different features could be documented even if plaque vulnerability and, particularly, calcifications occurred with a significantly less incidence than the same manifestations in smokers.

Moreover, it is worth noting that the degree and extension of coronary atherosclerosis in the population could undergo changes within a relatively short period of time [84]. These changes might be expected to parallel changes in risk factors in the population.

In conclusion, the wide spectrum of observations derived from findings in never smokers exposed is consistent with the statement that passive smoking increases the risk of cardiovascular events related to coronary circulation impairment.

Physiologic Parameters in Nonsmokers

Several physiologic parameters may influence coronary circulation in nonsmokers, primarily age and health status of the individuals.

Age

"A man is as old as his arteries"
Thomas Sydenham (1624 –1689) [86]

Age, particularly advancing age [87], has been identified as a major risk factor for coronary heart disease and an indicator of coronary plaque burden.

There is evidence that advancing age induces a large spectrum of changes in structural coats of the arteries addressed to fibrosclerotic process formation with consequent arterial hardening [88–92]. It is worth noting, however, that while intimal-media thickening is an age associated phenomenon that is unrelated to the pathophysiologic mechanisms of atherosclerosis, intimal thickening, in itself, is a risk factor for atherosclerosis. Therefore, all determinants, including passive smoking in nonsmokers, of atherosclerotic plaque formation or progression may induce changes in coronary circulation and, then, favor the appearance of coronary heart disease.

Coronary heart disease is a common occurrence of the elderly and some anatomo-functional characteristics related to the elderly may produce inconsistent data in interpreting those alterations due to passive smoking exposure from those due to advanced age, being the type of alterations similar in a large number of cases. Moreover, heart and cerebrovascular disease is the major cause of mortality and morbidity in the 65 and older age group [91].

Assessment of cardiovascular risk factors in nonsmokers is pertinent since elderly subjects may have a history of hypertension or diabetes mellitus usually associated with increased risk of atherosclerosis, whereas smoking, elevated cholesterol concentrations, and family history of cardiovascular disease appear to have much less significance [92]. Moreover, a previous study demonstrated that the poor prognosis of elderly patients with a previous myocardial infarction was not related to age but to gender and type of coronary risk factors associated [93]. Among these factors, systolic hypertension occurred most frequently with, however, no negative prognostic significance, unless when it was associated with diabetes mellitus or accompanying diastolic hypertension.

Statistical analysis of the role of different cardiovascular risk factors separately including also the age of the subjects by using Student's test could identify the possibility that each factor has a statistical significance. Instead, by using those statistical methods, which compare together statistical significance of different risk factors – and correctly this test must be used – a very interesting observation arises: in elderly patients each factor could induce changes in function and structure of the cardiovascular system including coronary circulation, although there will be evidence of prevailing effects of some of them rather than others. Therefore, it is hard to establish which of the observed alterations belong specifically to a factor and which to another. Moreover, all the alterations that one can observe as an effect of a single risk factor may be well related to the type of damage caused by the other factors.

Another most important problem is to define the age to which an individual shoud be considered as an elderly individual. Unfortunately, there is no specific biological determinant of a physiological age that can be applied appropriately to different subjects, and, therefore, this parameter is often based on physical appearance, considering that each individual displays biological age of his arteries. However, old people are, conventionally, individuals over 65 years.

Cardiovascular system in the elderly usually responds differently to passive smoking exposure limitedly to some parameters.

Autonomic nervous system, a structure influenced negatively by the exposure to passive smoking, feels the effects of aging. Primarily, phasic variation in heart rate accompanying respiration is attenuated with increasing age as a consequence of diminished vagal activity [94]. Also the sensitivity of baroreceptor reflex in elderly is impaired with an evident decreased function [95–96]. The baroreceptors are located in the wall of the aorta and respond to deformation of the arterial wall. The decrease in sensitivity of baroceptors would be mainly due to an increased aortic stiffness, although carotid sinus hypersensitivity may be increased [97–98]. Such a response is yet unclear and, therefore, it needs further investigation.

The effects of aging on the beta-adrenergic system have been also examined by an experimental study [99]. It demonstrated that the amount of isoproterenol - a chemical compound capable of increasing the heart rate significantly - needed to increase heart rate of 25 beats per minute increased with age and the amount of propranolol needed to block the heart rate response decreased with increasing age. Thus, the beta-adrenergic system appeared to be less sensitive to both agonist and antagonist drugs with a sensible imbalance in observed responses. A similar decreased sensitivity has been noted for the inotropic response to catecholamines [91]. Reduced sensitivity seemed to be related to catecholamine receptors that were unable to respond physiologically to binding of chemical substance with the receptor. From these observations, it emerges that age may alter the cardiovascular system through responses of different type, but, however, all capable of influencing coronary circulation and worsening coronary vasomotor tone during passive smoking exposure, being involved particularly changes in inotropic response and endothelial function.

Atherosclerotic changes are, usually, found in coronary and carotid arteries of old individuals who have not been exposed to passive smoking as a consequence of aging. These alterations are almost similar to those attributed to environmental tobacco smoke exposure.

In the elderly, artery wall elastic fibers are fragmented and reduced with an increase in collagen, so that the total content of elastin into the arterial wall is, usually, reduced by about one-third. Moreover, intima becomes thickened. With aging, deposits of lipids and calcium accumulate progressively into the media.

Finally, systolic blood pressure in older patients increases as a consequence of the changes in arterial structure but, at the same time, it promotes similar structural changes that can aggravate vascular alterations. Isolated systolic hypertension, that is the most common form of hypertension over age 50, even when it is mild in severity, usually is associated with a significant increase in cardiovascular disease risk [100-101]. Alterations sustained by isolated systolic hypertension can involve and impair coronary circulation in nonsmokers exposed to environmental tobacco although it is hard to establish their degree and extension.

Cardiovascular changes that may affect elderly people, even after chronic exposure to passive smoking, should be evaluated prudentially and, however, they would have less significance compared to those determined by other major coronary risk factors like combined systolic and diastolic blood pressure or diabetes mellitus [93].

Also children's exposure to passive smoking is worthwhile to be analyzed separately since the characteristics of the exposure and type of response may be different from those observed in adults and follow a way related to the functional characteristic of the cardiovascular system in infancy where coronary circulation may be, at a maximum, minimally involved.

At birth, the cardiovascular system undergoes those progressive changes that will be for the adult heart. Therefore, in children there are some characteristics that may be considered as an advantage compared to the adult heart and, on the contrary, others that may predispose a child's cardiovascular system more heavily to harmful effects of passive smoking exposure without a primary involvement of coronary arteries.

Initially, children display a heart rate considerably more elevated than that in adults. Such a factor is accompanied by an autonomic system response that differs from that of the adults since adults have, usually, a balanced autonomic system function. On the contrary, a sympathetic stimulation of the cardiovascular system is prevailing in children and pre-adolescents. This type of physiological response, age-related, makes the cardiovascular system susceptible to a major degree of damage from passive smoking exposure. Conversely, there are other age-related features that may reduce the harm from exposure to smoking like an usual absence of other major cardiovascular risk factors and atherosclerotic lesions, although fatty streaks may be seen early also in coronary artery vessels of children and adolescents.

For these reasons, children who are exposed to passive smoking are suffering particularly from respiratory symptoms [102] more than cardiovascular symptoms. Among respiratory symptoms, asthma and respiratory infections [103] are prevailing in children of parents who smoke compared to those living with nonsmoker parents. Moreover, there is a significant relationship between the incidence of respiratory diseases and the number of cigarettes smoked indoors.

Since environmental tobacco smoke causes primarily those alterations of the heart and blood vessels which are closely related to a progression of the atherosclerosis, it is easy to recognize the reasons for the reduced impairment of coronary circulation in children where atherosclerosis is, usually, far from being developed. However, children exposed to tobacco smoke [104] have been distinguished, and could be distinguished, from those non-exposed by the measurements of urinary cotinine concentrations. As described previously, measuring urinary concentrations of cotinine should be an effective method to assess involuntary smoking exposure.

Since there is evidence of an age-related damage from passive smoking, antismoking campaigns are addressed particularly to avoid children's exposure. The slogan "save the children from passive smoking" (figure 8.1.) is the campaign that we were beginning to launch. By pictures showing the innocence and impossibility of children to protect themselves against the harmful effects of passive smoking, there is a fair chance to obtain positive results in fighting passive smoking exposure. This could be a little battle to win a war – the war against smoking – since adults who live with children are, usually, susceptible to health problems that involve infancy.

Health Status of Exposed Nonsmokers

Health status of nonsmokers may influence strongly the responses of coronary circulation following environmental tobacco exposure.

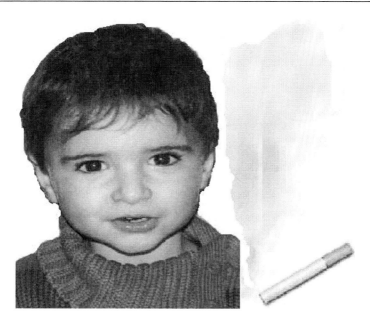

Figure 8.1. "Save the children from passive smoking". Campaign against Smoking: Little battles to win a war! From: Archilli E et al., 8th World Conference on Tobacco or Health. Building a Tobacco-Free World, Buenos Aires, Argentina, March 30 – April 3, 1992. Reproduced with Authors' permission.

Absence of chronic disease, particularly cardiovascular and metabolic disease, associated with an effective control of major coronary risk factors contribute to reduce either the negative effects of passive smoking exposure on coronary circulation of nonsmokers or the appearance of heart attacks.

There are a great number of factors that may be controlled by a correct lifestyle. Firstly, obesity is considered the number one health priority also in nonsmokers, and one of the major contributors to premature deaths and disability [105].

The most effective efforts in preventing obesity [106] must be addressed to children and adolescents since weight control may be obtained with more favorable outcome. Body mass index assessment is estimated to be a good measure of adiposity when this parameter exceeds its value.

Moreover, there is a strong link between obesity and metabolic factors and, consequently, between obesity and environmental tobacco smoke exposure (figure 8.2.).

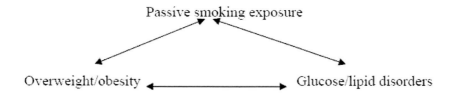

Figure 8.2. A close association links metabolic disorders, overweight and exposure to passive smoking.

Passive smoking exposure has been demonstrated also able to influence negatively lipid metabolism in children exposed passively to smoking since those living with parents who smoked had lower HDL-cholesterol concentrations [107].

A rich diet, and sedentary life also, should be avoided for reducing negative effects of passive smoking exposure on coronary circulation. Hypercaloric foods [108] associated with an excess of alcohol consumption make an individual particularly susceptible to develop coronary artery disease, the degree of which is influenced negatively by passive smoking.

As one can deduce, those changes in lifestyle that contribute to maintain the health of individuals could be achieved since findings would demonstrate their beneficial effects on the coronary damage caused by passive smoking exposure. Therefore, there is evidence that the old idiom " prevention is better than cure" could find its reason particularly in the control of lifestyle in those nonsmokers potentially exposed to passive smoking.

References

[1]   Ambrose GA, Barua RS. The pathophysiology of cigarette smoking and cardiovascular disease: an update. *J. Am. Coll. Cardiol.* 2004; 43: 1731 – 7.

[2]   Leone A. Cardiovascular damage from smoking: a fact or belief? *Int. J. Cardiol.* 1993; 38: 113 – 7.

[3]   Sherman CB. Health effects of cigarette smoking. *Clin. Chest. Med.* 1991; 12: 643 – 58.

[4]   Hammond EC, Garfinkel L. Coronary heart disease, stroke and aortic aneurysm. *Arch. Environ. Health.* 1969; 19: 167 – 82.

[5]   Peto R, Lopez AD, Boreham J, Thun M, Heath C. *Mortality from smoking in developed countries: 1950 – 2000.* Oxford: Oxford University Press, UK, 1994.

[6]   Fiore MC, Novotny TE, Pierce JP, Giovino GA, Hatziandreu EJ, Newcomb PA, Surawicz TS, Davis RM. Methods used to quit smoking in the United States. *JAMA.* 1990; 263: 2760 – 5.

[7]   Hughes JR, Gulliver SB, Fenwick JW, Valliere WA, Cruser K, Pepper S, Shea P, Solomon LJ, Flynn BS. Smoking cessation among self-quitters. *Health Psychol.* 1992; 11: 331 – 4.

[8]   Doll R, Peto R, Wheatley K, Gray R, Sutherland I. Mortality in relation to smoking: 40 years' observation on male British doctors. *BMJ.* 1994; 309: 901 – 10.

[9]   Hughes JR. Tobacco withdrawal in self-quitters. *J. Consult. Clin. Psychol.* 1992; 60: 689 – 97.

[10]   Russel MAH, Wilson C, Taylor C, Baker CD. Effect of general practitioners' advice against smoking. *BMJ.* 1979; 2: 231 – 5.

[11]   Raw M, Russel MAH. Rapid smoking, cue exposure and support in the modification of smoking. *Behav. Res. and Ther.* 1980; 18: 363 – 72.

[12]   Salonen JT. Stopping smoking and long-term mortality after acute myocardial infarction. *Br. Heart J.* 1980; 43: 463 – 9.

[13]   Kaplan GA, Keil JE. Socioeconomic factors and cardiovascular disease: a review of the literature. *Circulation.* 1993; 88: 1973 – 98.

[14] Penn A, Snyder CA. Inhalation of sidestream cigarette smoke accelerates development of arteriosclerotic plaque. *Circulation.* 1993; 88: 1820 – 5.

[15] Fiore MC. The new vital sign: assessing and documenting smoking status. *JAMA.* 1991; 266: 3183 – 4.

[16] Rosemberg L, Kaufman DW, Helmrich SP, Shapiro S. The risk of myocardial infarction after quitting smoking in men under 55 years of age. *N. Engl. J. Med.* 1985; 313: 1511 – 4.

[17] Birkui PJ. Some facts about the assistance to smokers at high risk in cardiology. In: *Tobacco and Health,* Slama K (ed.), Plenum Press, New York and London 1995; 431 – 4.

[18] Leone A. Relationship between cigarette smoking and other coronary risk factors in atherosclerosis: risk of cardiovascular disease and preventive measures. *Curr. Pharm. Design.* 2003; 9: 2417 – 23.

[19] Loewen GM, Romano CF. Lung cancer in women. *Psychoactive Drugs.* 1989; 21: 319 – 21.

[20] Cigarette smoking among adults – United States, 2000. *MMWR Morb. Mortal Wkly Rep.* 2002; 51: 642 – 5.

[21] Leone A, Lopez M. Role du tabac et de la contraception orale dans l'infarctus du myocarde de la femme. Description d'un cas. *Pathologica.* 1984; 76: 493 – 8.

[22] Leone A, Lopez M. Oral contraception, ovarian disorders and tobacco in myocardial infarction of woman. *Pathologica.* 1986; 78: 237 – 42.

[23] Doyle JT, Dawber TR, Kannel WB, Kinch SH, Kahn HA. The relationship of cigarette smoking to coronary heart disease. *JAMA.* 1964; 190: 886 – 90.

[24] Sparrow D, Dawber TR, Colton T. The influence of cigarette smoking on prognosis after a first myocardial infarction. *J. Chronic Dis.* 1978; 31: 425 – 32.

[25] Zhu BQ, Sun YP, Sievers RE, Isenberg WM, Glantz SA, Parmley WW. Passive smoking increases experimental atherosclerosis in cholesterol fed rabbits. *J. Am. Coll. Cardiol.* 1993; 21: 225 – 32.

[26] Haskell WL, Alderman EL, Fair JM, Maron DJ, Mackey SF, Superko HR, Williams PT, Johnstone IM, Champagne MA, Krauss RM. Effects of intensive multiple risk factor reduction on coronary atherosclerosis and clinical cardiac events in men and women with coronary artery disease. The Stanford Coronary Risk Intervention Project (SCRIP). *Circulation.* 1994; 89: 975 – 90.

[27] Rabkin SW. Effect of cigarette smoking cessation on risk factors for coronary atherosclerosis. A control clinical trial. *Atherosclerosis.* 1984; 53: 173 – 84.

[28] Allen SS, Hatsukami D, Gorsline J. Cholesterol changes in smoking cessation using the transdermal nicotine system. *Transdermal Nicotine Study Group. Prev. Med.* 1994; 23: 190 – 6.

[29] Wood D, De Backer G, Faergeman O, Graham I, Mancia G, Pyorala K. Prevention of coronary heart disease in clinical practice. Recommendations of the Second Joint Task Force of European and other Societies on Coronary Prevention. *Eur. Heart J.* 1998; 19: 1434 – 503.

[30] Ockene IS, Miller NH. Cigarette smoking, cardiovascular disease, and stroke: a statement for healthcare professionals from the American Heart Association. American Heart Association Task Force on Risk Reduction. *Circulation.* 1997; 96: 3243 – 7.

[31] Wells AJ. Heart disease from passive smoking in the workplace. *J. Am. Coll. Cardiol.* 1998; 31: 1 – 9.

[32] Penn A, Snyder CA. 1,3 butadiene, a vapor phase component of environmental tobacco smoke, accelerates arteriosclerotic plaque development. *Circulation.* 1996; 93: 552 – 7.

[33] Gidding SS, Morgan WW, Perry C, Isabel-Jones J, Bricker TJ, for the Committee on Atherosclerosis and Hypertension in Children, Council on Cardiovascular Disease in the Young, American Heart Association. Active and passive tobacco exposure: a serious pediatric health problem. *Circulation.* 1994; 90: 2581 – 90.

[34] LeVois ME, Layard MW. Publication bias in the environmental tobacco smoke/coronary heart disease epidemiologic literature. *Reg. Toxicol. Pharmacol.* 1995; 21: 184 – 91.

[35] Steenland K. Passive smoking and the risk of heart disease. *JAMA.* 1992; 267: 94 – 9.

[36] Taylor AE, Johnson DC, Kazemi H. Environmental tobacco smoke and cardiovascular disease. *Circulation.* 1992; 86: 699 – 702.

[37] Leone A. Biochemical markers of cardiovascular damage from tobacco smoke. *Curr. Pharm. Design.* 2005; 11: 2199 – 2208.

[38] US Department of Health and Human Services. The Health Consequences of Involuntary Smoking. A report of the Surgeon General. Rockville, Md: Centers for Disease Control, Center for Health Promotion and Education, Office on Smoking and Health, 1981; DHHS Publication No (CDC)87-8398.

[39] Fielding JE, Phenow KJ. Health effects of involuntary smoking. *N. Engl. J. Med.* 1988; 319: 1452 – 60.

[40] Leone A. Cigarette smoking and health of the heart. *J. Roy Soc. Health.* 1995; 115: 354 – 5.

[41] Leone A, Mori L, Bertanelli F, Fabiano P, Filippelli M. Indoor passive smoking: its effect on cardiac performance. *Int. J. Cardiol.* 1991; 8: 247 – 52.

[42] Otsuka R, Watanabe H, Hirata K, Tokai K, Muro T, Yoshiyama M, Takeuchi K, Yoshikawa J. Acute effects of passive smoking on the coronary circulation in healthy young adults. *JAMA.* 2001; 286: 436 – 41.

[43] Law MR, Morris JK, Wald NJ. Environmental tobacco smoke exposure and ischaemic heart disease: an evaluation of the evidence. *BMJ.* 1997; 315: 973 – 80.

[44] Gori GB. Environmental tobacco smoke and coronary heart syndromes: absence of an association. *Reg. Toxicol. Pharmacol.* 1995; 21: 281 – 95.

[45] Glantz SA, Parmley WW. Passive smoking and heart disease. Mechanisms and risk. *JAMA.* 1995; 273: 1047 – 53.

[46] Woodruff T, Rosebrook B, Pierce J, Glantz SA. Lower levels of cigarette consumption found in smoke-free workplaces in California. *Arch. Intern. Med.* 1993; 153: 1485 – 93.

[47] Siegel M. Involuntary smoking in the restaurant workplace: a review of employee exposure and health effects. *JAMA.* 1993; 270: 490 – 3.

[48] Willis GC. The reversibility of atherosclerosis. *Canad. MAJ.* 1957; 77: 106 – 9.

[49] Hodis HN. Reversibility of atherosclerosis-evolving perspectives from two arterial imaging clinical trials: the cholesterol lowering atherosclerosis regression study and the monitored atherosclerosis regression study. *J. Cardiovasc. Pharmacol.* 1995; 25: S25 – 31.

[50] Davignon J. Beneficial cardiovascular pleiotropic effects of statins. *Circulation.* 2004; 109: SIII39 – 43.

[51] Jeremias A, Huegel H, Lee DP, Hassan A, Wolf A, Yeung AC, Yock PG, Fitzgerald PJ. Spatial orientation of atherosclerotic plaque in non-branching coronary artery segments. *Atherosclerosis.* 2000; 152: 209 – 15.

[52] Worrel PC, Edwards R, Powell JT. Smoking markers as a reflection of smoking habit. *J. Smoking-Related Dis.* 1995; 6: 89 – 97.

[53] Apselhoff G, Ashton HM, Friedman H, Gerber N. The importance of measuring cotinine levels to identify smokers in clinical trials. *Clin. Pharmacol. Ther.* 1994; 56: 460 – 2.

[54] Benowitz NL. Cotinine as a biomarker of environmental tobacco smoke exposure. *Epidemiol. Rev.* 1996; 18: 188 – 204.

[55] Jarvis MJ, Tunstall-Pedoe H, Feyerabend C, Vesey C, Saloojee Y. Comparison of tests used to distinguish smokers from nonsmokers. *Am. J. Public Health.* 1987; 77: 1435 – 8.

[56] Giovino GA. Epidemiology of the tobacco use in the United States. *Oncogene.* 2002; 21: 7326 – 39.

[57] Powell JT. Vascular damage from smoking: disease mechanisms at the arterial wall. *Vasc. Med.* 1998; 3: 21 – 8.

[58] Tunstall-Pedoe H, Brown CA, Woodward M, Tavendale R. Passive smoking by self report and serum cotinine and the prevalence of respiratory and coronary heart disease in the Scottish heart health study. *J. Epidemiol. Community Health.* 1995; 49: 139 – 43.

[59] Doll R, Peto R. Mortality in relation to smoking: 20 years' observations on male British doctors. *BMJ.* 1976; 2: 1525 – 36.

[60] Helsing K, Sandler D, Comstock G, Chee E. Heart disease mortality in nonsmokers living with smokers. *Am. J. Epidemiol.* 1988; 127: 915 – 22.

[61] Hole D, Gillis C, Chopra C, Hawthorne VM. Passive smoking and cardiorespiratory health in a general population in the west of Scotland. *BMJ.* 1989; 299: 423 – 7.

[62] Hyrayama T. Passive smoking (letter). *NZ. Med. J.* 1990; 103: 54.

[63] Kawachi I, Colditz GA, Speizer FE, Manson JE, Stampfer MJ, Willet WC, Hennekens CH. A prospective study of passive smoking and coronary heart disease. *Circulation.* 1997; 95: 2374 – 9.

[64] Dobson AJ, Alexander HM, Heller RF, Lloyd DM. Passive smoking and the risk of heart attack or coronary death. *Med. J. Aust.* 1991; 154: 793 – 7.

[65] Muscat JE, Wynder EL. Exposure to environmental tobacco smoke and the risk of heart attack. *Int. J. Epidemiol.* 1995; 24: 715 – 9.

[66] He Y, Lam TH, Li LS, Li LS, Du RY, Jia GL, Huang J, Zheng J. The number of stenotic coronary arteries and passive smoking exposure from husband in lifelong non-smoking women in Xi'an, China. *Atherosclerosis.* 1996; 127: 229 – 38.

[67] Wells AJ. Passive smoking as a cause of heart disease. *J. Am. Coll. Cardiol.* 1994; 24: 546 – 54.

[68] Law MR, Hackshaw AK. Environmental tobacco smoke. *Br. Med. Bull.* 1996; 52: 22 – 34.

[69] Hutchenson S. L-arginine restores normal endothelium: mediated relaxation in hypercholesterolemic rabbits exposed to environmental tobacco smoke. *J. Am. Coll. Cardiol.* 1996; 39A (abstract).

[70] Valkonen M, Kuusi T. Passive smoking induces atherogenic changes in low-density lipoprotein. *Circulation.* 1998; 97: 2012 – 6.

[71] Strachan DP. Predictors of death from aortic aneurysm among middle-aged men: the Whitehall Study. *Br. J. Surg.* 1991; 78: 401 – 4.

[72] Deanfield J. Passive smoking and early arterial damage. *Eur. Heart J.* 1996; 17: 645 – 6.

[73] Celermajer DS, Sorensen KE, Georgakopoulos D, Bull C, Thomas O, Robinson J, Deanfield JE. Cigarette smoking is associated with dose-related and potentially reversible impairment of endothelium-dependent dilation in healthy young adults. *Circulation.* 1993; 88: 2149 – 55.

[74] Giannini D, Leone A, DiBisceglie D, Nuti M, Strata G, Buttitta F, Masserini L, Balbarini A. The effects of acute passive smoking exposure on endothelium-dependent brachial artery dilation in healthy individuals. *Angiology.* 2007; 58: 211 – 7.

[75] Ayres SM, Mueller HS, Gregory JJ, Giannelli S Jr, Penny JL. Systemic and myocardial hemodynamic responses to relatively small concentrations of carboxyhemoglobin (COHB). *Arch. Environ. Health.* 1969; 18: 699 – 709.

[76] Aronow WS, Rokaw SN. Carboxyhemoglobin caused by smoking nonnicotine cigarettes. Effects in angina pectoris. *Circulation.* 1971; 44: 782 – 8.

[77] Aronow WS, Harris CN, Isbell MW, Rokaw SN, Imparato B. Effects of freeway travel on angina pectoris. *Ann. Intern. Med.* 1972; 77: 669 – 76.

[78] Anderson EW, Andelman RJ, Strauch JM, Fortuin NJ, Knelson JH. Effect of low-level carbon monoxide exposure on onset and duration of angina pectoris. A study in ten patients with ischemic heart disease. *Ann. Intern. Med.* 1973; 79: 46 – 50.

[79] Aronow WS. Aggravation of angina pectoris by two percent carboxyhemoglobin. *Am. Heart J.* 1981; 101: 154 – 7.

[80] Adams KF, Koch G, Chatterjee B, Goldstein GM, O'Neil JJ, Bromberg PA, Sheps DS. Acute elevation of blood carboxyhemoglobin to 6% impairs exercise performance and aggravates symptoms in patients with ischemic heart disease. *J. Am. Coll. Cardiol.* 1988; 12: 900 – 9.

[81] Leone A, Bertanelli F, Mori L, Fabiano P, Bertoncini G. Ventricular arrhythmias by passive smoke in patients with pre-existing myocardial infarction. *J. Am. Coll. Cardiol.* 1992; 19: 256A.

[82] Sheps DS, Herbst MC, Hinderliter AL, Adams KF, Ekelund LG, O'Neil JJ, Goldstein GM, Bromberg PA, Dalton JL, Ballenger MN. Production of arrhythmias by elevated carboxyhemoglobin in patients with coronary artery disease. *Ann. Intern. Med.* 1990; 113: 343 – 51.

[83] Allred EN, Bleecker ER, Chaitman BR, Dahms TE, Gottlieb SO, Hackney JD, Pagano M, Selvester RH, Walden SM, Warren J. Short-term effects of carbon monoxide exposure on the exercise performance of subjects with coronary artery disease. *N. Engl. J. Med.* 1989; 321: 1426 – 32.

[84] Solberg LA, Strong JP. Risk factors and atherosclerotic lesions. A review of autopsy studies. *Arteriosclerosis.* 1983; 3: 187 – 98.

[85] Strong JP, Richards ML. Cigarette smoking and atherosclerosis in autopsied men. *Atherosclerosis.* 1976; 23: 451 – 76.

[86] Garrison FH. On Thomas Sydenham (1624 – 1689). Bull NY Acad Med 1928; 4: 993.

[87] Grundy SM. Age as a risk factor: you are as old as your arteries. *Am. J. Cardiol.* 1999; 83: 1455 – 7.

[88] Naijar SS, Scuteri A, Lakatta EG. Arterial aging: is it an immutable cardiovascular risk factor? *Hypertension.* 2005; 46: 454 – 62.

[89] Lakatta EG, Levy D. Arterial and cardiac aging: major shareholders in cardiovascular disease enterprises: part I: aging arteries: a "set-up" for vascular disease. *Circulation.* 2003; 107: 139 – 46.

[90] Lakatta EG. Central arterial aging and the epidemic of systolic hypertension and atherosclerosis. *JASH.* 2007; 1: 302 – 40.

[91] Weisfeldt ML. Aging of the cardiovascular system. *N Engl J Med* 1980; 303: 1172 – 4.

[92] Kannel WB, Gordon T. Evaluation of cardiovascular risk in the elderly: the Framingham Study. *Bull. N.Y. Acad. Med.* 1978; 54: 573 – 91.

[93] Bertoncini G, Bertanelli F, Leone A. Coronary risk factors in acute myocardial infarction (AMI) of elderly with and without hypertension. *AJH.* 1999; 12: 197A.

[94] Davies HEF. Respiratory change in heart rate, sinus arrhythmias in the elderly. *Gerontol. Clin.* 1975; 17: 96 – 100.

[95] Gribbin B, Pickering TG, Sleight P, Peto R. Effect of age and high blood pressure on baroreflex sensitivity in man. *Circ. Res.* 1971; 29: 424 – 31.

[96] Rothbaum DA, Shaw DJ, Angell CS, Shock NW. Cardiac performance in the unanesthetized senescent male rat. *J. Gerontol.* 1973; 28: 287 – 92.

[97] Ritch AES. The significance of carotid sinus hypersensitivity in the elderly. *Gerontol. Clin.* 1975; 17: 146 – 53.

[98] Smiddy J, Lewis HD Jr, Dunn M. The effect of carotid massage in older men. *J. Gerontol.* 1972; 27: 209 – 11.

[99] Vestal RE, Wood AJJ, Shand DG. Reduced beta-adrenoreceptor sensitivity in the elderly. *Clin. Pharmacol. Ther.* 1979; 26: 181 – 6.

[100] Franklin SS, Larson MG, Khan SA, Wong ND, Leip EP, Kannel WB, Levy D. Does the relation of blood pressure to coronary heart disease risk change with aging? The Framingham Heart Study. *Circulation.* 2001; 103: 1245 – 9.

[101] Sesso HD, Stampfer MJ, Rosner B, Hennekens CH, Graziano MJ, Manson JAE, Glynn RJ. Systolic and diastolic blood pressure, pulse pressure, and mean arterial pressure as predictors of cardiovascular disease risk in men. *Hypertension.* 2000; 36: 801 – 7

[102] Shima M, Adachi M. Effects of environmental tobacco smoke on serum levels of acute phase proteins in schoolchildren. *Prev. Med.* 1996; 25: 617 – 24.

[103] Rossier ML, Fernandez Vega M, Villalba Caloca J, Letama CM, Flores Sanchez S. Frequency of acute respiratory infections in children of parents who smoke and children of nonsmoking parents. In Tobacco and Health, Slama K (ed.,) Plenum Press, New York, 1995; 537 – 9.

[104] Bakoula CG, Kafritsa YJ, Kavadias GD, Lazopoulou DD, Theodoridou MC, Maravelias KP, Matsaniotis NS. Objective passive-smoking indicators and respiratory morbidity in young children. *Lancet.* 1995; 346: 280 – 1.

[105] Himes JD, Dietz WH. Guidelines for overweight in adolescent preventive service: recommendations from an expert committee. *Am. J. Clin. Nutr.* 1994; 59: 307 – 16.

[106] Pietrobelli A, Faith MS, Allison DB, Gallagher D, Chiumello G, Heymsfield SB. Body mass index as a measure of adiposity among children and adolescents: a validation study. *J. Pediatr.* 1998; 132: 204 – 10.

[107] Neufeld EJ, Mietus-Snyder M, Beise AS, Backer AL, Newburger JW. Passive cigarette smoking and reduced HDL cholesterol levels in children with high-risk lipid profiles. *Circulation.* 1997; 96: 1403 – 7.

[108] Block G, Dresser CM, Hartman AM, Carrol MD. Nutrient sources in the American diet: Quantitative data from the NHANES II Survey. II. Macronutrients and fats. *Am. J. Epidemiol.* 1985; 122: 27 – 40.

Chapter IX

Coronary Circulation in Smokers

Abstract

Coronary artery alterations in smokers involve both epicardial vessels and small intramyocardial vessels. Alterations are strongly related to atherosclerosis either macroscopically or microscopically.

Atherosclerotic plaque with a different degree of luminal narrowing, possible superimposed thrombus and/or erosion and plaque rupture, is the basic lesion of coronary arteries of smokers. Compared to atherosclerotic lesions of nonsmokers, there is evidence of a greater amount of calcium deposits and advanced fibrous-hyaline thickening of both epicardial and intramyocardial arteries in smokers. Moreover, lesions are strongly related to the number of cigarettes smoked for what concerns their degree and extension.

Finally, a few smokers display normal or nearly normal coronary arteries.

Keywords: Smoker, coronary artery, atherosclerotic plaque, complicated plaque, thrombus, plaque erosion, fatty streak, platelets, coagulation-fibrinolysis, thrombin, fibrin, fibrinogen, plasminogen, plasmin, nicotine, carbon monoxide, hyaline thickening, coronary wall.

In smokers, four main clinico-pathological disorders related to coronary circulation changes may be observed (table 9.1.): angina pectoris, acute myocardial infarction, sudden death, and ischemic cardiomyopathy. Their appearance may be either acute or chronical and it is also documented experimentally.

Table 9.1. Types of coronary heart disease more frequently observed in smokers

Ischemic heart disease	Main clinical characteristic
Angina pectoris	Stable
	Unstable
	Variant
Myocardial infarction	NonSTEMI (nonST-segment elevation)
	STEMI (ST-segment elevation)
Sudden death	Heart failure
Ischemic cardiomyopathy	Arrhythmias
	Heart failure associted with arrhythmias

Both functional and, particularly, structural changes in coronary arteries may cause ischemic heart attacks, although minimal or no coronary luminal reduction due to atherosclerosis in smokers as well as in nonsmokers has been described [1]. Even small [2-4], the number of necropsy cases had been previously documented and patent coronary arteries in patients affected by ischemic heart disease described also angiographically [2, 5–10]. However, these characteristics of coronary circulation are an exception to the rule since severe coronary alterations are usually observed in smokers [11].

There is evidence that mortality and morbidity related to coronary heart disease increase proportionately with the number of smoked cigarettes [12–15] since coronary damage is related to the amount of tobacco smoke compounds inhaled actively and their concentrations reached into the blood. Moreover, cigarette smoking is addictive because of the nicotine, and nicotine withdrawal is responsible for difficulties in stopping smoking. Since a large number of physiopathological changes at any level of atherosclerotic plaque formation occurs as a consequence of cigarette smoking, such a fact can explain the strong relationship existing between coronary artery alterations due to smoking and increased incidence in coronary artery disease.

Analyzing the references on the relationship between cigarette smoking and cardivascular system, one can see that they are timely dated and follow, as rate, only those related to cancer in smokers. That should be a confirmation of the attention given to the phenomenon as well as the potential harm of smoking on heart and coronary circulation.

Several biological parameters are involved severely in the coronary circulation changes which, however, are finally represented by an atherosclerotic plaque of different degree, extension, and vulnerability. Although endothelial dysfunction seems to be the triggering mechanism of coronary damage in active smokers, as described in chapter 4, there are other parameters like platelets, fibrinogen and coagulation-fibrinolysis chain equally involved early. Changes in their function that smoking produces allows the building of the "main street" through which coronary damage occurs.

Platelets

Platelets are blood cells that maintain primary hemostasis by forming the hemostatic plug which occludes sites of arterial wall damaged by different types of harmful factors.

Platelets are small, anuclear cells of a diameter from 2 to 4 microns derived by fragmentation of megacaryocytes. Therefore, since DNA is a substance nuclear- structured, platelets have only a poor amount of RNA and ribosomes and, consequently, limited metabolic functions that may be potentiated by an increase in platelet number.

When harmful stimuli of different type, particularly mechanical or biological factors, destroy these cells, their function is deeply altered. Therefore, platelets, under these occurrences, increase not only the number but, simultaneously, exalt their properties of aggregation and adhesiveness. In so doing, the "white head", formed to repair an altered arterial wall, consists primarily, if not exclusively, of an amount of aggregated platelets [16].

Usually, platelet deposition occurs locally and not diffusely. Mechanical or metabolic factors like blood turbulence or chemical stimuli can enhance the degree of adhesiveness [17–19]. Moreover, increased platelet activity has been associated with the development of atherosclerotic plaques, also vulnerable plaques, and has been identified as a factor responsible for sudden coronary death [20].

Plasma catecholamines are metabolites able to increase platelet adhesiveness and aggregation. Since cigarette smoking is a strong factor of catecholamine production and release [21-22], there is evidence that cigarette smoking may also promote platelet aggregation indirectly in this way. Also, thrombin is an effective agonist of platelet aggregation [23]. Thrombin stimulates platelet shape change and both primary and secondary aggregation [24] and, metabolically, inhibits the increase in platelet cyclic adenosine monophosphate concentration induced by prostaglandins, particularly prostacyclin [25]. Moreover, thrombin is a basic factor in coagulation-fibrinolysis cascade, as it will be described.

Stimulated blood platelets damage the endothelium of the coronary vessels and facilitate the development of the atherosclerotic process [26–27].

Physiopathologically [28–30], platelet aggregation is determined by three main mechanisms (table 9.2.): platelet adenosine-diphosphate (ADP) release, arachidonic acid metabolism activation, and platelet activating factor (PAF) production.

Table 9.2. Main mechanisms responsible for platelet aggregation

1.	Platelet-ADP release
2.	Arachidonic acid metabolism
3.	PAF production

The first mechanism of platelet aggregation is, usually, triggered by platelet agonists like ADP, thrombin at a low concentration and low concentration in collagen. ADP release forms both endoperoxides from arachidonic acid and thromboxane-A2 (TXA2). Arachidonic endoperoxides and TXA2 exit from the platelets and then develop their vasoconstrictor action.

The second mechanism of aggregation consists of a direct activation of arachidonic acid due to the combined action of thrombin, collagen, epinephrine and exogenous arachidonic acid with consequent production of endoperoxides and TXA2. This pathway is, usually, inhibited by aspirin and, generally, by cyclooxygenase inhibitors.

The third mechanism involves PAF produced mainly by a large variety of cells including neutrophils, eosinophils, monocytes, mast cells, and endothelial cells, which are factors that mediate the inflammatory process [31–32].

By these main mechanisms, that follow phosphate metabolic chain activation, platelets increase their degree of aggregation and adhesiveness on an injured vascular wall to impede its bleeding.

From these observations, it emerges that changes in functional properties of platelets are particularly induced by biological factors that involve coagulation-fibrinolysis cascade mainly through thrombin participation, adrenergic stimulation with catecholamine release, endothelial cell and endothelial metabolite interaction and different metabolic pathways. There is evidence that these factors are directly and indirectly stimulated by cigarette smoking which, therefore, may activate the circle of coronary artery damage, explaining also the early intervention of platelet changes in current smokers.

Platelets in smokers are, usually, maximally activated [27] since toxic compounds of tobacco do that according to chronic smoking habit of the smoker. Therefore, increased platelet aggregation and adhesiveness is one of the first parameters which may be documented as an effect of tobacco smoke.

Biochemically, experimental studies conducted by administration of cigarette-smoking extract would demonstrate that compounds of tobacco smoke induced changes in platelet function with an increase of PAF by a negative interaction with plasma enzyme PAF acetylhydrolase [33]. This enzyme is specific to reduce PAF function and, therefore, impedes platelet aggregations. Consequently, smoking compounds exert pro-aggregatory effects on platelets [34] that potentiate those due to underlying endothelial dysfunction caused by smoking itself on coronary circulation.

Since the changes of platelet function play a chronic effect due to smoking habit of active smokers, there is evidence that active smokers are predisposed heavily to the development of coronary atherosclerosis.

Moreover, experimental findings conducted in active smokers concluded that also short-term exposure to smoking products [35] induced morphological changes in endothelial cells with the appearance of anuclear endothelial cell carcasses in the blood. These constituents would be a toxic manifestation to smoking chemicals and have pro-atherosclerotic effects which potentiate platelet effects.

Thrombus formation as a result of changed platelet function in smokers needs some explanations since such an occurrence may be seen during atherosclerotic plaque formation or complication of a developed plaque.

Various mechanisms contribute to thrombus development in smokers. Firstly, studies would suggest that platelet aggregation in vitro would be increased as an effect of a single cigarette smoked [36–37]. It is worth noting that platelet aggregation raises as an effect of adrenergic stimulation, and nicotine induces catecholamine release whereas carbon monoxide damages particularly the structure of the arterial wall [38].

Platelet thrombi in smokers reduce coronary blood flow, although cyclic changes in reduction have been described [20]. Indeed, initially platelet thrombi are unstable and, consequently, they may disappear with possibly transient increase in coronary blood flow. Conversely, elevated release of catecholamines would induce and maintain the impairment in coronary blood flow [39]. However, nicotine [20] administered intravenously or through the smoke of a cigarette exacerbates the formation of platelet-mediated thrombi in experimental findings. Moreover, since initially platelet-thrombi are loose, they can be carried distally into small coronary arteries causing severe changes in coronary blood flow.

Instability in platelet thrombi-adhesion to the arterial wall is greater in the smokers when it is compared to other occurrences since platelets are chronically but also acutely stimulated from smoking cigarettes and such an event makes current smokers, particularly heavy smokers, at a high risk of thrombo-embolic complications.

Most thrombi are composed mainly of platelets and fibrin in variable proportion and often develop at the site of non-flow-limiting coronary stenosis [40]. When this event occurs in smokers, coronary blood flow could precipitate dramatically if, simultaneously, arterial narrowings exist.

Also, old thrombi often superimposed to an atherosclerotic plaque have been observed and, particularly in women, these thrombi are prevailing on an erose plaque [41-42]. However, it emerges [43] that both old and fresh platelet-thrombi may induce acute coronary syndromes in current smokers.

In conclusion, either clinico-pathological or experimental studies demonstrate undoubtedly smokers' vulnerability towards platelet alterations.

Fibrinogen

Current smokers have higher fibrinogen levels that correlate with the number of cigarettes smoked. It is worth noting that toxics of tobacco smoke increase their harmful effects proportionately to the amount of smoking tobacco consumption.

High fibrinogen levels determine an increase in blood viscosity and may also play a direct role in atherogenesis and platelet aggregation.

Plasma fibrinogen is an independent predictor of cardiovascular disease including coronary heart disease [44–45] with a risk value actually estimated equal to that of the major coronary risk factors.

In smokers, plasma fibrinogen may promote coronary heart disease by several mechanisms primarily atherogenesis, thrombogenesis and increased blood viscosity. In so doing, elevated fibrinogen levels potentiate the effects of platelets and may reduce blood flow [46] particularly through an increase in thrombogenesis independently from the action of other coronary risk factors.

Increased plasma fibrinogen levels found in smokers would be a consequence of an elevated synthesis of this substance in the liver, without an increased catabolism, associated with a series of processes related to inflammation.

A previous study would seem to demonstrate this statement although indirectly [47]. Current smokers had an elevated synthesis of fibrinogen when compared to non-smokers. Conversely, when smokers stopped smoking for two weeks, a reduced synthesis of fibrinogen associated with decrease in its blood concentrations was observed. All together, these data documented that cigarette smoking was the factor which caused these changes.

Increased plasma viscosity and erythrocyte sedimentation rate, which are two biological parameters depending closely on plasma fibrinogen levels, increased their values in current smokers [45]. Moreover, these parameters decreased when also fibrinogen reduced its blood levels [48–49]. From these observations, the role of those factors usually involved in inflammation seems to emerge further.

Fibrinogen levels increase not only with smoking but also in women using contraceptives – we studied a young woman, who smoked a great number of cigarettes and also used oral contraceptives. She was suffering from angina pectoris and developed a fatal myocardial infarction. At the autopsy, severe multiple coronary lumen narrowings with superimposed occlusive thrombi were found [50] – and in diabetic patients, where a decrease in physical activity [51] is experienced regularly.

On the contrary, lipid disorders correlate poorly with fibrinogen levels. Therefore, smokers could display either a risk due to the action of fibrinogen alone or associated with other major coronary risk factors different from lipids, or a potentiated risk due to combined action of fibrinogen with possibly associated factors added to the strong role of lipid disorders. All together, they lead to atherosclerotic coronary lesions

Coagulation-Fibrinolysis Cascade

This hematologic parameter plays a crucial role in contributing to atherosclerotic plaque formation as well as its complication since it is the biochemical substrate that permits the final step to be reached for those factors which are able to trigger the atherosclerotic mechanism. Indeed, various components of coagulation-fibrinolysis cascade are found in the specific structure of the plaque and thrombus formation.

Studies [52–55] identify a large series of changes in chemical metabolites of hemostasis that can cause primarily platelet adhesiveness and aggregation, leukocyte count changes, fibrinogen level increase, plasma viscosity and T-cell function alterations, and all these factors are influenced heavily by cigarette smoking.

Physiologically, the main mechanisms of coagulation-fibrinolysis are the result of an interaction of different factors as table 9.3 shows. Blood vessel, platelet, and plasma factors' combined activity play a basic role for the formation and dissolution of a blood clot, the first step of which recognizes initially, as previously mentioned, a mechanism of vasoconstriction that reduces blood flow to the injured site. However, the exact mechanism by which blood coagulation is initiated is not yet well established, and newer chemical components are, always, found to be involved in the mechanism of coagulation.

Two pathways lead to the formation of a fibrin clot: 1. Intrinsic pathway and 2. Extrinsic pathway. A similar mechanism of vasoconstriction initiates these processes that converge together to clot formation. Then, clot lysis is activated by plasmatic factors generically named the fibrinolytic system.

Chemically, the blood coagulation system is a proteolyitic enzyme cascade [56-58]. Enzymes are present in the plasma as inactive zymogens which on activation undergo lytic cleavage to release active metabolites. The final production of thrombin as a result of both intrinsic and extrinsic pathways, converts soluble fibrinogen into fibrin. Thrombin, as just described, is also a strong platelet agonist.

Table 9.3. Main factors interacting in blood coagulation-fibrinolysis

Steps	Results
1. Platelets	Increased adhesiveness/aggregation
2. Thrombin	Unstable and transient platelet plug
3. Fibrinogen + platelet interaction	Platelet clumping
4. Platelet release of chemical factors adenosine-5-diphosphate (ADP), TXA2, serotonin, phospholipids, lipoproteins	Coagulation-fibrinolysis cascade
5. Fibrinogen to fibrin	Fibrin mesh
6. Plasminogen to plasmin	Clot dissolution and lysis

The phases that follow clot formation are physiologically characterized by clot dissolution and lysis as an effect of plasmin derived from activated plasminogen.

The whole coagulation-fibrinolysis cascade is regulated to avoid the hemorrhage and maintain vessel lumen patency. Cigarette smoking particularly potentiates fibrin clot formation with possible appearance of atherothrombotic manifestations [59–60].

Intracoronary thrombosis results from the action of thrombogenic stimuli that are triggered by chemical components of cigarette smoking particularly nicotine and carbon monoxide. These substances activate metabolic pathways related to endothelial function, platelet function, plasma fibrinogen level and coagulation-fibrinolysis cascade up to a break-down directed toward hard clot formation.

Features of Coronary Alterations

It is known that the relationship between cigarette smoking and coronary atherosclerosis is timely dated. A large spectrum of alterations characterize coronary the circulation of a current smoker although severe coronary lesions usually may be documented as prevailing patterns.

Smoking is causally associated with all the major vascular diseases like stroke, abdominal aortic aneurysm, systemic atherosclerosis [61], but coronary circulation and the heart are involved with a greater incidence severely either as a result of functional disorders induced by both forms of smoking, active smoking and passive smoking [62], or structurally.

Figure 9.1 analyzes the main characteristics of epicardial coronary arteries in smokers.

Autopsy studies [11, 63–64] show a clear prevalence of atherosclerotic lesions in the coronary arteries of smokers. All observations demonstrated an increased degree of atherosclerosis either macroscopically or histologically more frequent than three times in smokers when they were compared to those who had no history of smoking. Also, experimentally [65], coronary changes were observed as related to the number of cigarettes smoked.

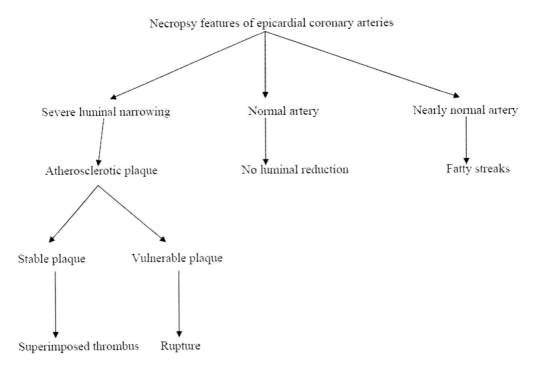

Figure 9.1. Epicardial coronary arteries may display three main types of alterations associated with different pathological features going from severe anatomical lesions to nearly normal or normal artery wall , although severe structural disorders are prevailing.

Every segment of coronary arteries could be affected by alterations: either epicardial arteries or small intramyocardial arteries. Indeed, different types of anatomical changes were described.

Macroscopic changes, which were significantly prevailing with age, consisted particularly of fibrous thickening of the arterial wall and its consequent hardening. The evidence that older individuals displayed more severe coronary wall alterations could be due to three main factors: number of cigarettes smoked, time duration of smoking habit, and changes of arterial structure linked to the age. However, statistical correction of different possible influencing factors documented undoubtedly a significant prevalence of atherosclerotic alterations in current smokers particularly if heavy smokers. Calcifications, independent from an individuals' age, may be seen frequently.

Microscopically, arterial wall fibrous thickening, atherosclerotic plaque variable in extension and type, arterial luminal narrowings, and calcifications are the main features described in the coronary circulation of smokers. Atherosclerotic plaque usually shows a superimposed thrombus, that determines different levels of arterial narrowings, or a vulnerable plaque undergone erosion and consequent rupture may be often seen. Calcium deposits are distributed irregularly with a prevalence along the major axis of the plaque. Such an event contributes to reduce actively vasomotor tone in coronary vessels.

A factor worth noting is the prevailing location of the atherosclerotic lesions. Both coronary districts, left side and right side, are involved in what concerns coronary alterations, although changes localized on the left descending coronary artery are, usually, more proximal than those belonging to other coronary arteries [66].

A few other explanations are necessary for fibrous thickening of coronary arteries [65]. It is a hyaline thickening which consists of an association of intracellular changes with extracellular matrix which give a homogeneous glassy appearance in histologic sections. There is no specific factor that permits one to recognize the pathogenesis of the alteration when it has developed. Conversely, when hyalinosis affects a vascular district, identifying its causal mechanism would be of basic importance since those factors able to induce hyalinosis could be fought. Unfortunately, one can observe the phenomenon when it reaches a well-established level with no possibility to determine the causative factor. Therefore, attributing generically the appearance of hyalinosis to tobacco toxics is without a specific demonstration unless the fact that never smokers do not show fibrous-hyaline thickening in the coronary artery wall while they display the other coronary alterations when ischemic heart disease occurs. Moreover, the development of all other alterations described above well correlate their appearance with smoking.

Carbon monoxide, the main factor responsible for carboxyhemoglobin concentrations, and nicotine may act together since carbon monoxide induces changes in cell permeability [67] and nicotine increases free fatty acid concentrations and epinephrine release [68].

Several other chemicals of burned tobacco may have an atherogenic effect on coronary vessels although there is no significative evidence of experimental atherosclerosis fully related to tobacco chemicals different from nicotine and carbon monoxide.

In conclusion, both autopsy observations in humans and experimental findings identify that atherosclerotic lesions are most severe and extensive in smokers, particularly heavy smokers, even if there are a few cases where coronary arteries are normal or nearly normal displaying only minimal coronary changes. Isolated fibrous-hyaline thickening of coronary wall, particularly in epicardial coronary arteries, could be interpreted as a precursor of more severe lesions that will develop in coronary circulation.

References

[1]   Eliot RS, Baroldi G, Leone A. Necropsy studies in myocardial infarction with minimal or no coronary luminal reduction due to atherosclerosis. *Circulation.* 1974; 49: 1127 – 31.

[2]   Eliot RS, Bratt GT. The paradox of myocardial ischemia and necrosis in young women with normal coronary arteriograms – relationship to anomalous hemoglobin-oxygen dissociation. *Am. J. Cardiol.* 1969; 23: 633 – 8.

[3]   Gross H, Stenberg WH. Myocardial infarction without significant lesions of coronary arteries. *Arch. Intern. Med.* 1939; 64: 249 – 67.

[4]   Friedberg CK, Horn H. Acute myocardial infarction not due to coronary artery occlusion. *JAMA.* 1939; 112: 1675 – 9.

[5]   Soloff LA. Clinical significance of the angiographic demonstration of coronary atherosclerosis. *Am. Heart J.* 1972; 83: 727 – 31.

[6]   Sidd JJ, Kemp HG, Gorlin R. Acute myocardial infarction in a nineteen-year-old student in the absence of coronary obstructive disease. *N. Engl. J. Med.* 1970; 282: 1306 – 7.

[7]   Nizet PM, Robertson L. Normal coronary arteriograms following myocardial infarction in a 17-year-old boy. *Am. J. Cardiol.* 1971; 28: 715 – 7.

[8]   James TN. Angina without coronary disease (sic). *Circulation.* 1970; 42: 189 – 91.

[9]   Heras M, Sanz G, Roig E, Perez-Villa F, Recasens L, Serra A, Betriu A. Endothelial dysfunction of the non-infarct related, angiographically normal, coronary artery in patients with an acute myocardial infarction. *Eur. Heart J.* 1996; 17: 715 – 20.

[10]   Cianflone D, Lanza GA, Maseri A. Microvascular angina in patients with normal coronary arteries and with other ischaemic syndromes. *Eur. Heart J.* 1995; 16: 96 – 103.

[11]   Auerbach O, Carter HW, Garfinkel R, Hammond EC. Cigarette smoking and coronary artery disease. A macroscopic and microscopic study. *Chest.* 1976; 70: 697 – 705.

[12]   Hammond EC. Smoking in relation to death rates of 1 million men and women: Epidemiologic approaches to the study of the cancer and other chronic diseases. *Natl. Cancer Inst. Monogr.* 1966; 19: 127 – 204.

[13]   Kahn HA. The Dorn study of smoking and mortality among U.S. veterans: Report of 8½ years of observation. *Natl. Cancer Inst. Monogr.* 1966; 19: 1 – 125.

[14]   Doyle JT, Dawber TR, Kannel WB. The relationship of cigarette smoking to coronary heart disease: The second report of the combined experience of the Albany, N.Y., and the Framingham, Mass., studies. *JAMA.* 1964; 190: 886 – 90.

[15]   Weir JM, Dann JE Jr. Smoking and mortality: A prospective study. *Cancer.* 1970; 25: 105 – 12.

[16]   Poole JCF, French JE. Thrombosis. *J. Atherosclerosis Res.* 1961; 1 : 251 – 82.

[17]   McDonald L, Edgill M. Changes in coagulability of the blood during various phases of ischaemic heart disease. *Lancet.* 1959; 1: 1115 – 8.

[18]   Mustard JF, Murphy EA. Effect of smoking on blood coagulation and platelet survival in man. *BMJ.* 1963; 1: 846 – 9.

[19]   O'Brien JR. The mechanism and prevention of platelet adhesion and aggregation considered in relation to arterial thrombosis. *Blood.* 1964; 24: 309 – 14.

[20]   Folts JD, Bonebrake FC. The effects of cigarette smoke and nicotine on platelet thrombus formation in stenosed dog coronary arteries: inhibition with phentolamine. *Circulation.* 1982; 65: 465 – 70.

[21]   Robson RH, Fluck DC. Smoking and catecholamines and c-AMP concentrations in the coronary circulation of man and the effect of oxprenolol. *Eur. J. Clin. Pharmacol.* 1977; 12 : 81 – 7.

[22]   De Lorgeril M, Reinharz A, Busslinger B, Reber G, Righetti A. Acute influence of cigarette smoke in platelets, catecholamines and neurophysins in the normal condition of daily life. *Eur. Heart J.* 1985; 6: 1063 – 8.

[23]   Berndt MC, Gregory C, Dowden G, Castaldi PA. Thrombin interactions with platelet membrane proteins. *Ann. N.Y. Acad. Sci.* 1986; 485: 374 – 86.

[24]   Holmsen H. The platelet: its membrane, physiology, and biochemistry. *Clin. Haematol.* 1972; 1: 235 - 66.

[25] Aktories K, Jakobs KH. Ni-mediated inhibition of human platelet adenylate cyclase by thrombin. *Eur. J. Biochem.* 1984; 145: 333 – 8.

[26] Pittilo RM, Mackie IJ, Rowles PM, Machine SJ, Woolf N. Effects of cigarette smoking on the ultrastructure of rat thoracic aorta and its ability to produce prostacyclin. *Throm. Haemost.* 1982; 48: 173 – 6.

[27] Burghuber O, Punzengruber C, Sinzinger H, Haber P, Silberbauer K. Platelet sensitivity to prostacyclin in smokers and non-smokers. *Chest.* 1986; 90: 34 – 8.

[28] Moncada S, Vane JR. Pharmacology and endogenous roles of prostaglandin endoperoxides, thromboxane A2, and prostacyclin. *Pharmacol. Rev.* 1978; 30: 293 – 331.

[29] Perret B, Chap HJ, Douste-Blazy L. Asymmetric distribution of arachidonic acid in the plasma membrane of human platelets. A determination using purified phospholipases and a rapid method for membrane isolation. *Biochim. Biophys. Acta.* 1979; 556: 434 – 46.

[30] Vargaftig BB, Chara M, Benveniste J. Present concepts on the mechanisms of platelet aggregation. *Biochem. Pharmacol.* 1981; 30: 263 – 71.

[31] Hanahan DJ, Demopoulos CA, Liehr J, Pinckard RN. Identification of platelet activating factor isolated from rabbit basophils as acetyl glyceril ether phosphorylcholine. *J. Biol. Chem.* 1980; 255: 5514 – 6.

[32] Hanahan DJ. Platelet activating factor: A biologically active phosphoglyceride. *Annu. Rev. Biochem.* 1986; 55: 483 – 509.

[33] Miyaura S, Eguchi H, Johnson JM. Effect of a cigarette smoke extract on the metabolism of the proinflammatory autacoid, platelet-activating factor. *Circ. Res.* 1992; 70: 341 – 7.

[34] Davis JW, Shelton L, Eigenberg DA, Hignite CE, Watanabe IS. Effects of tobacco and non-tobacco cigarette smoking on endothelium and platelets. *Clin. Pharmacol. Ther.* 1985; 37: 529 – 33.

[35] Prerovsky I, Hladovec J. Suppression of the desquamating effect of smoking in the human endothelium by hydroxyethylrutosides. *Blood Vessels.* 1979; 16: 239 – 40.

[36] Grignani G, Gamba G, Ascari E. Cigarette-smoking effect on platelet function. *Thromb. Haemostas.* 1977; 37: 423 – 8.

[37] Levine PH. An acute effect of cigarette smoking on platelet function – a possible link between smoking and arterial thrombosis. *Circulation.* 1973; 48: 619 – 23.

[38] Leone A. Relationship between cigarette smoking and other coronary risk factors in atherosclerosis: risk of cardiovascular disease and preventive measures. *Curr. Pharm. Design.* 2003; 9: 2417 – 23.

[39] Folts JD. Platelet aggregation in stenosed coronary or cerebral arteries: a mechanism for sudden death? *Wis. Med. J.* 1980; 79: 24 – 6.

[40] Maseri A. From syndromes to specific disease mechanisms. The search for the causes of myocardial infarction. *Ital. Heart J.* 2000; 1: 253 – 7.

[41] Burke AP, Farb A, Malcom GT, Liang YH, Smialek J, Virmani R. Coronary risk factors and plaque morphology in men with coronary disease who died suddenly. *N. Engl. J. Med.* 1997; 336: 1276 – 82.

[42] Burke AP, Farb A, Malcom GT, Liang YH, Smialek J, Virmani R. Effect of risk factors on the mechanism of acute thrombosis and sudden coronary death in women. *Circulation.* 1998; 97: 2110 – 6.

[43] Rival J, Riddle JM, Stein PD. Effects of chronic smoking on platelet function. *Thromb. Res.* 1987; 45: 75 – 85.

[44] Maresca G, Di Blasio A, Marchioli R, Di Minno G. Measuring plasma fibrinogen to predict stroke and myocardial infarction: an update. *Arterioscler. Thromb. Vasc. Biol.* 1999; 19: 1368 – 77.

[45] Danesh J, Collins R, Appleby P, Peto R. Association of fibrinogen, C-reactive protein, albumin, or leukocyte count with coronary heart disease. *JAMA.* 1998; 279: 1477 – 82.

[46] Kannel WB, D'Agostino RB, Belanger AJ. Fibrinogen, cigarette smoking, and risk of cardiovascular disease: insights from the Framingham Study. *Am. Heart J.* 1987; 113: 1006 – 10.

[47] Hunter KA, Garlick PJ, Broom I, Anderson SE, McNurlan MA. Effects of smoking and abstension from smoking on fibrinogen synthesis in humans. *Clin. Sci.* 2001; 100: 459 – 65.

[48] Lowe GDO, Lee AJ, Rumley A, Smith WCS, Tunstall-Pedoe HD. Epidemiology of haematocrit, white cell count, red cell aggregation and fibrinogen: the Glasgow MONICA study. *Clin. Hemorheology.* 1992; 12: 535 – 44.

[49] Rothwell M, Rampling MW, Cholerton S, Server PS. Haemorheological changes in the short term after abstension from tobacco by cigarette smokers. *Br. J. Haematol.* 1991; 79: 500 – 3.

[50] Leone A, Lopez M. Role du tabac et de la contraception orale dans l'infarctus du myocarde de la femme. Description d'un cas. *Pathologica.* 1984; 76 : 493 – 8.

[51] Abramson JL, Vaccarino V. Relationship between physical activity and inflammation among apparently healthy middle-aged and older US adults. *Arch. Intern. Med.* 2002; 162: 1286 – 92.

[52] Imaizumi T, Satoh K, Yoshida H, Kawamura Y, Hiramoto M, Takamatsu S. Effect of cigarette smoking on the levels of platelet-activating factor-like lipid(s) in plasma lipoproteins: *Atherosclerosis.* 1991; 87: 47 – 55.

[53] Becker C, Dubin T. Activation of factor XII glycoprotein by tobacco. *J. Exp. Med.* 1977; 146: 457 – 67.

[54] Saba S, Mason R. Some effects of nicotine on platelets. *Thromb. Res.* 1975; 7: 819 – 24.

[55] FitzGerald GA, Oates JA, Novak J. Cigarette smoking and hemostatic function. *Am. Heart J.* 1988; 115: 267 – 71.

[56] Howell WH. Theories of blood coagulation. *Physiol. Rev.* 1935; 15: 435 – 70.

[57] Mcfarlane RG. An enzyme cascade in the blood clotting mechanism and its function as a biochemical amplifier. *Nature.* 1964; 202: 498 – 9.

[58] Davie EW, Ratnoff ED. Waterfall sequence for intensive blood clotting. *Science.* 1964; 145: 1310 – 2.

[59] Wald NJ, Hackshaw AK. Cigarette smoking: an epidemiological overview. *Br. Med. Bull.* 1996; 52: 3 – 11.

[60] Leone A. Smoking, haemostatic factors, and cardiovascular risk. *Curr. Pharm. Design.* 2007; 13: 1661 – 7.

[61] Powell JW. Vascular damage from smoking: disease mechanisms at the arterial wall. *Vasc. Med.* 1998; 3: 21 – 8.

[62] Barnoya J, Glantz S. Cardiovascular effects of secondhand smoke: nearly as large as smoking. *Circulation.* 2005; 111: 2684 – 98.

[63] Strong JP, Richards ML, McGill HC Jr. On the association of cigarette smoking with coronary and aortic arteriosclerosis. *J. Atheroscler. Res.* 1969; 10: 303 – 17.

[64] Strong JP, Richards ML. Cigarette smoking and atherosclerosis in autopsied men. *Atherosclerosis.* 1976; 23: 451 – 76.

[65] Auerbach O, Hammond EC, Garfinkel L. Thickness of walls of myocardial arterioles in relation to smoking and age: Findings in men and dogs. *Arch. Environ. Health.* 1971; 22: 20 – 7.

[66] Leone A, Lopez M. Myocardial infarction and coronary damage in the smokers: histopathologic features. XII Interamerican Congress of Cardiology, Vancouver, Canada, 1985, Abstract Book.

[67] Astrup P, Kjeldsen K, Wanstrup J. The effects of exposure to carbon monoxide, hypoxia and hyperoxia on the development of experimental atherosclerosis in rabbits. In: Jones RJ (ed.), *Proceedings of the Second International Symposium on Atherosclerosis.* Springer Verlag, New York, NY, USA, 1970; 108 – 11.

[68] Hill P, Wynder EL. Smoking and cardiovascular disease: effect of nicotine on the serum epinephrine and corticoids. *Am. Heart J.* 1974; 87: 491 – 6.

Chapter X

Comparison of Coronary Lesions in Nonsmokers and Smokers

Abstract

Some crucial observations arise from the comparison of coronary alterations between smokers and nonsmokers. There is evidence that clinically smokers, particularly those suffering from an ischemic heart disease, show a higher incidence of coronary events than nonsmokers, and such an occurrence is supported by a major development in pathological alterations of coronary vessels observed in the first group of individuals.

Structurally, coronary arteries of smokers compared to those of nonsmokers show the following characteristics: 1. An increase in size, extension, and instability of atherosclerotic plaque. That may cause a more frequent appearance of complications as well as greater reduction in coronary blood flow. 2. A major incidence of thrombosis, often old thrombi superimposed to plaque, but also fresh thrombi that may give embolization distally. 3. A major amount and number of calcium deposits on the arterial wall of the coronary arteries. 4. A significantly major development in collateral coronary circulation since this parameter increases as much as coronary stenosis is severe.

Keywords: Atherosclerotic plaque, coronary narrowing, thrombosis, platelet, calcium deposits, calcification, coronary collateral(s), nonsmoker(s), smoker(s), comparison, myocardial infarction, reinfarction, unstable angina, sudden death.

There is evidence that ischemic heart disease in nonsmokers and smokers displays similar characteristics for what concerns clinical patterns, although a different degree of coronary alterations and prognosis have been documented often for the two groups. Moreover, as just described, patients who continue smoking after a coronary event have at follow-up a worsened prognosis compared to those who stopped smoking [1]. A significantly higher incidence of reinfarctions [2] was seen in the smokers compared to those who stopped smoking after their infarction and, then, could be identified as past-smokers.

For smokers who survived a first myocardial infarction, greater mortality was supported in other studies. Pohjola et al. [3] in findings on 648 men who survived one year after myocardial infarction, reported that age-adjusted deaths in the next 4 years were 2.3 times greater for continuing smokers than for non-smokers. In those who stopped smoking after their infarction , the risk was almost identical with that of non-smokers.

The Framingham study [4] documented that those individuals who stopped smoking after a heart attack had a death rate 6 years later that was 62 percent less than that of those subjects who continued to smoke, despite the fact that both smokers and non-smokers still continued to have an equal number of nonfatal heart attacks.

Wilhelmsson et al. [5] studied 564 male patients who survived a first acute myocardial infarction and whose smoking habits were measured three months after enrolling in the study. Results showed a halving of cardiovascular mortality and nonfatal myocardial infarctions over a 2-year period in those who stopped smoking.

Daly et al. [6], Jenkins et al. [7], and Vlietstra et al.'s [8] observations were similar, although differing in number with regard to mortality, reinfarction and smoking habits of studied individuals.

Among ischemic heart diseases, acute myocardial infarction, reinfarction and chronic stable angina [9], where, usually, there is pathogenetic evidence of coronary atherosclerosis progression, are more closely related to cigarette smoking in current smokers than sudden coronary death and coronary vasospasm [10], where functional disorders are more frequently involved. About vasospasm, it emerges that past smokers or never smokers with normal or nearly normal coronary arteries may also be affected by this functional disorder [11] determined, certainly, by a larger number of factors which may be different and not always related to cigarette smoking.

Histopathologic findings [12–13] conducted on necropsy material showed more advanced narrowing of coronary arteries in smokers, particularly heavy smokers, when compared to nonsmokers. Smoking seemed to promote the formation of fatty plaques on the surface of blood vessels and also thickening of the small coronary arteries.

An increased frequency of restenosis has been, also, found in patients who continued to smoke after percutaneous transluminal coronary angioplasty [14]. Such a feature will be widely described in chapter 12.

From these statements, it emerges that also in smokers there is a difference in the degree of pathology when continuing smokers are compared to stopping smokers with similar coronary artery disease. Such an observation gives evidence to the fact that an increased progression in structural alterations occurs in coronary circulation when smoking is continued. Therefore, difference in the degree and, sometimes, type of coronary circulation changes usually affect smokers more heavily than nonsmokers.

Alterations of Smokers Versus Nonsmokers

Atherosclerotic Plaque

Atherosclerotic plaque, as mentioned in Chapter 7, consists, histologically, of a great amount of lipid material, intimal smooth muscle cells and macrophages localized in the intimal coat which are associated with an accumulation of connective tissue including collagen, elastic fibers, and proteoglycans. Intracellular and extracellular lipid deposits complete non-complicated plaque composition. Superimposed partially or totally occluding thrombi or distally embolization may occur when a complicated plaque exists. There is evidence that all components of an atherosclerotic plaque belong to those metabolites and cellular material that are strongly stimulated by chemical compounds of cigarette smoking, particularly nicotine and carbon monoxide. Therefore, it emerges easily that smoking stimulates atherosclerotic damage formation and, consequently, smokers should have more pronounced atherosclerosis than nonsmokers. Both clinical and experimental results give evidence of that.

Among smokers, the composition of the plaque usually has cellular and metabolic material in varying proportions and, therefore, a wide spectrum of lesions may be seen. Such a feature makes smokers differently susceptible to coronary heart disease. The risk of an ischemic event is particularly higher in young smokers, where other major coronary risk factors had not yet caused coronary alterations. On the contrary, old people often have an appearance of coronary artery changes which may be a result of the combined influence of several coronary risk factors, and cigarette smoking damage, when present, often undertakes a feature of irreversibility.

At the autopsy [12–13], the degree of coronary atherosclerosis is greater in smokers than in nonsmokers with a percent rate of mortality in smokers from 70 to 200 times higher than nonsmokers. Changes in this rate may be seen when there is a combination among the different major coronary risk factors which could change the incidence of coronary events also in those nonsmokers who have no coronary lesion caused by smoking exposure.

Histologically, a heterogeneity of morphologic lesions in coronary circulation have been described with regard to atherosclerotic plaque.

For many years, nicotine has been identified as a promotor of the development of atherosclerotic lesions in smokers since it caused necrosis and calcifications of the medial coat particularly of medium-large size arteries with the appearance of the Monckeberg type arteriosclerosis [15]. This pathologic pattern, however, differs remarkably from the atherosclerotic lesion.

Nicotine is also responsible for enhanced lipid accumulation in the coronary artery wall and impaired oxygen supply to the heart because of its vasoconstrictory effects mediated directly by the chemical itself and indirectly by sympathetic and adrenergic stimulation.

On the contrary, coronary circulation changes in smokers seem to be particularly a consequence of carbon monoxide toxicity.

Intimal and subintimal injuries of the arterial wall indistinguishable from atherosclerosis are produced in experimental animal models by carbon monoxide [16], which is one of the most toxic compounds of cigarette smoking.

Morphologically, the primary effect of carbon monoxide on the cardiovascular system consists of an increased endothelial permeability, that leads to subendothelial edema easily identifiable histologically since empty spaces exist between any cells and the contiguous ones. This histopathologic change, that involves also myocardial structure, has been considered as a phenomenon of early atherosclerotic alterations and is rather frequent in the coronary arteries and heart muscle of smokers who have undergone ischemic events.

Experimentally, it may be observed in that cardiac pattern defined as smoke cardiomyopathy [17].

Carboxyhemoglobin concentrations higher than 5 percent usually found in smokers would be responsible for both early atherosclerotic changes and atherosclerosis progression.

It is worth noting that carbon monoxide and nicotine usually have synergistic effects that potentiate the result of the coronary alterations in smokers producing an atherosclerotic plaque more evident as extension and type as well as earlier than similar changes observed in the coronary circulation of the nonsmokers.

Thrombosis

Thrombosis is the most severe occurrence that complicates an atherosclerotic plaque. Smokers rather than nonsmokers have all those physiopathological factors able to determine a thrombus formation in coronary arteries. Nonsmokers also can display coronary thrombosis in the absence of cigarette smoking although at a lower rate. When thrombus occurs in nonsmokers, it depends most often on interference of the other major coronary risk factors. However, thrombosis in nonsmokers is, absolutely, less frequent and extensive than that observed in smokers.

Of the many factors which are able to cause thrombi formation, undoubtedly platelet activation, pre-existing vessel stenosis and injury or plaque disruption play a crucial role in development of thrombosis. Authors [18] studied habitual smokers with stable coronary disease, who had taken aspirin immediately before and 5 minutes after smoking two cigarettes each. Compared with before smoking, morphometrically measured platelet thrombus formation on arterial media significantly increased after smoking. Plasma epinephrine also increased more than twofold after smoking as well as whole blood platelet aggregation to thrombin. These results, both physiopathologically and statistically well conducted, would suggest that smoking-induced platelet thrombosis plays a crucial role in acute coronary events in smokers usually not protected, notwithstanding administered aspirin. Moreover, adrenergic-system stimulation simultaneously would enhance pro-thrombotic effects of cigarette smoking.

There is evidence, moreover, that a lot of other parameters (table 10.1.) may increase thrombi formation [19]. Parameters involve various pathways which, all together, interact to produce those biochemical alterations that may lead to the formation of thrombi.

As one can see from the analysis of table 10.1, all listed parameters influenced by smoking may lead to thrombi formation although with a different role, pathway, and activity.

Platelet response and survival appear to be adversely affected by chronic smoking since increased platelet aggregation and adhesiveness have been shown after smoking [20]. Platelet adhesiveness to endothelium, as previously described, is a step that follows endothelial dysfunction caused by cigarette smoking and comes before thrombus formation. Since thrombi formation is, usually, a chronic process that develops through different phases, assessing early endothelial dysfunction in smokers or nonsmokers exposed to tobacco smoking may help to detect, and then to prevent, heart and coronary vessel damage. Simultaneously, decreased endothelium-prostacyclin, that is a potent inhibitor of platelet aggregation [21], enhances platelet aggregation and thrombus formation progression. Moreover, a platelet agonist like thromboxane further stimulates the previous pathways.

Table 10.1. Main parameters changed by cigarette smoking to cause thrombus formation

Hematologic parameters	Increased LDL-Cholesterol
	Decreased HDL-Cholesterol
	Increased plasma fibrinogen
	Increased glucose concentration
	Increased factor VII
	Decreased plasminogen level
Hormonal parameters	Increased plasma catecholamine release
	Increased cortisol production
	Decreased serum estrogen level
Cellular parameters	Increased platelet aggregation
	Increased platelet adhesiveness
	Increased platelet-thromboxane
	Decreased endothelial-prostacyclin
	Change in blood cell count
	Increased reactive C-protein

For smokers, identifying changes in some hemo-coagulative parameters [22–23] like fibrinogen, factor VII, plasminogen and others, up to a degree significantly higher than that seen for never smokers is a further, although indirect, evidence of why smoke thrombosis may reach a significantly more severe and extensive level in coronary arteries.

Finally, lipid metabolism disorder, which has been frequently observed in smokers, is a factor that potentiates coronary artery changes [24–27].

In conclusion, thrombosis may be considered a result of two interrelated phases. A first phase consists of platelet activation following an endothelial injury particularly induced by chemical compounds of cigarette smoking, whereas a second phase involves almost completely coagulation-fibrinolysis system. Smoking and coronary thrombosis are linked by a large series of factors which are able to stimulate both steps of the phenomenon. Functional and cellular mechanisms are primarily activated, although coagulation-fibrinolysis changes follow closely and are prolonged in time.

Coronary Narrowings

The number, degree and extension of coronary narrowings play a crucial role in influencing coronary circulation. Narrowings are the major anatomical determinants of coronary blood flow impairment, and tobacco smoking is often quoted as one of the major risk factors for developing coronary narrowing. Usually, smokers have a twice greater chance to undergo heart attacks than nonsmokers and such an occurence is related strongly to anatomical characteristics of coronary arteries since coronary atherosclerosis progresses much more rapidly in smokers than in nonsmokers [28]. Findings [28] underlined that, angiographically, new coronary lesions, which narrowed coronary artery lumen, developed in more than half of the placebo-treated smokers compared with less than one quarter of the placebo-treated nonsmokers. However, several other angiographic studies did not reach the same conclusions [29–36] with one finding exception [37]. The different conclusions reached by these reports may be explained by the fact that study protocols used most often varied from one finding to the other, different endpoints were estimated, and also different attention to the results carried out, prevailing clinical outcomes in some studies and epidemiologic observations in others, although coronary atherosclerosis progression was the common benchmark of every study.

Necropsy studies, which provide more reliable meaning to the results, demonstrate undoubtedly a significantly major extension of coronary narrowings in smokers when they were compared to similar nonsmoking individuals [12, 13]. Particularly, Leone et al. conducted pathological findings of 80 autopsy cases of patients aged from 48 to 78 years who died from an acute myocardial infarction. Sixty-eight subjects, who were 85 percent of the whole study material, were smokers and 12, the 15 percent, were nonsmokers. Coronary arteries of both smokers and nonsmokers displayed multiple narrowings, occlusive thrombi and calcium deposits. However, the extension of alterations involved all three major coronary vessels of smokers, but, at a maximum, two coronary arteries in nonsmokers. From these data, there is evidence of a greater number of coronary narrowings in smokers simultaneously to a major involvement of the coronary arteries, and such an observation permits one to understand well the reasons for the major severity of damage and consequent heavier impairment in coronary circulation.

Studies in animal models, carefully conducted, provided a remarkably precise meaning of the role of coronary narrowings. Different papers [38–42] generally concluded that in normal dogs maximal coronary blood flow begins to decline when percent diameter narrowing in a short coronary segment reached up to 45 percent and impairment was more significant as coronary stenoses progressed in degree.

Moreover, there is evidence that coronary narrowings, that in the past had been identified as having a fixed diameter, demonstrate, on the contrary, to be dynamic structures capable of active responses. It is worth noting that coronary obstructions produced by the atherosclerotic process dilate in response to nitroglycerin whereas, in susceptible patients, stenotic segments can constrict after infusion of ergonovine [43–44]. These features of coronary narrowings suggest that coronary blood flow, which is severely impaired in stenotic coronary vessels with no development in coronary collaterals, may change under functional factors [45] that, however, may be strongly influenced by cigarette smoking.

Number, degree, type and extension of narrowings are the major determinants of coronary blood flow reduction. Therefore, the knowledge of their greater severity in smokers contributes to explain why a smoker is more susceptible to coronary events than a nonsmoker. As mentioned, the latter may reach the same results observed in smokers as a consequence of interaction among other major coronary risk factors that, however, are often present in smokers too. Thus, cigarette smoking acts as a causative effect of damage also on those factors.

Table 10.2 summarizes the main differences which may be observed for coronary narrowings of smokers and nonsmokers.

Finally, since vulnerable plaques may be identified more easily when the number of coronary stenoses increase, one can deduce the potential harm that affect those individuals, like smokers, who have a greater number of coronary narrowings.

Table 10.2. Major differences in coronary narrowing of nonsmokers and smokers

Narrowing	Smokers	Nonsmokers
Number	Usually higher	Usually lower
Type	Concentric/eccentric	Concentric/eccentric
Superimposed thrombi	Frequent	Variable incidence
Extension	Higher	Lower
Vulnerable plaque	Frequent	Less frequent
Calcification	Most frequent	Frequent

Calcification

Calcification is a pathologic phenomenon characterized by calcium deposits in various tissues and organs of the body as a consequence of a metabolic disorder of the Ca-ion that precipitates to form encrusted crystals particularly on the arterial walls.

Calcium deposits on the coronary wall are a frequent observation of coronary damage caused cigarette smoking [13] and may be displayed also [17] in experimentally-induced smoke cardiomyopathy.

Morphologically, calcium deposits are usually seen in the atheromas of advanced coronary atherosclerosis together with lipid accumulation particularly as an effect of nicotine and carbon monoxide of burned cigarettes. Histologically, calcium deposits have a basophilic, amorphous granular appearance and may have intracellular, extracellular and both, intracellular and extracellular, localization. Usually, calcium crystals precipitate into altered cellular areas where they become encrusted deposits when accompanying changes in calcium metabolism, that cigarette smoking may induce, occur. These morphologic features are a frequent observation in coronary arteries and myocardium of animals or humans exposed to smoking [46]. The great majority of patients with acute coronary syndromes and at least moderate angiographic disease showed identifiable coronary calcium assessed by imaging techniques like electron-beam computed tomography (EBCT). On the contrary, those individuals with negative EBCTs had minimal or no atherosclerotic plaque formation.

Calcium could play a crucial role in regulating coronary blood flow either by acting as Ca-ion influencing the calcium channels or as a precipitate that determines artery wall hardening. The first parameter may be influenced functionally by cigarette smoking. Conversely, the latter is a result of those structural alterations of the arterial wall that characterize atherosclerotic lesions together with other major metabolic and cellular components under the effect of smoking.

The role of coronary calcium in determining ischemic heart disease is always better defined by several papers. Authors [47] identified a calcium score to assess coronary events and observed that electron beam CT coronary calcium score predicted ischemic heart events independently from standard risk factors.

Atherosclerotic calcification [48–49] begins as early as the second decade of life, just before fatty streak formation and microscopically crystalline calcium aggregates in the lipid core have been identified. Generally, calcium deposits characterize more frequently, and in a greater amount, either elderly or more advanced coronary lesions, particularly in smokers [13].

Calcium phosphate salt, which contains about 40 percent in weight of calcium, precipitates on the arterial wall by a mechanism almost identical to that demonstrated in active bone formation and remodeling [50–52].

Coronary remodeling associated with a progression of atherosclerosis is already a described phenomenon [53]. The luminal cross-sectional area and external vessel size become enlarged to compensate for increasing areas of mural atherosclerotic plaques [54–55].

Cigarette smoking that is able to induce changes in calcium metabolism and its physico-chemical properties favoring precipitation in coronary artery plaques aggravates pre-existing structural alterations of coronary arteries.

Finally, since coronary plaques are major in number, extension and degree of narrowing in smokers, as already described, there is evidence that a greater amount of calcium deposits, which are found, usually, in atherosclerotic plaque, characterize smokers compared with nonsmokers and a remodeling of coronary arteries is more frequent and severe in the first group of individuals with consequent significantly major impairment in coronary blood flow.

Coronary Collaterals

Coronary circulation, related to the development of collateral vessels in an attempt to improve, at a maximum, the supply in coronary blood flow reduced by stenoses, is a parameter to estimate carefully in smokers and nonsmokers since important differences have been documented in a varied number of events.

As mentioned, coronary collaterals, also defined as natural bypasses [56], are anastomotic vessel connections without an intervening capillary bed between portions of the same coronary artery and/or different coronary arteries. Therefore, coronary collaterals represent potentially an alternative way of blood supply to a specific myocardial area when the original coronary vessel cannot permit that because of coronary stenosis or occlusion of a different degree and severity [57–58].

Anatomical characteristics of coronary collateral circulation have been detailedly described in chapter 1.

Here, it is worth underlining the physiopathological role carried out by collaterals when major coronary risk factors including cigarette smoking trigger an ischemic mechanism.

When a sudden occlusion of a coronary artery already compromised by atherosclerotic lesions occurs, there is a dramatically strong reduction in coronary blood flow and development of related ischemia [59]. Often atherosclerosis plaque rupture with superimposed thrombosis is the main cause of the appearance of an acute coronary syndrome, usually unstable angina, acute myocardial infarction and cardiac sudden death [60]. Many factors of different type may be aggressive on a stable plaque increasing its vulnerability.

Those particularly involved in vulnerable plaque complication including mechanical, biological, cellular and hematologic factors are summarized in table 10.3. It is worth noting that they may trigger instability mechanisms acting isolatedly or, more often together.

Table 10.3. Main factors involved in atherosclerotic plaque instability

1. Plaque architecture	Thickness of fibrous cap
	Location of lipid core
	Calcium deposits
2. Mechanical factors	Shear stress
	Mechanical deformation
3. Extracellular matrix biology	Synthesis
	Degradation
4. Inflammatory phenomena	Biochemical markers
	Cellular markers
5. Hematologic factors	Coagulation cascade
	Thrombogenic factors
	Tissue factor
6. Major coronary risk factors	

Recently, a tissue factor, that is a potent initiator of the coagulation, has been identified as capable of determining atherosclerotic plaque thrombogenicity [60].

Cigarette smoking has been investigated by findings related to its potential role in coronary collateral circulation development [61-63].

Smoking and, to some extent, alcohol use were associated with collateral development in the coronary tree. Data would suggest that cigarette smoking, often associated with some specific lifestyle habits, may influence the development of coronary collaterals particularly in patients suffering from an ischemic heart disease. Such an assessment is well supported by the fact that coronary circulation of smokers is greatly impaired by a larger spectrum of anatomical alterations than that of nonsmokers.

References

[1]   Leone A. Cigarette smoking and health of the heart. *J. Roy Soc. Health.* 1995; 115: 354 – 5.

[2]   Leone A. Cardiovascular damage from smoking: a fact or belief? *Int. J. Cardiol.* 1993; 38: 113 – 7.

[3]   Pohjola S, Siltanen P, Romo M. Five-year survival of 728 patients after myocardial infarction. *Br. Heart J.* 1980; 43: 176 – 83.

[4]   Sparrow D, Dawber TR, Colton T. The influence of cigarette smoking on prognosis after a first myocardial infarction. *J. Chronic Dis.* 1978; 31: 425 – 32.

[5]   Wilhelmsson C, Vedin JA, Elmfeldt D, Tibblin J, Wilhelmsen L. Smoking and myocardial infarction. *Lancet.* 1975; i: 415 – 20.

[6]   Daly LE, Mulcahy R, Graham IM, Hickey N. Long-term effect on mortality of stopping smoking after unstable angina and myocardial infarction. *BMJ.* 1983; 287: 324 – 6.

[7]   Jenkins CD, Zyzanski SJ, Rosenman RH. Risk of new myocardial infarction in middleaged men with manifest coronary heart disease. *Circulation.* 1976; 53: 342 – 7.

[8]   Vlietstra RE, Kronmal RA, Oberman A. Stopping smoking improves survival in patients with angiographically-proven coronary artery disease. *Am. J. Cardiol.* 1982; 49: 984A.

[9]   Meinert CL, Forman S, Jacobs DR, Stamler J. Cigarette smoking as a risk factor in men with a prior history of myocardial infarction. *J .Chronic Dis.* 1979; 32: 415 – 25.

[10] Health or Smoking. Follow-up Report of the Royal College of Physicians. Pitman Publishing, London, UK, 1983.

[11] Sugiishi M, Takatsu F. Cigarette smoking is a major risk factor for coronary spasm. *Circulation.* 1993; 87: 76 – 9.

[12] Auerbach O, Carter HW, Garfinkel L, Hammond EC. Cigarette smoking and coronary heart disease, a macroscopic and microscopic study. *Chest.* 1976; 70: 697 – 705.

[13] Leone A, Bertanelli F, Mori L, Fabiano P, Battaglia A. Features of ischaemic cardiac pathology resulting from cigarette smoking. *J. Smoking-Related Dis.* 1994; 5: 109 – 14.

[14] Galan KM, Deligonul U, Kern MJ, Chaitman BR, Vandormael MG. Increased frequency of restenosis in patients continuing to smoke cigarettes after percutaneous transluminal coronary angioplasty. *Am. J. Cardiol.* 1988; 61: 260 – 3.

[15] Schievelbein H, Longdon V, Longdon W, Grumbach H, Remplik V, Schauer A, Immich H. Nicotine and arteriosclerosis. *Z. Klin. Chem.* 1970; 8: 190 – 6.

[16] Astrup P. Carbon monoxide, smoking, and cardiovascular disease. *Circulation.* 1973; 48: 1167 – 8.

[17] Lough J. Cardiomyopathy produced by cigarette smoke. Ultrastructural observations in guinea pigs. *Arch. Pathol. Lab. Med.* 1978; 102: 377 – 80.

[18] Hung J, Lam JY, Lacoste L, Letchacovski G. Cigarette smoking acutely increases platelet thrombus formation in patients with coronary artery disease taking aspirin. *Circulation.* 1995; 92:2432 – 6.

[19] Leone A. Biochemical markers of cardiovascular damge from tobacco smoke. *Curr. Pharm. Design.* 2005; 11: 2199 – 208.

[20] Meade TW, Imeson J, Stirling Y. Effects of changes in smoking and other characteristics on clotting factors and the risk of ischemic heart disease. *Lancet.* 1987; 2: 986 – 8.

[21] FitzGerald GA, Oates JA, Nowak J. Cigarette smoking and hemostatic function. *Am. Heart J.* 1988; 115: 267 – 71.

[22] Kannel WB, D'Agostino RB, Belanger AJ. Fibrinogen, cigarette smoking, and the risk of cardiovascular diseases: insights from the Framingham study. *Am. Heart J.* 1987; 113: 1006 – 10.

[23] Stone MC, Thorpe JM. Plasma-fibrinogen-a major coronary risk factor. *JR. Coll. Gen. Pract.* 1985; 35: 565 – 9.

[24] Craig WY, Palomaki GE, Haddow JE. Cigarette smoking and serum lipid and lipoprotein concentrations: an analysis of published data. *BMJ.* 1989; 298: 784 – 8.

[25] Fisher ER, Wholey M, Shoemaker R. Cigarette smoking and cholesterol atherosclerosis of rabbits. *Arch. Pathol.* 1974; 98: 418 – 21.

[26] Pedersen TR. Lowering cholesterol with drugs and diet. *N. Engl. J. Med.* 1995; 333: 1350 – 1.

[27] Ross R. The pathogenesis of atherosclerosis: A perspective for the 1990s. *Nature.* 1993; 362: 801 – 9.

[28] Waters D, Lesperance J, Gladstone P, Boccuzzi SJ, Cook T, Hudgin R, Krip G, Higginson L, for the CCAIT Study Group. Effects of cigarette smoking on the angiographic evolution of coronary atherosclerosis. A Canadian Coronary Atherosclerosis Intervention Trial (CCAIT) Substudy. *Circulation.* 1996; 94: 614 – 21.

[29] Bemis CE, Gorlin R, Kemp HG, Herman MV. Progression of coronary artery disease: a clinical arteriographic study. *Circulation.* 1973; 47: 455 – 64.

[30] Kramer JR, Matsuda Y, Mulligan JC, Aronow M, Proudfit WL. Progression of coronary atherosclerosis. *Circulation.* 1981; 63: 519 – 26.

[31] Vanhaecke J, Piessens J, Van de Werf F, Willems JL, De Geest H. Angiographic evolution of coronary atherosclerosis in non-operated patients. *Eur. Heart J.* 1983; 4: 547 – 56.

[32] Shea S, Sciacca RR, Esser P, Han J, Nichols AB. Progression of coronary atherosclerotic disease assessed by cinevideodensitometry: relation to clinical risk factors. *J. Am. Coll. Cardiol.* 1986; 8: 1325 – 31.

[33] Moise A, Theroux P, Taeymans Y, Waters DD, Lesperance J, Fines P, Descoings B, Robert P. Clinical and angiographic factors associated with progression of coronary artery disease. *J. Am. Coll. Cardiol.* 1984; 3: 659 – 67.

[34] Benchimol D, Benchimol H, Bonnet J, Dartigues JF, Couffinhal T, Bricaud H. Risk factors for progression of atherosclerosis six months after balloon angioplasty of coronary stenosis. *Am. J. Cardiol.* 1990; 65: 980 – 5.

[35] Alderman EL, Corley SD, Fisher LD, Chaitman BR, Faxon DP, Foster ED, Killip T, Sosa JA, Bourassa MG, and the CASS participating investigators and staff. Five-year angiographic follow-up of factors associated with progression of coronary artery disease in the Coronary Artery Surgery Study (CASS). *J. Am. Coll. Cardiol.* 1993; 22: 1141 – 54.

[36] Nobuyoshi M, Tanaka M, Nosaka H, Kimura T, Yokoi H, Hamasaki N, Kim K, Shindo T, Kimura K. Progression of coronary atherosclerosis: is coronary spasm related to progression? *J. Am. Coll. Cardiol.* 1991; 18: 904 – 10.

[37] Raichlen JS, Healy B, Achuff SC, Pearson TA. Importance of risk factors in the angiographic progression of coronary artery disease. *Am. J. Cardiol.* 1986; 57: 66 – 70.

[38] Shipley RE, Gregg DE. The effect of external constriction of a blood vessel on blood flow. *Am. J. Physiol.* 1944; 141: 289 – 96.

[39] Khouri EM, Gregg DE, Lowensohn HS. Flow in the major branches of the left coronary artery during experimental coronary insufficiency in the unanesthetized dog. *Circ. Res.* 1968; 23: 99 – 109.

[40] Arnett EN, Isner JM, Redwood DR, Kent DM, Baker WP, Ackerstein H, Roberts WC. Coronary artery narrowing in coronary heart disease: comparison of cineangiographic and necropsy findings. *Ann. Intern. Med.* 1979; 91: 350 – 6.

[41] Gould KL, Lipscomb K, Hamilton GW. Physiologic basis for assessing critical coronary stenosis. Instantaneous flow response and regional distribution during

coronary hyperemia as measures of coronary flow reserve. *Am. J. Cardiol.* 1974; 33: 87 – 94.

[42] Gould KL, Lipscomb K. Effects of coronary stenoses on coronary flow reserve and resistance. *Am. J. Cardiol.* 1974; 34: 48 – 55.

[43] Doerner TC, Brown GB, Bolson E, Frimer M, Dodge HT. Vasodilatory effects of nitroglycerin and nitroprusside in coronary arteries- a comparative analysis. *Am. J. Cardiol.* 1979; 43: 416A.

[44] Heupler FA Jr, Proudfit WL, Razavi M, Shirey EK, Greenstreet R, Sheldon WC. Ergonovine maleate provocative test for coronary arterial spasm. *Am. J. Cardiol.* 1978; 41: 631 – 40.

[45] Likoff M, Reichek N, Sutton MSJ, Makoviak J, Harken A. Epicardial mapping of segmental myocardial function: an echocardiographic method applicable in man. *Circulation.* 1982; 66: 1050 – 8.

[46] Schmermund A, Baumgart D, Gorge G, Seibel R, Gronemeyer D,Ge J, Haude M, Rumberger J, Erbel R. Coronary artery calcium in acute coronary syndromes. *Circulation.* 1997; 96: 1461 – 9.

[47] Arad Y, Goodman KJ, Roth M, Newstein D, Guerci AD. Coronary calcification, coronary disease risk factors, C-reactive protein, and atherosclerotic cardiovascular disease events. *J. Am. Coll. Cardiol.* 2005; 46: 158 – 65.

[48] Stary HC. The sequence of cell and matrix changes in atherosclerotic lesions of coronary arteries in the first forty years of life. *Eur. Heart J.* 1990; 11(suppl E): 3-19.

[49] Doherty TM, Detrano RC. Coronary arterial calcification as an active process: a new perspective on an old problem. *Calcif. Tissue Int.* 1994; 54: 224 - 30.

[50] Bostrom K, Watson KE, Horn S, Wortham C, Herman IM, Demer LL. Bone morphogenetic protein expression in human atherosclerotic lesions. *J. Clin. Invest.* 1993; 91: 1800 - 9.

[51] Schmid K, McSharry WO, Pameijer CH, Binette JP. Chemical and physicochemical studies on the mineral deposits of the human atherosclerotic aorta. *Atherosclerosis.* 1980; 37: 199-210.

[52] Anderson HC. Mechanism of mineral formation in bone. *Lab. Invest.* 1989; 60: 320 - 33.

[53] Gibbons GH, Dzau VJ. The emerging concept of vascular remodeling. *N. Engl. J. Med.* 1994; 330:1431-8.

[54] Glagov S, Weisenberg E, Zarins CK, Stankunavicius R, Kolettis GJ. Compensatory enlargement of human atherosclerotic coronary arteries. *N. Engl. J. Med.* 1987; 316: 1371-5.

[55] Clarkson TB, Prichard RW, Morgan TM, Petrick GS, Klein KP. Remodeling of coronary arteries in human and nonhuman primates. *JAMA.* 1994;271: 289 – 94.

[56] Koerselman J, van der Graaf Y, de Jaegere PPTh, Grobbee DE. Coronary Collaterals. An important and underexposed aspect of coronary artery disease. *Circulation.* 2003; 107: 2507 – 11.

[57] Sasayama S, Fujita M. Recent insights into coronary collateral circulation. *Circulation.* 1992, 85:1997-1204.

[58] Moritz AR, Beck CS. The production of a collateral circulation to the heart. Pathological anatomical study. *Am. Heart J.* 1935 – 7: 874 – 80.

[59] Oliver MF. Prevention of coronary heart disease – propaganda, promises, problems, and prospects. *Circulation.* 1986; 73: 1 – 9.

[60] Moons AH, Levi M, Peters RJ. Tissue factor and coronary artery disease. *Cardiovasc. Res.* 2002; 53: 313 – 25.

[61] Kyriakides ZS, Kremastinos DT, Michelakakis NA, Matsakas EP, Demovelis T, Toutouzas PK. Coronary collateral circulation in coronary artery disease and systemic hypertension. *Am. J. Cardiol.* 1991; 67: 687 – 90.

[62] Witte DR, Bots ML, Hoes AV, Grobbee DE. Cardiovascular mortality in Dutch men during 1996 European football championship: longitudinal population study. *BMJ.* 2000; 321: 1552 – 4.

[63] Koerselman J, de Jaegere PPTh, Verhaar MC, Grobbee DE, van der Graaf Y, and for the SMART Study Group. Coronary collateral circulation: The effects of smoking and alcohol. *Atherosclerosis.* 2007; 191: 191 – 8.

Chapter XI

Ischemic Heart Disease

Abstract

Ischemic heart disease is characterized by two types of events: a chronic event like stable angina pectoris, chronic postischemic cardiomyopathy associated or not with arrhythmias, and acute events, typically unstable angina, acute myocardial infarction, ventricular arrhythmias and sudden cardiac death.

Structural changes that affect the cardiovascular system as an effect of smoking do not differ from those attributable to the same disease caused by other factors, although some differences may be met in the development and manifestations of the lesion when both active or passive smoking are the responsible factors.

Coronary heart disease is a disorder strictly related to smoking. Coronary atherosclerosis affects mainly the coronary arteries of individuals suffering from chronic or acute ischemic heart disease. Moreover, focal intramyocardial areas of hemorrhage may be seen with a major incidence in myocardial infarctions of smokers. Severe coronary narrowings as well as vessel calcification also characterize a myocardial infarction from smoking. Therefore, finding focal hemorrhagic areas in the context of a necrosis, severe coronary narrowings and calcification can mean that smoking exposure has influenced myocardial changes with a high probability.

Other manifestations of coronary heart disease are sudden death and arrhythmias, particularly related to functional disorders induced by smoking exposure, as well as two types of cardiomyopathies: postischemic cardiomyopathy with progressive heart failure, and experimental cardiomyopathy described in different animal models as an event strictly related to smoking exposure.

Keywords: Smoking, coronary heart disease, stable angina, unstable angina, myocardial infarction, structural alterations, sudden death, arrhythmias, postischemic cardiomyopathy, heart enlargement, experimental cardiomyopathy, heart failure.

The purpose of this chapter is not to describe in detail the varied and complex patterns that characterize ischemic heart disease that is fully developed in specific textbooks of cardiovascular disease like Braunwald's Heart Disease [1], Hurst's the Heart [2], and others.

This chapter will focus on those characteristics of ischemic heart disease which can permit us to better understand the clinico-pathological correlations which exist between the appearance of ischemic heart disease and cigarette smoking particularly as a consequence of coronary circulation alterations.

Clinical manifestations of ischemic heart disease are similar for both nonsmokers and smokers, although some differences exist about the complications that may be associated with the underlying disease. Reinfarction, mortality, and reinfarction associated with mortality have been documented particularly in smokers [3–9], as described in the previous chapter. It is worth noting that progression of coronary atherosclerosis, developed with a significantly major incidence in smokers than that in nonsmokers, usually by the mechanism of plaque rupture and possible thrombosis, causes mainly unstable angina and myocardial infarction [10–12].

Most atherosclerosis progression occurs without associated symptoms, although, sometimes, there is evidence of an acute appearance of symptoms and, also, of sudden cardiac death. Moreover, increased newer plaque formation may explain why smokers develop ischemic heart disease more often and at a younger age compared with nonsmokers. Lesions at a high risk for plaque complications are those composed particularly [13] by elevated lipid content as well as thin fibrous cap that are specifically those alterations observed in smokers.

Ischemic heart disease continues to be a serious health problem [14] strongly related to cigarette smoking. Worldwide [15–16], more than 3 million people currently die each year from smoking, half of them before the age of 70 years, and that is an enormous human cost to which must be added the fact that more than one third have cardiovascular events, particularly of the ischemic type, that often determine permanent disability of affected individuals. Indeed, there are more than one billion smokers in the world with an increased/decreased/again increased smoking habit.

Two types of clinical manifestations, that may be also associated among themselves, characterize ischemic heart disease: chronic manifestations, the main patterns of which are stable angina and postischemic cardiomyopathy, and acute manifestations that group acute myocardial infarction, unstable angina and sudden cardiac death.

It is worth noting the role that cigarette smoking usually plays. Chronic disease is affected particularly by chronic exposure to cigarette smoking that causes progressive structural alterations in coronary circulation. The second group of disease often may recognize a functional mechanism induced acutely by cigarette smoking that may be superimposed to pre-existing structural coronary alterations. There is evidence, in the latter case, as a more complex and severe pathogenetic mechanism of lesion may be identified.

Coming straight to the point, the main features of the different manifestations of ischemic heart disease will be described.

Ischemic Heart Disease

A large series of epidemiological studies [17-29], most of them conducted also after chronic or acute exposure to passive smoking, support strongly statistical evidence that the smoking habit is followed by a significant increase in coronary events.

On the contrary, experimentally acute exposure to passive smoking can cause impairment in exercise tolerance for both healthy individuals and individuals with a pre-existing myocardial infarction [30].

Coronary heart disease recognizes a multifactorial etiology. Risk factors may play their effects isolatedly or with different combinations among themselves inducing myocardial hypoxia. It may result from either a fall in oxygen transportation to the heart by coronary arteries or an increased demand for oxygen by the cardiovascular system. Pathologically, a reduced availability in oxygen is responsible for an impairment in coronary blood flow with consequent myocardial ischemia.

Usually, myocardial ischemia develops as an effect of occlusion or narrowing of the lumen of one or more coronary arteries because of a progression or complication of atherosclerotic plaques.

Whatever factor may induce coronary artery disease, the types of pathological patterns observed are characterized by functional or structural alterations and clinical symptoms due to the specific disease without any identification of the causative factor, although from the analysis of the structural changes some features may be identified as related to smoking. That has been particularly documented by experimental findings conducted on animal models.

Table 11.1 analyzes the main mechanisms responsible for clinical events related to both chronic or acute patterns of ischemic heart disease.

Table 11.1. Types of coronary heart disease and main causative mechanisms

Type of event	Main mechanism
Chronic patterns:	
StableAngina	Fixed single or multiple coronary narrowings
Postischemic cardiomyopathy	Chronic and heavy hypoxia
Acute patterns:	
Unstable angina	Vasospasm
Myocardial infarction	Acute coronary occlusion
Sudden death	Increased sympathetic stimulation / life threatening ventricular arrhythmias
Arrhythmias (ventricular and atrial)	Increased sympathetic stimulation

Stable Angina

Stable angina may be defined as a clinical syndrome characterized by discomfort or pain in the chest, jaw, shoulder, back or arm. Usually, symptoms are precipitated or aggravated by physical or emotional exertion and relieved by nitroglycerin. Angina, preferably, occurs in individuals who are suffering from coronary artery disease affecting one or more large epicardial coronary arteries. Other cardiac or extracardiac causes (table 11.2.) may be responsible for the appearance of anginal symptoms. In these circumstances, coronary arteries of affected patients may be altered by atherosclerotic lesions or, more often, they may be normal or nearly normal, but an increased demand for oxygen by the heart not associated with a coronary flow capable to supply oxygenated blood to the cardiac muscle exists. Poor availability of oxygen due to a large series of factors that impede a stable link of the oxygen with hemoglobin, as in the presence of carboxyhemoglobin, may cause anginal symptoms.

Table 11.2. Main causes of stable angina

Cardiac factors	Coronary atherosclerosis
	Valvular heart disease
	Hypertrophic cardiomyopathy
	Uncontrolled hypertension
Extracardiac factors	Hematologic disorders
	Chest wall disorders
	Esophageal disorders
	Lung diseases
	Endocrine disorders
	Metabolic disorders
	Cerebrovascular disorders
	Nervous system disorders
	Toxics

A different type of almost constant coronary atherosclerosis with coronary narrowings of different degree, or single or multiple occlusions [31] of coronary vessel lumen, may be documented in the large majority of individuals affected by stable angina, although other possible mechanisms as a coronary vasospasm [32], acute thrombosis and platelet aggregation [33] can play a crucial role. Therefore, there is a strong relationship between cigarette smoking and stable angina, since the type of underlying coronary heart disease is coronary atherosclerosis with plaque progression, although plaque rupture, thrombosis and, sometimes, functional vasospasm mediated by catecholamine release may contribute to aggravate the clinical manifestations.. Moreover, about 90 percent of the hearts of patients suffering from angina showed, at the postmortem examination, different but severe degrees of coronary atherosclerosis [34–35].

Aronow [36] studied the effect of passive smoking on exercise-induced angina. Patients exposed to passive smoking had a larger increase in resting heart rate, systolic and diastolic blood pressure and venous carboxyhemoglobin as well as a greater reduction in heart rate and systolic blood pressure with a significant reduction of exercise duration. Leone and coworkers [30] in their observations concerning both healthy individuals and individuals with a pre-existing myocardial infarction, who were exposed acutely to passive smoking, reached similar conclusions. Moreover, Meinert and coworkers [37] identified cigarette smoking as a factor of progression of coronary atherosclerosis in patients with a pre-existing myocardial infarction.

Risk factors for stable angina are basically the same as risk factors for coronary heart disease. They are summarized in table 11.3.

Table 11.3. Main risk factors for stable angina

Hypertension (or uneffective control in blood pressure)
Lipid disorders
Smoking
Diabetes mellitus
Obesity
High salt intake
Male sex
Postmenopausal woman
Family history of ischemic heart disease
Low physical exercise

The first step to diagnose carefully stable angina is to recognize the characteristic of chest pain or discomfort. This symptom permits us to classify patients with stable angina into two groups: patients with typical chest pain and patients with atypical chest pain. It is worth noting that, usually, chest pain shows the same characteristics for the same patient who is able, therefore, to know the threshold of appearance of angina.

Five main parameters should be estimated for anginal chest pain: its location, quality, duration, triggering factor, and response to nitroglycerin.

It should be noted that angina is described as stable angina when it does not change characteristics for, at least, 60 days.

Cigarette smoking increases the risk of stable angina as well as changes in its threshold by multiple mechanisms that involve, at least, three factors: the level of structural alterations in coronary arteries – atherosclerotic plaque formation has been demonstrated to be the most important, sympathetic and adrenergic stimulation induced by nicotine followed by an increased demand for oxygen by the cardiac muscle, and, finally, increased carboxyhemoglobin concentrations and, consequently, reduced availability in oxyhemoglobin mediated basically by carbon monoxide.

Therefore, patients who suffer from stable angina must absolutely stop smoking since further observations on the role of smoking in patients with ischemic heart disease suggest such a behaviour.

Findings of Aronow [36] and Aronow et al. [38] showed that cigarette smoking decreases exercise tolerance in patients with angina pectoris. Allen et al. [39] also supplemented this observation by showing that in patients who smoked, ST-segment depression at the electrocardiogram performed by ambulatory monitoring, typically common during episodes of silent ischemia, occurred more commonly during smoking than nonsmoking periods.

Finally, for what concerns antianginal drugs, there is evidence that [40] smoking has a direct and adverse effects on the heart and interferes with the efficacy of all antianginal classes of drugs, particularly beta-blockers and calcium antagonists like nifedipine.

Postischemic Cardiomyopathy

This pathologic pattern is a clinical event characterized by symptoms of congestive heart failure and structural alterations usually characterized by degenerative lesions and fibrotic processes which are the result of a chronic repair following recurrent and acute hypoxic cardiovascular events due to coronary artery disease. Multiple areas of microfocal fibrosis or confluent massive fibrosis affect myocardium with impairment of cardiac function. A marked heart enlargement is a constant manifestation of this clinico-pathological picture.

Postischemic cardiomyopathy may follow an acute ischemic event, the manifestations of which continue chronically in the time as a consequence of coronary circulation impairment, or begins as a chronic manifestation linked to a repeated ischemic insult of hypoxic type. There is evidence, in case of chronic hypoxia, that a severe compromise of coronary circulation exists and cardiac muscle results in being chronically hypoperfused. Therefore, postischemic cardiomyopathy is a dilated cardiomyophathy where the degree of coronary narrowings and/or a previous ischemic event causing ventricular dysfunction are not able solely to be explained by the underlying ischemia [41]. The existence of such a condition leads one to hypothesize that other factors, particularly major coronary risk factors including cigarette smoking, may play a crucial role in maintaining and aggravating the disease by not only hypoxic mechanisms but also metabolic reactions.

Metabolic and functional responses capable of determining a normal heart function may be severely worsened also at rest, and a state of chronic inadequate nutrition characterize the myocardium with development of atrophic alterations. There is a decrease in size of myocardial fibers associated, however, with ventricular chambers enlargement. Histologically, the myocardial fibers [42] first become smaller and then completely disappear probably as a result of autolysis in various myocardial areas. These alterations associated with a variable development of multiple fibrotic zones determine a myocardial remodeling which is functionally uneffective.

Clinically, a progressive congestive heart failure is present in those individuals who are affected by the disease often associated with significant disability to develop their routine job.

The precise role that cigarette smoking plays in the context of postischemic cardiomyopathy is far from being clearly established. However, the severe compromise of coronary circulation due to cigarette smoking plays a crucial role in determining chronic hypoxia that is responsible for chronic inadequate nutrition for myocardial fibers. However, up till now, there is no certain evidence that toxic compounds of smoking can exert a direct damage on the myocardium to maintain this disease.

Unstable Angina

Unstable angina among the different pictures that characterize ischemic heart disease is undoubtedly one of the most serious events.

Unstable angina is a clinical syndrome where coronary alterations are often associated and may lead to cardiac death or non Q-wave myocardial infarction. Angiografically, findings show that a disruption of an athero-thrombotic plaque with a subsequent series of pathologic events able to impair, sometimes heavily, coronary blood flow may exist [43].

Clinically, chest pain in unstable angina is identical to that of stable angina, but sudden cardiac death, life-threatening ventricular arrhythmias or a recurrent myocardial infarction may affect individuals suffering from the first of the two syndromes [44–45].

Pathogenetically, among the possibly different causes capable of triggering unstable angina, all those determining reduced myocardial perfusion, coronary artery luminal narrowing with a nonocclusive fresh thrombus formed following plaque rupture or erosion play a crucial role. As just described, thrombus may embolize distally. Another frequent mechanism of coronary flow reduction is the coronary vasospasm, that has been more diffusely described in the chapter of this book on coronary atherosclerosis. Moreover, inflammatory phenomena [46–50] have been identified to play an even major role in causing biochemical and cellular changes able to trigger the coronary syndrome. Other factors, probably less important, related to external coronary mechanisms have been described for the pathogenesis of unstable angina. Table 11.4 lists the main pathogenetic mechanisms.

Table 11.4. Main pathogenetic mechanisms for the pathogenesis of unstable angina

Plaque rupture or erosion with subsequent fresh thrombus
Coronary segmental vasospasm
Inflammatory processes
Severe narrowing without spasm or thrombosis
External factors to coronary arteries

Cigarette smoking may cause unstable angina particularly by nicotine and carbon monoxide, which impair coronary circulation either by coronarogenic mechanisms related to atherosclerotic plaque formation and/or complication, or by a direct action on the heart muscle reducing oxygen availability and increasing cardiac demand in oxygen.

Acute Myocardial Infarction

Acute myocardial infarction is, absolutely, the most important heart disease since its incidence is worldwide significantly high [51–52] and prognosis varies widely according to a large series of factors, some of which well known nowadays, but some others yet in progress or obscure. Moreover, the outcome of the disease depends on triggering events and coronary circulation involvement. Alterations in some coronary arteries like left anterior descending artery or main left coronary artery may cause usually myocardial infarctions significantly more extensive which are characterized, usually, by poor long-term prognosis. On the contrary, sudden death, as an onset of an acute myocardial infarction, may occur independently from the coronary artery affected by lesions, although, even in this case, impairment in left coronary circulation usually plays a stronger role.

Acute myocardial infarction is also strictly related to the presence and combination of the major coronary risk factors including cigarette smoking, the effects of which involve not only coronary circulation but also directly the myocardium.

Another factor to be underlined is the age of affected individuals with prevailing acute myocardial infarction from the fifth to sixth decade of life, a period where the smoking habit, usually started in youth, is well established and there has been enough time to permit the harm from smoking on coronary circulation. Moreover, women smokers who use oral contraceptives or show ovarian disorders are at a high risk of developing an acute myocardial infarction associated with severe coronary artery alterations [53–54].

Pathologically, acute myocardial infarction is the necrosis of a portion of myocardium with total or partial loss in myocell function due to insufficient acute blood supply.

Necrosis may be well defined as a result of those morphologic changes which follow cell death in a living tissue or organ with partial or total loss in their function. Usually, histologic changes in death cells may be documented a few hour later from injury action.

All infarcts of the heart muscle belong to the group of necrotic lesions, but not all cardiac necroses are necessarily infarcts. It should be noted that necrosis from an infarct recognizes a coronarogenic origin with partial or total vessel occlusion either of structural or functional type, while there is evidence of other cardiac alterations characterized by a typical necrosis where coronary circulation maintains its integrity and is also able to provide an adequate blood flow to the heart. Therefore, two types of necrosis may develop as a consequence of smoking exposure: coronarogenic necrosis, that is an ischemic necrosis, and non-coronarogenic necrosis.

Myocardial necrosis is the most serious alteration that nicotine and carbon monoxide of smoking can cause. The pathogenetic mechanism which causes cardiac cell necrosis, anyhow it is produced, consists of a hypoxia due to two main, often associated, factors: reduced coronary blood flow as a consequence of alterations in the coronary tree, and/or a direct hypoxic action due to chemicals of tobacco smoke. Therefore, an acute vascular mechanism characterized by thrombo-atherosclerotic occlusion may induce cell death, and this is the typical myocardial infarct as, usually, defined by pathologists, as well as a myocardial necrosis like that induced by electrolyte disequilibrium, vasopressor amines and smoking chemicals [55–56].

Macroscopic and microscopic characteristics of myocardial infarction [57] have been well described for a long time and their feature is common whatever the triggering mechanism, although, histologically, some patterns, which would seem to be associated with cigarette smoking, may be observed in both smoker individuals and individuals exposed passively to smoking [58-59].

The main gross and microscopic changes of a myocardium affected by an infarct may be seen in tables 11.5 and figure 11.1 to 11.3. Usually, pathological alterations may be documented after 6 to twelve hours from the onset of the disease. Therefore, the clinical symptoms of myocardial infarction may be also lacking in the case of sudden coronary death occurring before the appearance of pathologic alterations. In this case, great difficulties exist in establshing the true cause of death in an individual who does not yet show heart alterations at the autopsy. However, evidence of major coronary risk factors associated with pre-existing symptoms related to coronary involvement could suggest a possible acute myocardial infarction, although histochemical procedures do not permit us to assess certainly the type of myocardial alterations necessary to carry out a precise diagnosis.

Table 11.5. Gross changes in acute myocardial infarction

Appearance time	Progression of the lesions
6-12 hours to 3-4 days	Pale and dry myocardium with red focal hemorrhagic areas.
4 to 8 days	Peripheral yellow zone extending into the dry myocardium where a well-defined border health/altered myocardium is seen.
8 to 12 days	Reduced myocardial wall thickness; yellow surface of infarct surronded by a red-purple depressed zone.
1 month	Red-purple material extends into infarct area.
2 to 3 months	Formation of a gray, firm scar at the infarct area (healed infarct).

Briefly, gross changes in acute myocardial infarction are the result of necrotic phenomena with a loss of myocardial structure of the affected area followed by processes of repair with formation of a firm and gray scar due to myocardial fibrosis.

These alterations may involve transmurally myocardium or, conversely, be localized into subendocardium. Transmural infarcts usually affect the free wall of the left ventricle massively and often involve also interventricular septum limitedly to its anterior two third. Sometimes, there is an extension of anterior myocardial, transmural infarction to the right ventricle although more rarely to myocardium of corresponding atrium. Therefore, transmural infarction extends from the endocardium to the epicardium reaching a size largely variable according to the degree of coronary alterations and occurrence of occlusion. Sudden coronary narrowing, particularly when it is totally occluding vessel lumen, originates, often, extensive and massive infarctions with a significant heart dysfunction.

Figures 11.1 and 11.2 show a macroscopic pattern of a myocardial infarction and a postmortem coronary angiography where a mild coronary narrowing may be seen.

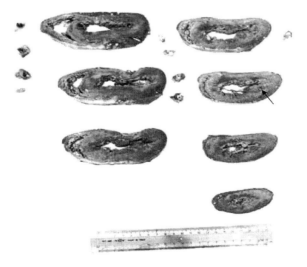

Figure 11.1. Postmortem examination of the heart by the technique of Roussy and Ameuille [62]. The heart is cut into 6 to 7 slices of approximately 1 cm of thickness together with coronary artery. Myocardial alterations are, then, established and measured. There is a massive area of myocardial infarction (pale white color, arrow!) involving anterior and lateral free wall of the left ventricle in a 67-year-old man who was a heavy smoker.

As one can see, macroscopic alterations may be easily examined by this method of investigation since myocardial mass is completely exposed and, then, measures concerning ventricular wall thickness carried out to establish gross characteristics of ventricular walls and septum as well as possible enlargement of cardiac chambers that are parameters linked to the involvement of coronary circulation.

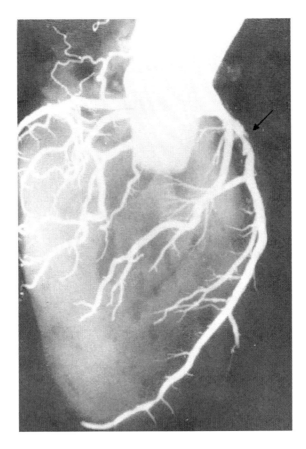

Figure 11.2. Postmortem coronary angiography. There is evidence of a mild coronary stenosis (arrow!) on the first portion of the left anterior coronary artery with poor development in coronary collaterals. Notwithstanding the mild degree of coronary stenosis, this patient developed a fatal myocardial infarction.

From these observations, it emerges that a wide spectrum of coronary patterns which may go from severe and multiple stenoses to nearly normal or normal coronary arteries have been documented, also macroscopically, in patients with an acute myocardial infarction.

The main histologic features of an acute myocardial infarction are summarized in figure 11.3. There is evidence that the first phase of cellular damage is followed by the intervention of a wide series of reactive phenomena that lead to healed infarction, which is the final step of the process.

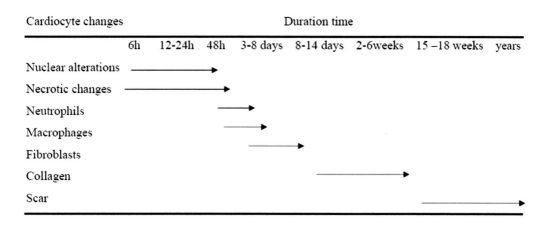

Figure 11.3. Histopathologic features and evolution of human myocardial infarct. There is evidence that a fixed and stable scar remains in affected myocardium.

Microscopic changes of a myocardial infarction follow a well-defined pathway.

The first two to three days from the onset of the disease, necrotic phenomena with myocell fragmentation and nuclear disappearance may be seen. They are followed by the appearance of polimorphonuclear infiltrates. Then, during the next 4 to 10 days a granulation tissue into the area of infarct tends to form, and finally, after two to three months, a firm scar completes the healing process.

Neutrophil polymorphonuclears are the main characteristic living cells of the early stage that reach the dead zone of an infarct. However, these cells too become rapidly necrotic and their breaking really initiates all those repairing processes which lead to a fibrous scar formation since a large amount of active enzymes and chemical substances deriving from polymorphonuclear degeneration clean up the infarct zone from necrotic material.

Necrotic fibers may show different histologic patterns attributed to different pathogenetic mechanisms. There is evidence of a coagulation necrosis that is the typical vascular necrosis due to coronary occlusion and, then, markedly coronary blood flow impairment. A second pattern of acute ischemic cell damage is the contract band necrosis. In this case, cardiocytes are hypercontracted and have a more intense stain due to their eosinophilia. Mechanisms related to reperfusion or sympathetic phenomena have been hypothesized to explain this pattern. Finally, myocytolisis is characterized by progressive lysis of myofibrils producing a clear vacuolation of sarcoplasm with possible leaving of empty sarcolemmal sheaths. Figure 11.4 shows a typical histologic pattern of an acute myocardial infarct where coagulation necrosis and myocytolysis associated with wide zones of initial fibrosis may be seen.

Coronary arteries may show different degrees of narrowing, complete occlusions due to old thrombi, atherosclerothic plaque rupture with fresh thrombi superimposed and calcifications. However, myocardial infarcts with minimal or no coronary luminal reduction due to atherosclerosis at the necropsy have been described, and among these patients with myocardial infarction there were also smokers [58].

From these structurally basic alterations of a myocardial infarct, differences due to smoking exposure have been described [59-60].

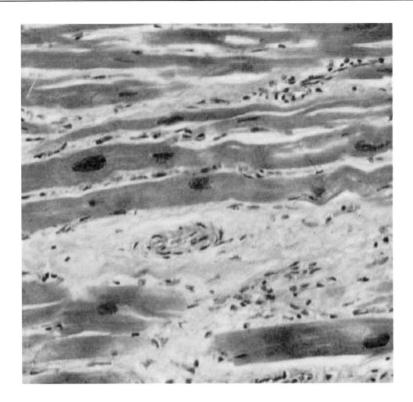

Figure 11.4. Myocardial infarction of 4 to 6 day-old. Several cardiocytes show focal or total lysis; many cardiocyte nuclei are intact, but there are cardiac fibers with disappearance of the nuclei; a central zone with polymorphonuclear infiltration and granulation tissue formation may be also seen. (Reproduced, with permission, from: Passive Smoking and Cardiovascular Pathology: Mechanisms and Physiopathological Bases of Damage, A. Leone ed., Nova Science Publishers, Inc. New York, 2007).

Smoking exposure causes hemorrhagic microfocal infiltrates in the area affected by myocardial infarct with a major rate. This occurrence could be due to a direct effect of carbon monoxide on cardiac cells similarly to what has been demonstrated for the experimental cardiomyopathy from smoking. Moreover, in necropsy studies [59-60] the finding of more advanced narrowings of coronary arteries characterized the smokers, particularly heavy smokers, when compared with nonsmokers exposed passively to smoking or, even more, non exposed never smokers.

A major incidence of thickening of the small coronary vessels and calcifications affected particularly both smokers and nonsmokers who were exposed to environmental tobacco products. It is known that a rise in intracellular calcium concentrations [61] with consequent calcification phenomena activates some enzyme chains that induce heavy cell injury until cell death with complete loss of its function.

As one can see, smoking may cause myocardial infarction particularly as a consequence of development, progression and complication of an atherosclerotic lesion. Moreover, structural alterations observed in both myocardial cells and coronary arteries are usually heavier than those in nonexposed never smokers affected by the ischemic event.

Establishing these facts, there is evidence that coronary circulation of smokers with an acute myocardial infarction is more severely impaired when it is compared to that of similar individuals who are nonsmokers, as almost all the findings undoubtedly seem to demonstrate.

Ventricular Arrhythmias

The appearance of ventricular arrhythmias, particularly life-threatening ventricular arrhythmias in individuals suffering from ischemic heart disease is a frequent observation and has been well demonstrated to be related either to active smoking or passive smoking exposure [63–64].

The crucial role played by smoking for the appearance of these arrhythmias has been unequivocally proven in a man with a previous myocardial infarction who displayed experimentally identical ventricular arrhythmias [64] during exercise stress testing performed twice in the same environment polluted by carbon monoxide at 35 ppm/air concentration whereas the same occurrence did not take place when exercise was performed in the same environment not polluted by cigarette smoking.

Functional disorders , basically linked with sympathetic stimulation, may be the factors responsible for rhythm disorders, although severe structural alterations in coronary circulation play a crucial role.

Sudden Cardiac Death

Sudden cardiac death is an unexpected natural death due to cardiac events within a short time period from the onset of symptoms in an individual previously in a healthy state or without any prior condition that could be identified as potentially fatal [65–66].

Sudden cardiac death is, usually, triggered by ventricular arrhythmias [67–68] that are commonly produced by sympathetic and adrenergic stimulation. Nicotine derived from cigarette smoking increases catecholamine release which is potentially an arrhythmogenic factor [69].

A strong evidence, however, of the role played by cigarette smoking in causing coronary sudden death is yet far to be reached. Reports [70-73] underline a strong role, whereas others do not identify proven results [74–75].

Among findings that would identify smoking as an independent risk factor of sudden cardiac death, there is the study of Goldenberg et al. [70]. Authors enrolled more than 3,000 individuals who were affected by coronary artery disease. Everyone in the study had either had a heart attack or anginal pain. Enrolled individuals were followed up for an average of about 8 years. It was found that current smokers were more than twice affected by sudden cardiac death during the follow-up than people who were never smokers. Moreover, former smokers had a similar risk of sudden death as individuals who had never smoked. Therefore, the risk of sudden cardiac death disappears when smokers quit smoking. Toxic effects of smoking, particularly attributed to nicotine, would play a crucial role. However, various other mechanisms such as increased platelet adhesiveness, decreased ventricular fibrillation threshold, increased heart rate and blood pressure, elevated carboxyhemoglobin concentration and coronary vasospasm are possible determinants of cardiac sudden death as a consequence of cigarette smoking. Figure 11.5 shows life-threatening ventricular arrhythmias in a heavy smoker admitted to a Coronary Care Unit for an acute myocardial infarction. Sudden cardiac death could be triggered by this or similar rhythm disorder.

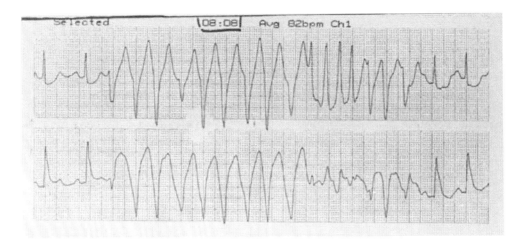

Figure 11.5. Electrocardiographic monitoring in a heavy smoker with an acute myocardial infarction. One can see life-threatening ventricular arrhythmias like those able to cause sudden cardiac death.

Other large-scale findings [74–75] did not demonstrate, however, a direct relationship between smoking alone and sudden death, but, conversely, a relationship existed between all major risk factors including cigarette smoking and the cardiac event.

From these observations, particularly related to possible effects of cigarette smoking on the appearance of sudden death, there emerges a significant concept: the evidence that disorders more specifically related to functional effects of toxic compounds of cigarette smoking more than a structural damage of coronary circulation, which, however, exists and, sometimes, of severe degree, may cause more easily the occurrence of sudden cardiac death.

Therefore, changes in lifestyle, particularly for those individuals who suffer from an ischemic heart disease or have a family history for this event and major coronary risk factors including cigarette smoking, are recommended to control the appearance of cardiac sudden death.

References

[1]   *Braunwald's Heart Disease – A Textbook of Cardiovascular Medicine.* Zipes DP, Libby P, Bonow RO, Braunwald E (eds.), 7th edition, Elsevier Saunders, Philadelphia, Penn, USA, 2005.

[2]   *Hurst's The Heart.* Fuster V, Alexander RW, O'Rourke RA (eds.), 11th edition, The McGraw-Hill Companies, Inc. New York, NY, USA, 2004.

[3] Leone A. Cardiovascular damage from smoking: a fact or belief? *Int. J. Cardiol.* 1993; 38: 113 – 7.

[4] Pohjola S, Siltanen P, Romo M. Five-year survival of 728 patients after myocardial infarction. *Br. Heart J.* 1980; 43: 176 – 83.

[5] Sparrow D, Dawber TR, Colton T. The influence of cigarette smoking on prognosis after a first myocardial infarction. *J. Chronic Dis.* 1978; 31: 425 – 32.

[6] Wilhelmsson C, Vedin JA, Elmfeldt D, Tibblin J, Wilhelmsen L. Smoking and myocardial infarction. *Lancet.* 1975; i: 415 – 20.

[7] Daly LE, Mulcahy R, Graham IM, Hickey N. Long-term effect on mortality of stopping smoking after unstable angina and myocardial infarction. *BMJ.* 1983; 287: 324 – 6.

[8] Jenkins CD, Zyzanski SJ, Rosenman RH. Risk of new myocardial infarction in middleaged men with manifest coronary heart disease. *Circulation.* 1976; 53: 342 – 7.

[9] Vlietstra RE, Kronmal RA, Oberman A. Stopping smoking improves survival in patients with angiographically-proven coronary artery disease. *Am. J. Cardiol.* 1982; 49: 984A.

[10] Buja LM, Willerson JT. Clinicopathologic correlates of acute ischemic heart disease syndromes. *Am. J. Cardiol.* 1981; 47: 343 – 56.

[11] Moise A, Theroux P, Taeymans Y, Descoings B, Lesperance J, Waters DD, Pelletier GB, Bourassa MG. Unstable angina and progression of coronary atherosclerosis. *N. Engl. J. Med.* 1983; 309: 685 – 9.

[12] Ambrose JA, Tannenbaum MA, Alexopoulos D, Hjemdahl-Monsen CE, Leavy J, Weiss M, Borrico S, Gorlin R, Fuster V. Angiographic progression of coronary artery disease and the development of myocardial infarction. *J Am Coll Cardiol* 1988; 12: 56 – 62.

[13] Falk E. Why do plaques rupture? *Circulation.* 1992; 86 (Suppl III): III30 – 42.

[14] Gibbons RJ, Abrams J, Chatterjee K, Daley J, Deedwania P, Douglas JS, Ferguson B Jr, Fihn SD, Fraker TD, Gardin JM, O'Rourke RA, Pasternak RC, Williams SV. Guidelines for the management of patients with chronic stable angina :A report of the ACC/AHA Task Force on Practice Guidelines (Committee on the Management of Patients with Chronic Stable Angina). *J. Am. Coll. Cardiol.* 2003; 41: 159 – 168.

[15] Peto R, Lopez AD, Boreham J, Thun M, Heath C. *Mortality from smoking in developed countries: 1950 – 2000.* Oxford, UK: University Press 1994.

[16] Wald NJ, Hackshaw AK. Cigarette smoking: an epidemiological overview. *Br. Med. Bull.* 1996; 52: 3 – 11.

[17] Sherman CB. Health effects of cigarette smoking. *Clin. Chest Med.* 1991; 12: 643 – 58.

[18] Thun M, Henley J, Apicella L. Epidemiologic studies of fatal and nonfatal cardiovascular disease and ETS exposure from spousal smoking. *Environ. Health Perspect.* 1999; 107S: 841 – 6.

[19] Wells AJ. Passive smoking as a cause of heart disease. *J. Am. Coll. Cardiol.* 1994; 24: 546 – 54.

[20] Doll R, Peto R. Mortality in relation to smoking: 20 years' observations on male British doctors. *BMJ.* 1976; 2: 1525 – 36.

[21] Steenland K. Passive smoking and the risk of the heart disease. *JAMA.* 1992; 267: 94 – 9.

[22] Kawachi I, Colditz GA, Speizer FE, Manson JE, Stampfer MG, Willet W, Hennekens C. A prospective study of passive smoking and coronary heart disease. *Circulation.* 1997; 95: 2374 – 9.

[23] Helsing K, Sandler D, Comstock G, Chee E. Heart disease mortality in nonsmokers living with smokers. *Am. J. Epidemiol.* 1988; 127: 915 – 22.

[24] Hole D, Gillis C, Chopra C, Hawthorne VM. Passive smoking and cardiorespiratory health in a general population in the west of Scotland. *BMJ.* 1989; 299: 423 – 7.

[25] LeVois ME, Layard MW. Publication bias in the environmental tobacco smoke/coronary heart disease epidemiologic literature. *Regul. Toxicol. Pharmacol.* 1995; 21: 184 – 91.

[26] Steenland K, Thun M, Lally C, Heath C Jr. Environmental tobacco smoke and coronary heart disease in the American Cancer Society CPS-II cohort. *Circulation.* 1996; 94: 622 – 8.

[27] Dobson AJ, Alexander HM, Heller RF, Lloyd DM. Passive smoking and the risk of heart attack or coronary death. *Med. J. Aust.* 1991; 154: 793 – 7.

[28] Muscat JE, Wynder EL. Exposure to environmental tobacco smoke and the risk of heart attack. *Int. J. Epidemiol.* 1995; 24: 715 – 9.

[29] He Y, Lam TH, Li LS, Du RY, Jia GL, Huang JY, Zheng JS. Passive smoking at work as a risk factor for coronary heart disease in Chinese women who have never smoked. *BMJ.* 1994; 308: 380 – 4.

[30] Leone A, Mori L, Bertanelli F, Fabiano P, Filippelli M. Indoor passive smoking: its effect on cardiac performance. *Int. J. Cardiol.* 1991; 33: 247 – 52.

[31] Blumgart HL, Schlesinger MJ, Davis D. Studies on the relation of the clinical manifestations of angina pectoris, coronary thrombosis, and myocardial infarction to the pathologic findings. *Am. Heart J.* 1940; 19: 1 – 91.

[32] Maseri A, Severi S, De Nes M, L'Abbate A, Chierchia S, Marzilli M, Ballestra AM, Parodi O, Biagini A, Distante A. Variant angina: one aspect of a continuous spectrum of vasospastic myocardial ischemia. Pathogenetic mechanisms, estimated incidence, clinical and coronarographic findings in 138 patients. *Am. J. Cardiol.* 1978; 42: 1019 – 35.

[33] Folts JD, Crowell EB, Rowe G. Platelet aggregation in partially obstructed vessels and its elimination with aspirin. *Circulation.* 1976; 54: 365 – 70.

[34] Blumgart HL, Pitt B, Zoll PM, Freiman DG. Anatomic factors influencing the locations of coronary occlusions and development of collateral coronary circulation. In: *The Etiology of myocardial infarction*, James TN and Keys JW (eds.), Little, Brown, Boston, Mass, USA, 1963; 327 – 37.

[35] Blumgart HL, Zoll PM, Wessler S. Angina pectoris; clinical pathologic study of 177 cases. *Trans Ass. Amer. Physicians.* 1950; 63: 262 – 7.

[36] Aronow WS. Effect of passive smoking on angina pectoris. *N. Engl. J. Med.* 1978; 299: 21 – 4.

[37] Meinert CL, Forman S, Jacobs DR, Stamler J. Cigarette smoking as a risk factor in men with a prior history of myocardial infarction. *J. Chronic Dis.* 1979; 32: 415 – 25.

[38] Aronow WS, Kaplan MA, Jacob D. Tobacco: a precipitating factor in angina pectoris. *Ann. Intern. Med.* 1968; 69: 529 – 35.

[39] Allen RD, Gettes LS, Phalan C, Avington MD. Painless ST-segment depression in patients with angina pectoris. Correlation with daily activities and cigarette smoking. *Chest.* 1976; 69: 467 – 73.

[40] Deanfield J, Wright C, Krikler S, Ribeiro P, Fox K. Cigarette smoking and the treatment of angina with propranolol, atenolol, and nifedipine. *N. Engl. J. Med.* 1984; 310: 951 – 4.

[41] Richardson P, McKenna WJ, Bristow MR, Maisch B, Mautner B, O'Connel J, Olsen E, Thiene G, Goodwin J, Gyarfas I, Martin I, Nordet P. Report of the 1995 World Health Organization/International Society and Federation of Cardiology. Task Force on the definition and classification of cardiomyopathies. *Circulation.* 1996; 93: 841 – 2.

[42] Karsner H, Saphir O, Todd TW. The state of the cardiac muscle in hypertrophy and atrophy. *Am. J. Path. Bact.* 1925; 1: 351 – 71.

[43] Waters DD. Diagnosis and management of patients with unstable angina. In: Fuster V, Alexander RW, O'Rourke RA (eds.), *Hurst's The Heart*, 10th ed, McGraw-Hill, New York, NY, USA 2001; 1237 – 74.

[44] Boden WE, O'Rourke RA, Teo KK, Hartigan PM, Maron DJ, Kostuk WJ, Knudtson M, Dada M, Casperson P, Harris CL, Chaitman BR, Shaw L, Gosselin G, Nawaz S, Title LM, Gau G, Blaustein AS, Booth DC, Bates ER, Spertus JA, Berman DS, Mancini GB, Weintraub WS; COURAGE Trial Research Group. Optimal Medical Therapy with or without PCI for Stable Coronary Disease. *N. Engl. J. Med.* 2007; 356: 1503 – 16.

[45] Braunwald E, Antman EM, Beasley JW, Califf R, Cheitlin M, Hochman J, Jones R, Kereiakes D, Kupersmith J, Levin T, Pepine C, Schaeffer J, Smith E, Steward D, Theroux P, Gibbons R, Antman E, Alpert J, Faxon D, Fuster V, Gregoratos G, Hiratzka L, Jacobs A, Smith S. ACC/AHA 2002 guideline update for the management of patients with unstable angina and non-ST-segment elevation myocardial infarction-summary article. A report of the American College of Cardiology/American Heart Association task force on practice guidelines (Committee on the Management of Patients With Unstable Angina). *J. Am. Coll. Cardiol.* 2002; 40: 1366 – 74.

[46] Blake GJ, Ridker PM. Novel clinical markers of vascular wall inflammation. *Circ. Res.* 2001; 89: 763 – 71.

[47] Ridker PM, Stampfer MJ, Rifai N. Novel risk factors for systemic atherosclerosis: A comparison of C-reactive protein, fibrinogen, homocysteine, lipoprotein(a), and standard cholesterol screening as predictors of peripheral arterial disease. *JAMA.* 2001; 2835: 2481 – 5.

[48] Vorchheimer DA, Fuster V. Inflammatory markers in coronary artery disease: Let prevention douse the flames. *JAMA.* 2001; 286: 2154 – 6.

[49] Ridker PM, Glynn RJ, Hennekens CH. C-reactive protein adds to the predictive value of total and HDL cholesterol in determining risk of first myocardial infarction. *Circulation.* 1998; 97: 2007 – 11.

[50] Blake GJ, Ridker PM. C-reactive protein and other inflammatory markers in acute coronary syndromes. *J. Am. Coll. Cardiol.* 2003; 141: L23 –L305.

[51] World Health Statistics Annuals. WHO Report, Geneva, Switzerland, 1965 – 77.

[52] Walker WJ. Changing U.S. lifestyle and declining vascular mortality – a retrospective. *N. Engl. J. Med.* 1983; 308: 649 – 51.

[53] Leone A, Lopez M. Role du tabac et de la contraception orale dans l'infarctus du myocarde de la femme. Description d'un cas. *Pathologica.* 1984; 76 : 493 – 8.

[54] Leone A, Lopez M. Oral contraception, ovarian disorders and tobacco in myocardial infarction of woman. *Pathologica.* 1986; 78: 237 – 42.

[55] Bajusz E. The terminal electrolyte-shift mechanism in heart muscle; its significance in the pathogenesis and prevention of necrotizing cardiomyopathies. In: Bajusz E (ed.), *Electrolytes and Cardiovascular Diseases*, Vol 1; Karger, Basel, Sw, 1965.

[56] Bajusz E, Jasmin G. Observations on histochemical differential-diagnosis between primary and secondary cardiomyopathies. *Am. Heart J.* 1965; 69: 83 – 92.

[57] Mallory GK, White PD, Salcedo-Salgar J. The speed of healing of myocardial infarction. A study of the pathologic anatomy in seventy-two cases. *Am. Heart J.* 1939; 18: 647 – 71.

[58] Eliot RS, Baroldi G, Leone A. Necropsy studies in myocardial infarction with minimal or no coronary luminal reduction due to atherosclerosis. *Circulation.* 1974; 49: 1127 – 31.

[59] Leone A, Bertanelli F, Mori L, Fabiano P, Battaglia A. Features of ischaemic cardiac pathology from cigarette smoking. *J. Smoking-Related Dis.* 1994; 5: 109 – 14.

[60] Auerbach O, Carter HW, Garfinkel L, Hammond EC. Cigarette smoking and coronary heart disease, a macroscopic and microscopic study. *Chest.* 1976; 70: 697 – 705.

[61] Trump BJ, Berezesky I. The reactions of cells to lethal injury: oncosis and necrosis- the role of calcium. In Lockshin RA et al. (eds.). *When cells die – A comprehensive evaluation of apoptosis and programmed cell death.* Wiley-Liss, New York, NY, USA, 1998; 57 – 96.

[62] Roussy G, Ameuille P. *Techniques des autopsies et des recherches anatomo-pathologiques à l'Amphithèatre.* O Doin et Fils, Paris, France,1910.

[63] Leone A, Bertanelli F, Mori L, Fabiano P, Bertoncini G. Ventricular arrhythmias by passive smoke in patients with pre-existing myocardial infarction. *J. Am. Coll. Cardiol.* 1992; 19: 256A.

[64] Leone A. Passive smoking causes cardiac alterations in post-MI subjects. *Int. J. Smoking Cessation.* 1996; 3(4): 42 – 3.

[65] Kannel WB, Cupples LA, D'Agostino RB. Sudden death risk in overt coronary heart disease : the Framingham study. *Am. Heart J.* 1987; 113: 799 – 804.

[66] Zheng ZJ, Croft JB, Giles WH, Mensah GA. Sudden cardiac death in the United States, 1989 to 1998. *Circulation.* 2001; 104: 2158 – 63.

[67] Wilhelmsen I, Wedel H, Tibbin G. Multivariate analysis of risk factors for coronary heart disease. *Circulation.* 1973; 48: 950 – 8.

[68] Schlant RC, Forman S, Stamler J, Canner PL, for the Coronary Drug Project Research Group. The natural history of coronary heart disease: prognostic factors after recovery from myocardial infarction in 2789 men: the 5 year findings of the Coronary Drug Project. *Circulation.* 1982; 66: 401 – 14.

[69] Sugishi M, Faminaro T. Cigarette smoking is a major risk for coronary spasm. *Circulation.* 1993; 87: 76 – 9.

[70] Goldenberg I, Jonas M, Tenenbaum A, Boyko V, Matetzky S, Shotan A, Behar S, Reicher-Reiss H, for the Bezafibrate Infarction Prevention Study Group. Current

Smoking, Smoking Cessation, and the Risk of Sudden Cardiac Death in Patients with Coronary Artery Disease. *Arch. Intern. Med.* 2003; 163: 2301 – 5.

[71]   Burke AP, Farb A, Malcom GT, Liang Y, Smialek J, Virmani R. Coronary risk factors and plaque morphology in men with coronary disease who died suddenly. *N. Engl. J. Med.* 1997; 336: 1276 – 82.

[72]   Kannel WB. Update on the role of cigarette smoking in coronary artery disease. *Am. Heart J.* 1981; 101: 319 – 28.

[73]   Hallstrom AP, Cobb LA, Ray R. Smoking as a risk factor for recurrence of sudden cardiac arrest. *N. Engl. J. Med.* 1986; 314: 271 – 5.

[74]   Hinkle LE Jr. Short-term risk factors for sudden death. *Ann. N.Y. Acad. Sci.* 1982; 382: 22 – 38.

[75]   Kagan A, Yano K, Reed DM, MacLean CJ. Predictors of sudden cardiac death among Hawaiian-Japanese men. *Am. J. Epidemiol.* 1989; 130: 268 – 77.

Chapter XII

Coronary Surgery and Smoking

Abstract

The role of cigarette smoking in coronary circulation after revascularization procedures either of the surgical type like CABGS or hemodynamic type like PTCA is controversial and, therefore, no unanimous opinions on the subject exist.

Statistical observations selected by using multivariate analysis would indicate that cigarette smoking induces early and more frequent restenosis of coronary arteries at the site of intervention as well as myocardial infarction and, therefore, creates the need to repeat invasive procedures. Such a fact would be responsible for an enormous increase in costs and, particularly, of delay in interventions for those people suffering from ischemic heart disease who do not smoke or stopped smoking.

Stopping smoking is, therefore, an imperative act to do in an attempt to maintain the improvement in coronary circulation that revascularization procedures usually determine.

Keywords: Coronary artery bypass graft, CABGS, percutaneous transluminal coronary angioplasty, PTCA, coronary stenosis, restenosis, cigarette smoking, ischemic heart disease, surgical technique, hemodynamic technique.

Assessing the role of cigarette smoking in influencing the results of coronary surgery as well as the behaviour of a smoker following surgical procedures is a subject of greatest importance since an open debate still exists between researchers who recommend coronary surgery in continuing smokers and researchers who deny the intervention. That, since it would seem that continuing smokers may be early affected again by those alterations displayed before surgery.

The relationship between coronary surgery and major coronary risk factors as well as the outcome of postsurgical patients affected by major coronary risk factors has not yet been fully clarified, although it is a very promising expanding view. Inconsistent data would demonstrate an improvement in life quality of postsurgical patients although not associated with a better long-term prognosis, except for those cases who had successful revascularization of the left coronary tree [1].

The most largely used surgical technique for coronary arteries consists of coronary artery bypass graft surgery (CABGS). However, other invasive non-surgical procedures performed hemodynamically like percutaneous transluminal coronary angioplasty (PTCA) are widely used to correct coronary stenoses and, then, improve coronary blood flow. Even if, strictly speaking, the latter procedure cannot be considered as a surgical intervention, its diffuse application in coronary stenotic alterations as well as relationship with major coronary risk factors including cigarette smoking justifies its description in this chapter where the effects of cigarette smoking in surgical and post-surgical coronary patients will be discussed.

Therefore, CABGS and PTCA will be the subject of this chapter.

CABGS

Coronary revascularization has been conducted in almost all coronary patients who needed to improve coronary blood flow compromised by single or multiple coronary atherosclerotic narrowings or coronary vessel complete occlusion due to thrombi.

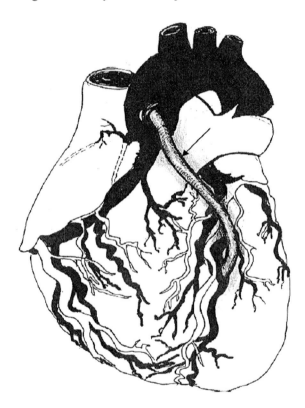

Figure 12.1. Schematic view of coronary artery bypass graft surgery (CABGS). An arterial or venous graft leads blood directly (arrow!) from the aorta down to a significant coronary artery stenosis or occlusion determining a coronary revascularization.

The crucial role is to identify those patients who may obtain significant benefits from CABGS. Bypass surgery (figure 12.1.) has become a common surgical procedure used to divert blood around blocked arteries in the heart. More than 200,000 undergo CABGS each year in the United States [1–3] with, usually, a significant improvement in the blood flow due to the newer route built over the occluded artery.

Main indication for CABGS are debilitating chest pain caused by severe and often multiple narrowings of the coronary arteries without any relief after medical drug administration, severe ventricular dysfunction, life-threatening ventricular arrhythmias not responsive to antiarrhythmic therapy, and inappropriate or previous unsuccessful PTCA.

There is evidence that CABGS does not cure the underlying coronary artery disease but improves coronary circulation. Therefore changes in lifestyle as well as correction of major coronary risk factors, as recommended in table 12.1, must be associated with the surgical procedure.

Table 12.1. Main coronary risk factors to be corrected after successful CABGS

Cigarette smoking
Lipid disorders
Hypertension
Diabetes mellitus
Excess body weight
Sedentary habit
Dietary imbalance
Electrolyte imbalance

Smoking cessation seems to reduce mortality after CABGS [4]. Moreover, results strongly indicated that continuing smokers after CABGS had a markedly elevated risk of premature death and a higher rate of repeated revascularization procedures compared with those patients who stopped smoking. Therefore, authors recommended smoking cessation after CABGS and encouraged clinicians to start or continue smoking cessation programs in order to help patients stop smoking [5].

Other reports [6–7], however, indicated that current smokers had fewer adverse events at the time of coronary revascularization than nonsmokers and smoking demonstrated to have beneficial effects even on thrombolytic therapy after an acute myocardial infarction.

These findings were conducted on study material extremely heterogeneous with different baseline characteristics. However, after statistical adjustment for all clinical baseline parameters, these findings showed no significant difference in mortality between smokers and nonsmokers. According to other findings [8], results could be explained by the fact that many smokers tend to die after an acute myocardial infarction before having the chance to undergo CABGS. However, a paper [9] showed a greater number of reinfarctions but not death in continuing smokers when they were compared with similar individuals who stopped smoking. Probably, patients with a previous myocardial infarction, who do not undergo a reinfarction, die for the myocardial infarction itself. It remains to be established if CABGS would result in a longer survival in these individuals.

When the follow-up period in continuing smokers after CABGS is lengthened, a closer negative relationship seems to link CABGS and cigarette smoking [10]. Authors studied 450 patients who had undergone venous CABGS and were followed up for a long-term period (15 years). They concluded that results showed smoking cessation after CABGS could have significant beneficial effects on clinical events linked to ischemic heart disease including acute myocardial infarction and death.

Indeed, there is evidence of a strongly negative association between smoking and myocardial infarction in men and also in women [11–19], although results that support such a statement extended to cigarette smoking and CABGS are yet inconsistent. Increasing the number of large-scale findings and, particularly, prolonged time of follow-up could better clarify the precise relationship. Analyzing, however, statistically, the different findings, less evidence that cigarette smoking worsens both short and long-term results of CABGS would exist.

Recently, a controversial debate about whether smokers and, particularly continuing smokers after an acute myocardial infarction, should undergo CABGS as nonsmokers [20–21], exists and proposals have been supported to hold smokers accountable for heart disease costs [22]. It is worth noting that taking a position on this subject is very hard since, ethically, it is not easy to deny those medico-surgical procedures, which could save the life, to an individual due to the fact that he is a smoker. So arguing, the smoking habit should be strongly fought [23] before the appearance of damage that cigarette smoking certainly will cause.

In summary, although there is strong evidence that cigarette smoking is strictly related to the progression of coronary artery disease, incidence of cardiac death and increased incidence of myocardial infarction as well as reinfarction, the crucial role that it plays towards CABGS is yet to be fully demonstrated even if promising results would identify a negative association and, therefore, show the need to stop smoking before and after coronary surgery.

PTCA

This invasive hemodynamic technique is the most widely used since its procedure and description by Gruentzig et al. [24]. Its beneficial results, when successfully performed, are to cause a coronary revascularization with a good degree of improvement in coronary blood flow without surgical procedures that require cardiopulmonary bypass and cardioplegia.

Progresses in technology as well as operator experience have improved the results obtained by PTCA [24–27] including a decline in complications and increase in difficult cases to treat.

The main indications for PTCA are summarized in table 12.2.

More than 650,000 PTCA are performed yearly in the United States and, worldwide, the number of interventions increases continuously with more always better results. Therefore, establishing the relationship that exists between cigarette smoking and short and long-term results observed after PTCA is a crucial demand but not an academic curiosity.

There is evidence that the major limitation of PTCA, when complications during the procedure do not occur, is the high incidence of restenosis with a rate from 30 to 40 percent and, moreover, within the first 4 to 6 months [28–30].

Some major risk factors like unstable angina, diabetes mellitus and lipid metabolism disorders [31–33] have been recognized as playing a crucial role in PTCA restenosis. For what concerns cigarette smoking, no unanimous opinions exist.

Table 12.2. Main clinical indications to PTCA

Stable angina	
Unstable angina	
Anginal equivalents/syndromes (dyspnea, life-threatening arrhythmias, recurrent syncope)	
Acute myocardial infarction	
Evidence of reversible ischemia by:	Resting electrocardiogram
	Exercise stress testing
	Holter monitoring
	Stress echocardiography

Findings of Kotamaki et al. [34] conducted in continuing smokers who had undergone PTCA concluded that two factors influenced negatively the short and long-term prognosis: high levels of endothelin which were associated with luminal narrowing after angioplasty and dilated stenoses located on the left anterior descending coronary artery. On the contrary, cigarette smoking could not be identified as a risk factor for restenosis after PTCA. Similar results were reported by Macdonald et al. [35] and Foley et al. [36] who identified only a lower restenosis incidence after PTCA. These two studies, however, did not monitor fully the smoking habit of treated individuals.

On the contrary, Taira et al. [37] found that quality-of-life benefits related to successful PTCA diminished in continuing smokers when they were compared with similar individuals who stopped smoking.

An excellent editorial of Hasdai and Holmes [38] published in the European Heart Journal, underlines that a lot of patients continue to smoke after their PTCA. In a group of 1,169 patients who were smokers at the time of PTCA [6], 734, or 63 percent of the population, continued to smoke after the intervention. Authors observed also that cessation of cigarette smoking was a difficult challenge for the patient after percutaneous coronary angioplasty, since patients who had a successful PTCA were, generally, predisposed to repeat it if necessary [39]. Avoiding the complex surgical procedures makes the patients free to not change their lifestyle [40–42] and, consequently, smoking habit. On the contrary, risk factor modification, including cigarette smoking, should be considered as a basic necessity of coronary revascularization.

In conclusion, coronary circulation is positively influenced by revascularization procedures with a significant increase in coronary blood flow.

Despite no unanimous conclusions on the role played by cigarette smoking after hemodynamic or surgical revascularization, statistical data would indicate that patients who continue to smoke or begin to smoke again after CABGS or PTCA have more elevated risks not only of an acute myocardial infarction but also coronary restenosis and reappearance of clinical symptoms of ischemic heart disease often needing a new revascularization when they are compared with never smokers or pastsmokers.

References

[1]   Eagle KA, Guyton RA, Davidoff R, Ewy GA, Fonger J, Gardner TJ, Gott JP, Herrmann HC, Marlow RA, Nugent W, O'Connor JT, Orszulak TA, Rieselbach RE, Winters WL, Yusuf S. ACC/AHA guidelines for coronary artery bypass graft surgery: executive summary and recommendations. A report of the American College of Cardiology/American Heart Association Task Force on Practice Guidelines (Committee to Revise the 1991 Guidelines for Coronary Artery Bypass Graft Surgery). *Circulation.* 1999;100: 1464 – 80.

[2]   Rihal CS, Raco DL, Gersh BJ, Yusuf S. Indications for coronary artery bypass surgery and percutaneous coronary intervention in chronic stable angina: review of the evidence and methodological considerations. *Circulation.* 2003; 108: 2439 – 45.

[3]   Arima M, Kanoh T, Suzuki T, Kuremoto K, Tanimoto K, Oigawa T, Matsuda S. Serial angiographic follow-up beyond 10 years after coronary artery bypass grafting. *Circ. J.* 2005; 69: 896 – 902.

[4]   van Domburg RT, Meeter K, van Berkel DFM, Veldkamp RF, van Herwerden LA, Bogers Ad JJC. Smoking cessation reduces mortality after coronary artery bypass surgery: a 20-year follow-up study. *J. Am. Coll. Cardiol.* 2000; 36: 878 – 83.

[5]   Raw M, McNiell A, West M. Smoking cessation: evidence based recommendations for the healthcare system. *BMJ.* 1999; 318: 182 – 5.

[6]   Hasdai D, Garratt KN, Grill DE, Lerman A, Holmes DR Jr. Effects of smoking status on the long-term outcome after successful percutaneous coronary revascularization. *N. Engl. J. Med.* 1997; 336: 755 – 61.

[7]   Barbash GI, Reiner J, White HD, Wilcox RG, Armstrong PW, Sadowsky Z, Morris D, Aylward P, Woodlief LH, Topol EJ. Evaluation of paradoxic beneficial effects of smoking in patients receiving thrombolytic therapy for acute myocardial infarction: mechanism of the "smoker's paradox" from the GUSTO-I trial with angiographic insights. Global Utilization of Streptokinase and Tissue-Plasminogen Activator for Occluded Coronary Arteries. *J. Am. Coll. Cardiol.* 1995; 26: 1222 – 9.

[8]   Schatzkin A, Cupples LA, Heeren T, Morelock S, Kannel WB. Sudden death in the Framingham Heart Study. Differences in incidence and risk factors by sex and coronary disease status. *Am. J. Epidemiol.* 1984; 120: 888 – 99.

[9]   Leone A. Cardiovascular damage from smoking: a fact or belief? *Int. J. Cardiol.* 1993; 38: 113 – 7.

[10]   Voors AA, van Brussel BL, Thijs Plokker HW, Ernst SMPG, Ernst NM, Koomen EM, Tijssen JGP, Vermeulen FEE. Smoking and cardiac events after venous coronary bypass surgery. *Circulation.* 1996; 93: 42 – 7.

[11]   Pohjola S, Siltanen P, Romo M. Five-year survival of 728 patients after myocardial infarction. *Br. Heart J.* 1980; 43: 176 – 83.

[12]   Sparrow D, Dawber TR, Colton T. The influence of cigarette smoking on prognosis after a first myocardial infarction. *J. Chronic. Dis.* 1978; 31: 425 – 32.

[13]   Wilhelmsson C, Vedin JA, Elmfeldt D, Tibblin J, Wilhelmsen L. Smoking and myocardial infarction. *Lancet.* 1975; i: 415 – 20.

[14] Daly LE, Mulcahy R, Graham IM, Hickey N. Long-term effect on mortality of stopping smoking after unstable angina and myocardial infarction. *BMJ.* 1983; 287: 324 – 6.

[15] Jenkins CD, Zyzanski SJ, Rosenman RH. Risk of new myocardial infarction in middleaged men with manifest coronary heart disease. *Circulation.* 1976; 53: 342 – 7.

[16] Vlietstra RE, Kronmal RA, Oberman A. Stopping smoking improves survival in patients with angiographically-proven coronary artery disease. *Am. J. Cardiol.* 1982; 49: 984A.

[17] Hermanson B, Omenn GS, Kronmal RA, Gersh BJ, for Participants in the Coronary Artery Surgery Study. Beneficial six-year outcome of smoking cessation in older men and women with coronary artery disease. *N. Engl. J. Med.* 1988; 319: 1365 – 9.

[18] Cavender JB, Rogers WJ, Fisher LD, Gersh BJ, Coggin CJ, Meyers WO, for the CASS Investigators. Effects of smoking on survival and morbidity in patients randomized to medical or surgical therapy in the Coronary Artery Surgery Study (CASS): 10-year follow-up. *J. Am. Coll. Cardiol.* 1992; 20: 287 – 94.

[19] Rosemberg L, Kaufman DW, Helmrich SP, Shapiro S. The risk of myocardial infarction after quitting smoking in men under 55 years of age. *N. Engl. J. Med.* 1985; 313: 1511 – 4.

[20] Underwood MJ, Bailey JS. Should smokers be offered coronary bypass surgery? *BMJ.* 1993; 306: 1047 – 50.

[21] Powell JT, Greenhalgh RM. Arterial bypass and smokers. *BMJ.* 1994; 308: 607 – 8.

[22] Kaesemeyer WH. Holding smokers accountable for heart disease costs. *Circulation.* 1994; 90: 1029 – 32.

[23] Archilli E, Novelli S, Romiti I, Musetti M, Leone A. Campaign against smoking: Little battles to win a war! 8th World Conference on Tobacco and Health. Building a Tobacco-free World. Buenos Aires, Argentina 1992, March 30 – April 3, Abstract Book; 1992.

[24] Gruentzig A. Transluminal dilatation of coronary artery stenosis. *Lancet* 1978; 1: 263

[25] Gruentzig AR, Senning A, Siegenthaler WE. Non-operative dilatation of coronary artery stenoses. Percutaneous transluminal coronary angioplasty. *N. Engl. J. Med.* 1979; 301: 61 – 8.

[26] Gruentzig AR, King SB III, Schlumpf M, Siegenthaler W. Long-term follow-up after percutaneous transluminal coronary angioplasty: the early Zurich experience. *N. Engl. J. Med.* 1987; 316: 1127 – 32.

[27] Gruentzig AR. Percutaneous transluminal coronary angioplasty: six years' experience. *Am. Heart J.* 1984; 107: 818 – 9.

[28] Serruys PW, Luijten HE, Beatt KJ, Geuskens R, de Feyter PJ, van den Brand M, Reiber JH, ten Katen HJ, van Es GA, Hugenholtz PG. Incidence of restenosis after successful coronary angioplasty: a time-related phenomenon. A quantitative angiographic study in 342 consecutive patients at 1, 2, 3, and 4 months. *Circulation.* 1988; 77: 361 – 71.

[29] Hirshfeld JW Jr, Schwartz JS, Jugo R, Macdonald RG, Goldberg S, Savage MP, Bass TA, Vetrovec G, Cowley M, Taussig AS. Restenosis after coronary angioplasty: a multivariate statistical model to relate lesion and procedure variables to restenosis. The M –HEART Investigators. *J. Am. Coll. Cardiol.* 1991; 18: 647 – 56.

[30] Beatt KJ, Serruys PW, Luijten HE, Rensing BJ, Suryapranata H, de Feyter PJ, van der Brand M, Laarman GJ, Roelandt J. Restenosis after coronary angioplasty: the paradox of increased lumen diameter and restenosis. *J. Am. Coll. Cardiol.* 1992; 19: 258 – 66.

[31] Weintraub WS, Kosinski AS, Brown CL III, King SB III. Can restenosis after coronary angioplasty be predicted from clinical variables? *J. Am. Coll. Cardiol.* 1993; 21: 6 – 14.

[32] Hearn JA, Donohue BC, Ba'albaki H, Douglas JS, King SB III, Lembo NJ, Roubin GS, Sgoutas DS. Usefulness of serum lipoprotein(a) as a predictor of restenosis after percutaneous transluminal coronary angioplasty. *Am. J. Cardiol.* 1992; 69: 736 – 9.

[33] Daida H, Lee YJ, Yokoi H, Kanoh T, Ishiwata S, Kato S, Nishikawa H, Takatsu F, Kato H, Kutsumi Y, for L-ART Group. Prevention of restenosis after percutaneous transluminal coronary angioplasty by reducing lipoprotein(a) levels with low-density lipoprotein apheresis. Low-density Lipoprotein Apheresis Angioplasty Restenosis Trial (L-ART) Group. *Am. J. Cardiol.* 1994; 73: 1037 – 40.

[34] Kotamaki M, Laustiola K, Syvanne M, Heikkila J. Influence of continued smoking and some biological risk factors on restenosis after percutaneous transluminal coronary angioplasty. *J. Intern. Med.* 1996; 240: 293 – 301.

[35] Macdonald RG, Henderson MA, Hirshfeld JW Jr, Goldberg SH, Bass T, Vetrovec G, Cowley M, Taussig A, Whitworth H, Margolis JR. Patient-related variables and restenosis after percutaneous transluminal coronary angioplasty- a report from the M-HEART Group. *Am. J. Cardiol.* 1990; 66: 926 – 31.

[36] Foley JB, Penn IM, Brown RIG, Murray-Parsons N, White J, Galligan L, Mac Donald C. Safety, success and restenosis after elective coronary implantation of the Palmaz-Schatz stent in 100 patients at a single center. *Am. Heart J.* 1993; 125: 686 – 94.

[37] Taira DA, Seto TB, Ho KKL, Krumholz HM, Cutlip DE, Berezin R, Kuntz RE, Cohen DJ. Impact of smoking on health-related quality of life after percutaneous coronary revascularization. *Circulation.* 2000; 102: 1369 – 74.

[38] Hasdai D, Holmes DR Jr. Smoking and outcome after PTCA. *Eur. Heart J.* 1997; 18: 1520 – 2.

[39] Gulanick M, Maito A. Patients' reactions to angioplasty: realistic or not? *Am. J. Crit. Care.* 1994; 3: 368 – 73.

[40] Crouse GR III, Hagaman AP. Smoking cessation in relation to cardiac procedures. *Am. J. Epidemiol.* 1991; 134: 699 – 703.

[41] McKenna KT, Maas F, McEniery PT. Coronary risk factors status after percutaneous transluminal coronary angioplasty. *Heart Lung.* 1995; 24: 207 – 12.

[42] Bliley AV, Ferrans CE, Quality of life after coronary angioplasty. *Heart Lung.* 1993; 22: 193 – 9.

Final Remarks

The main statements that can be deduced when an analysis that involves various and multifactorial characteristics related to coronary circulation in smokers and nonsmokers is carried out should provide, at least, three types of results: proven results, which should be easily identifiable and repeatable; results needing further observations to be confirmed or rejected; and results certainly rejected.

Such a concept, characterized by an evident logic, really finds a limited control since a wide spectrum of responses, interactions and baseline features influence coronary circulation providing not yet unanimous data. This assessment is more easily attributable to the effects of cigarette smoking, which exerts a different role according to various characteristics like number of smoked cigarettes and, consequently toxic concentrations of tobacco chemicals, type of exposure to smoking, health status of individuals exposed, and so on.

Indeed, some proven concepts deriving from both clinical and experimental findings conducted on coronary circulation of smokers, nonsmokers not exposed to smoke, past-smokers not exposed and smoke-exposed past-smokers may be rationally supported.

1. The anatomy of coronary arteries has a shape that may be influenced by a great number of factors including cigarette smoking. Particularly, epicardial medium-size coronary arteries undergo those changes consisting of endothelial dysfunction as well as platelet adhesiveness increase up to the formation of an atherosclerotic plaque and its complications. That is an effect of chemical compounds of cigarette smoking. Therefore, epicardial coronary arteries develop mainly structural alterations due to chronic smoking even if the starting mechanism of a lesion may be of the functional type. Conversely, intramyocardial small coronary arteries feel the effects of cigarette smoking displayed on coronary circulation but also a direct effect of smoking compounds on the cardiac muscle. The latter causes increased oxygen demand, increased heart inotropism and increased working. Finally, the type of coronary artery distribution into the atria associated with the smaller thickness of atrial mass explains the relatively weak damage induced by cigarette smoking on atrial circulation.

From these observations, there is evidence that cigarette smoking has harmful properties built specifically to induce coronary circulation changes particularly in epicardial arteries.

2. Endothelial dysfunction caused by smoking exposure, either active or passive exposure, is an event that influences negatively coronary circulation. Many findings seem to identify endothelial dysfunction as the first determinant of inducing those complex changes

that lead to atherosclerotic plaque formation as well as complications. Smoking would seem to induce endothelial alterations earlier, and also with a major incidence, than the other coronary risk factors. Moreover, some of these may be strongly potentiated by cigarette smoking without any evidence of the contrary. Functional disorders due to smoking, therefore, trigger those changes that will be responsible for the appearance of structural alterations in the coronary circulation of the smoker. Similar changes in nonsmokers may occur particularly as an effect of other major coronary risk factors although, however, with a lesser incidence.

3. Interaction between smoking and other cardiovascular stimulating factors, like catecholamine release and sympathetic stimulation, causes heavy functional and structural changes of coronary circulation. Functional changes which involve initially endothelium and platelet function develop transiently for a limited time up to trigger those cellular and metabolic reactions that will determine structural alterations. Structural alterations of coronary arteries recognize a first phase of reversibility of the lesions followed by irreversibility, in time, of them. The latter is produced and, particularly, maintained by the continuative action of cigarette smoking in the absence of quitting smoking.

4. The features of atherosclerotic plaques are the strongest determinants of the differences in coronary circulation between nonsmokers and smokers. Smoker's plaque is most often a vulnerable plaque, determines heavier luminal narrowings, affects a major number of coronary arteries with appearance of three vessel disease, and, finally, shows a greater amount of calcium deposits and lipids.

5. Plaque complications occur more frequently as a consequence of a multifactorial involvement including endothelium, adrenal and sympathetic stimulation, platelet function changes, inflammatory processes and coagulation-fibrinolysis cascade activation up to a level of clot formation in coronary circulation of the smoker when compared with that of a nonsmoker. Simultaneously all those mechanisms responsible for clot lysis are impaired in smokers.

6. A significant impairment of coronary circulation in smokers is also indirectly documented by the possibility to reproduce identical life-threatening ventricular arrhythmias in individuals with a previous myocardial infarction after undergoing exercise stress testing in a smoke-polluted environment.

7. Angiographically, there is evidence of a major progression of atherosclerotic lesions in smokers when they were compared with nonsmokers.

8. Narrowing mechanism of coronary circulation may follow different ways in pre-menopausal female smokers who uses oral contraception when compared with pre-menopausal female smokers who do not use them, pre-menopausal nonsmoking women who use contraception and, generically, post-menopasal women. There is evidence of coronary damage of the thrombogenic type that affects pre-menopausal female smokers who use contraceptive drugs when compared with non users or women in post-menopause. The increased incidence of coronary circulation alterations in postmenopausal women recognizes particularly a thrombotic mechanism of lesion appearance similar to what occurs in men rather than a thrombogenic mechanism.

9. A major incidence of complications has been identified in smokers suffering from ischemic heart disease than that in nonsmokers. Particularly, findings on stable angina well

documented myocardial function impairment related to coronary atherosclerosis progression and acceleration.

10. Invasive and/or surgical coronary revascularization procedures in smokers with ischemic heart disease are characterized by a higher appearance of coronary restenosis if compared with the results obtained in similar individuals who do not smoke.

There is evidence, therefore, that a decalogue to be kept in mind may be formulated to define the difference in coronary circulation between nonsmokers and smokers. Examining smokers, the decalogue is as follows:

1. Coronary artery anatomy is structurally influenced by smoking.
2. Endothelial dysfunction is strongly related to smoking.
3. Coronary responses are functionally promoted by smoke compounds.
4. Atherosclerotic plaque development may be a close result of smoking.
5. Smoking promotes plaque complications.
6. Smoking is associated with angiographic evidence of coronary atherosclerosis progression.
7. Smoking is often associated with life-threatening ventricular arrhythmias.
8. Smoking may induce both thrombogenic and thrombotic damages.
9. Ischemic heart disease atherosclerotic complications are prevailing in smokers.
10. Successful coronary revascularization may fail in smokers.

In conclusion, there are many observations that indicate cigarette smoking is a factor strongly associated with a markedly strong increase of coronary circulation impairment, although some papers disagree with that. Negative results of cardiovascular damage from cigarette smoking cannot be denied in view of the greatest number of findings that conclude for that. Paraphrasing Albert Einstein, who affirmed "God does not play dice with the universe" to interpret physical phenomena which regulate it, one can support with no doubt that "smoking does not play dice with the cardiovascular system," in the sense that alterations of coronary circulation from cigarette smoking exist and cannot be linked to the fate since a large number of findings document also their reproducibility in a majority of individuals.

Index

D

E

G

H

M

N

O

T